Textbook on NURSING FOUNDATION for PB BSc Nursing

Textbook on
NURSING FOUNDATION
for PB BSc Nursing

I Clement
Doctor of Philosophy in Nursing (PhD) MSc Nursing (Medical Surgical Nursing)
MA (Sociology) MA (Child Care and Education)
Postgraduate Diploma in Hospital Administration
Principal
VSS College of Nursing
Nagadevanahalli
Bengaluru, Karnataka, India

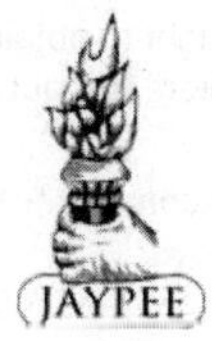

The Health Sciences Publisher

New Delhi | London | Philadelphia | Panama

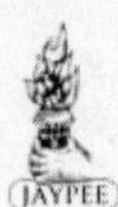

Jaypee Brothers Medical Publishers (P) Ltd

Headquarters

Jaypee Brothers Medical Publishers (P) Ltd
4838/24, Ansari Road, Daryaganj
New Delhi 110 002, India
Phone: +91-11-43574357
Fax: +91-11-43574314
Email: jaypee@jaypeebrothers.com

Overseas Offices

J.P. Medical Ltd
83 Victoria Street, London
SW1H 0HW (UK)
Phone: +44 20 3170 8910
Fax: +44 (0)20 3008 6180
Email: info@jpmedpub.com

Jaypee Medical Inc
The Bourse
111 South Independence Mall East
Suite 835, Philadelphia, PA 19106, USA
Phone: +1 267-519-9789
Email: jpmed.us@gmail.com

Jaypee Brothers Medical Publishers (P) Ltd
Bhotahity, Kathmandu, Nepal
Phone: +977-9741283608
Email: kathmandu@jaypeebrothers.com

Jaypee-Highlights Medical Publishers Inc
City of Knowledge, Bld. 237, Clayton
Panama City, Panama
Phone: +1 507-301-0496
Fax: +1 507-301-0499
Email: cservice@jphmedical.com

Jaypee Brothers Medical Publishers (P) Ltd
17/1-B Babar Road, Block-B, Shaymali
Mohammadpur, Dhaka-1207
Bangladesh
Mobile: +08801912003485
Email: jaypeedhaka@gmail.com

Website: www.jaypeebrothers.com
Website: www.jaypeedigital.com

Inquiries for bulk sales may be solicited at: jaypee@jaypeebrothers.com

Textbook on Nursing Foundation for PB BSc Nursing

First Edition: **2015**

ISBN: 978-93-5152-959-0

Printed at Rajkamal Electric Press, Plot No. 2, Phase-IV, Kundli, Haryana.

PREFACE

It gives me immense pleasure to complete this *Textbook on Nursing Foundation for PB BSc Nursing*. First and foremost I thank God, for his immeasurable blessing on me to complete this task. Basically, this book surrounds the sound knowledge on basic care in nursing. Gaining knowledge on this nursing foundation forms pillar for budding post basic nurses. Main aim of this book is to inculcate concept of nursing care, that is, primarily to assist the patient to function independently when the patient lacks knowledge, physical strength, or the will to act for himself as he would ordinarily act in health, and carry out prescribed therapy, maintain patient's physical, psychological, spiritual, cultural and social health. This function is found to be complex but creative, therefore, there is a need to provide adequate opportunity for the application of the practical knowledge and skill on physical, biological, and social sciences and the development of skills based on them. This book has good essence of content prepared as per the Indian Nursing Council syllabus. It has 7 sections with 31 chapters illustrated in simple English easy-to-grasp. Each chapter is narrated with adequate tables and diagrams, and has previous years question papers attached, which will help the students to get the concept about questions asked for the examinations. With this book, each student will gain good knowledge, develop positive attitude towards nursing care and practice the quality nursing care. I wish all the best for budding post basic nurses!

I Clement

ACKNOWLEDGMENTS

I am thankful to the Almighty, who strengthens me with his abundant blessing through innumerable means, helping me in all my accomplishments. My heartfelt thanks to Shri Sommana, Former Minister of Karnataka and Chairman of VSS Group of Institutions, for his constant support and encouragement. My sincere thanks to my guru Dr BT Basavanthappa, Principal, Raja Rajeshwari College of Nursing, Bengaluru, Karnataka, India and Professor PV Ramachandran, Chairman, College of Nursing, Sri Ramachandra University, Chennai, Tamil Nadu, India, a great philosopher and internationally renowned teacher of nursing, who helped me in discovering the world of knowledge. I am thankful to Ms Shylaja Sommana, Managing Directors Dr BS Naveen, Dr BS Arun and Ms Divya from VSS Group of Institutions, Bengaluru, for their support and encouragement. I am also grateful to Dr BC Bhagavan, Syndicate Member of RGUHS, Bengaluru, Professor, Department of Surgery, Kempagowda Institute of Medical Sciences, Bengaluru, and Dr Aswathnarayanan MLA, Chairman, Padmashree Group of Institutions, Bengaluru. Special thanks to Dr TV Ramakrishnan (Professor of Anesthesiology and Head of Clinical Services, Department of Accident and Emergency Medicine, Sri Ramachandra University, Chennai); Dr Jeyaseelan Manickam Devadassan (Syndicate Member, The Tamil Nadu Dr MGR Medical University, Chennai and Dean, Annai JKK Samporani Ammal College of Nursing, Erode, Tamil Nadu); Dr Tamilmani (Principal, Annai JKK Samporani Ammal College of Nursing); Professor Mrs Jessie Sudarsanum (Head, Department of Medical Surgical Nursing, Annai JKK Samporani Ammal College of Nursing), and all my teachers and students.

I convey my sincere thanks to my beloved parents, brothers and sisters and my wife Nisha Clement, for her continuous support and constant encouragement in each step of my life. I take this opportunity to thank my little ones, Cibin, Cynthia and Cavin. I extend thanks to my beloved friend and brother Mr Regi T Kurien, USA.

Special thanks to Shri Jitendar P Vij (Group Chairman), Mr Ankit Vij (Group President), Mr Tarun Duneja (Director–Publishing), Mr KK Raman (Production Manager) and Mr Rajesh Sharma (Production Coordinator) M/s Jaypee Brothers Medical Publishers (P) Ltd, New Delhi. Mr Venugopal V (Regional Manager, Bengaluru Branch), Mr Santhosh Kumar (Author Coordinator), Ms Sajini SV (Team Head) and other staff members of M/s Jaypee Brothers Medical Publisher (P) Ltd, Bengaluru branch.

SYLLABUS

PB BSc (N): NURSING FOUNDATION

COURSE DESCRIPTION

This course will help students develop an understanding of the philosophy, objectives and responsibilities of nursing as a profession. The purpose of the course is to orient to the current concepts involved in the practice of nursing and developments in the nursing profession.

OBJECTIVES

At the end of the course, the student will:

1. Identify professional aspects of nursing.
2. Explain theories of nursing.
3. Identify ethical aspects of nursing profession.
4. Utilize steps of nursing process.
5. Identify the role of the nursing in various levels of health services.
6. Appreciate the significance of quality assurance in nursing.
7. Explain current trends in health and nursing.

COURSE CONTENTS

UNIT I

1. Development of nursing as a profession.
2. Its philosophy.
3. Objectives and responsibilities of a graduate nurse.
4. Trends influencing nursing practice.
5. Expanded role of the nurse.
6. Development of nursing education in India and trends in nursing education.

UNIT II

1. Ethical, legal and other issues in nursing.
2. Concepts of health and illness, effects on the person.
3. Stress and adaptation.
4. Health care concept and nursing care concept.
5. Developmental concept, needs, roles and problems of the development stages of individual—newborn, infant, toddler, pre-adolescent, adolescent, adulthood, middle-age, old age.

UNIT III

1. Theory of nursing practice.
2. Metaparadigm of nursing—characterized by four central concepts, i.e. nurse, person (client/patient), health and environment.

UNIT IV

1. Nursing process.
2. Assessment: Tools for assessment, methods, recording.
3. Planning: Techniques for planning care, types of care plans.
4. Implementation of care, recording.
5. Evaluation: Tools for evaluation, process of evaluation.

UNIT V

1. Quality assurance: Nursing standards, nursing audit, total quality management.
2. Role of council and professional bodies in maintenance of standards.

UNIT VI

Primary health care concept:

1. Community-oriented nursing.
2. Holistic nursing.
3. Primary nursing.

Family-oriented nursing concept:

1. Problem-oriented nursing.
2. Progressive patient care.
3. Team nursing.

CONTENTS

SECTION I: BASIC CONCEPTS OF NURSING

SECTION II: HEALTH AND NURSING CARE DELIVERY

SECTION III: NURSING THEORIES

SECTION IV: NURSING PROCESS APPLICATION

SECTION V: QUALITY PATIENT CARE

SECTION VI: COMMUNITY HEALTH CARE

SECTION VII: WASTE MANAGEMENT

SECTION I
Basic Concepts of Nursing

GLOSSARY

1. **Models:** These are graphic or symbolic representations of phenomena that objectify and present certain perspectives or points of view about nature or function or both.
2. **Concept:** These are the elements or components of a phenomenon necessary to understand the phenomenon and derived from impressions the human mind receives about phenomena through sensing the human environment.
3. **Philosophy:** It is statement of belief and values about human being and their world.
4. **Theory:** It refers to a set of logically interrelated concepts, statements, propositions and definitions, which have been derived from philosophical beliefs of scientific data and from which questions or hypothesis can be deduced, tested and verified.
5. **Health:** A state of physical, mental and social well-being and the absence of disease or other disorders. It involves constant change and adaptation to stress.
6. **Community:** A group of inhabitants living together in a somewhat localized area under the same general regulations and having common interests, functions, needs and organizations.
7. **Nursing:** It is an art, science and profession by which we render, serve to human being to help to regain or to keep a normal state of body and mind and when it cannot accomplish this, it help for the relief from physical pain, mental anxiety or spiritual discomfort.
8. **Community health:** Public community health is a science and art of preventing disease, prolonging life and promoting health and efficiency through organized effort.
9. **Community health nursing:** This is a synthesis of nursing and public health practice applied for promoting and preserving the health of people. The practice is general and compressive. It is not limited to a particular age group or diagnosis, and continuing, not episodic.
10. **Profession:** It is an occupation with moral principles that are devoted to thc human and social welfare. The service is based on specialized knowledge and skill developed in a scientific and learned manner.

11. **Career planning:** The process of establishing career objectives and determining appropriate educational and developmental programs to further develop the skills required to achieve short- or long-term career objectives.
12. **Ethics:** Refer to the study of philosophical ideas of right and wrong behavior.
13. **Expanded role:** This role of nursing means enlargement of nurse role with the bonders of nurse.
14. **Empathy:** Intellectual and emotional awareness and understanding of another persons thoughts, behaviors and feelings.
15. **Nurse anesthetics:** A nurse who completed the course of study in an anesthesia school and carries out preoperative status of clients.
16. **Nurse practitioner:** He/she is a nurse who has completed either as certificate program or a Master's degree in a specialty and is also certified by the appropriate specialty organization. Nurse practitioner is skilled at making nursing assessments, performing physical examination, counseling, teaching and treating minor and self-limiting illness.
17. **Professional conduct:** This is behaving with a real sense of dignity and respect for the service given for the patient and for them with whom one works.
18. **Sympathy:** It is balancing someone's feeling especially in sorrow or trouble.

CHAPTER

1

Introduction to Nursing

INTRODUCTION

Nursing has been called the oldest of the arts and the youngest of the profession. The word nurse evolved from the Latin word nutritious, which means nourishing. The roots of medicine and nursing are intertwining and found in mythology, ancient eastern and western cultures and religion.

Nursing is defined by various authors at various times. Henderson says "Nursing is primarily assisting the individuals (sick or well) in the performances of those activities, contributing or its recovery (or to a peaceful death) that he would perform unaided, if he had the necessary strength, will or knowledge.

The unique contribution of nursing is to help the individual to be independent or such assistance as soon as possible.

Nursing, besides being a honorable profession, is one of the oldest arts and an essential modern occupation. Nursing is one of the greatest of humanitarian services and all people whether ill or well, rich or poor, literate or illiterate, young or old, at work or at play, in or out of hospital, are in some way or other, directly or indirectly closely associated with it. Nursing has its own body of knowledge scientifically based and humanitarianism that promises expanded benefits to people and society. It assists the individual or family to achieve their potential for self-direction for health.

DEFINITION

1. **The International Council of Nurses** defines "Nursing is to assist the individual, sick or well in the performance of those activities contributing to health or to its recovery (or to peaceful death) that he would perform unaided if he had the necessary strength, will or knowledge".
2. **Florence Nightingale:** Nursing defined as the act of utilizing the environment of the patient to assist him in his recovery.
3. **Canadian Nurses Association 1987:** Nursing practice is a dynamic, caring and helping relationship in which the nurse assists the client to achieve and obtain optimal health.
4. **American Nurses Association:** Nursing practice is direct goal oriented and adaptable to service the needs of the individual, the family and community during health and illness.

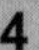

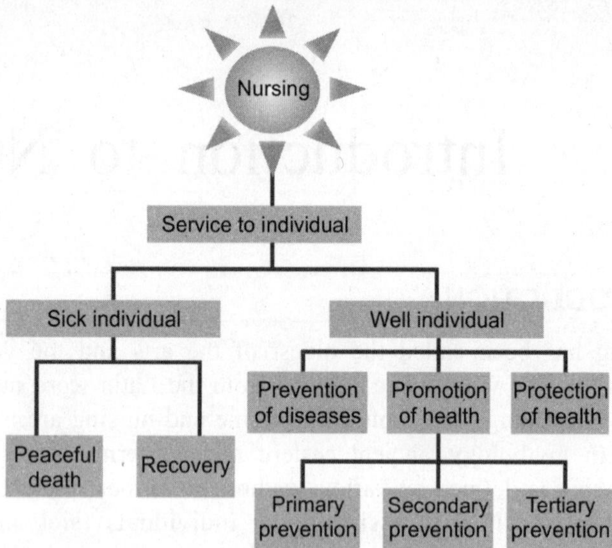

Figure 1.1: Definition of nursing

HISTORICAL DEVELOPMENT OF NURSING IN INDIA

1905: Association of Nursing Superintendents was constituted/formed.

1908: Trained Nurses Association of India was established/formed.

1909: Bombay Presidency Nursing Association was formed. Missionary Nurses North India Board set up under Medical Missionary Association of India.

1911: The South Indian Board was established Trained Nurses Association of India (TNAI) affiliated to International Council of Nurses.

1912: The First Nurses Registration Act was enacted in Madras Presidency.

1930: The Christian Nurses Auxilliary formed by the missionary nurses.

1934: The Bengal Nurses Act was enacted for the nurses, midwives and health visitors (HV) of undivided Bengal.

1936: The Mid India Board of Education affiliated to Christian Nurses League, Christian Nurses Auxilliary Association was affiliated to TNAI.

1941: Standardized pay scales and terms of services were established in Chennai. State Nursing Superintendent, appointed at state level (Chennai).

1942: The Auxiliary Nursing Service (ANS) was established. One Nursing Superintendent was appointed as nursing advisor at Directorate General of Health Services (DGHS), Government of India, to organize nursing services.

1943: Establishment of School of Nursing Administration for Military Nursing Services Health Survey and Development Committees (Bhore) constituted by Government of India. Study groups worked on proposal for university education in nursing in India. Christian Medical College (CMC) Vellore and Madras General Hospital started courses to train nursing tutors. Commissioned rank was given to the Indian Military Nursing sisters.

1946: Bhore Committee submitted report, recommendations made on improvement of various aspects of nursing profession: Nursing education, working conditions, nursing services in hospital and community and deputing nurses for higher education to abroad, etc. Establishment of the College of Nursing at Delhi (now Rajkumari Amrit Kaur College of Nursing) under the Union Ministry of Health to start university nursing education program for the first time in India leading to Bachelor's degree in nursing, i.e. BSc (Hons.) Nursing.

1947: Indian Nursing Council Act was passed (31.12.1947) on the basis of recommendations of Bhore Committee. Degree program for nursing started in Vellore.

1948: The first meeting of Indian Nursing Council (INC) was held.

1950: The INC took decision to establish Auxiliary Nurse Midwife (ANM) program to meet the requirement of workers in nursing.

1951: Establishment of urban field teaching center is started at College of Nursing, Delhi in collaboration with existing Medical Center Hospital (MCH) centers of Municipal Corporation, Delhi for teaching of Urban Community Health Nursing.

1952: Establishment of residential field teaching center for teaching Community Health Nursing in the rural area under College of Nursing, Delhi in collaboration with Primary Health Center, Najafgarh.

1953: Ms Edith M Buchanan, Vice-Principal, Rajkumari Amrit Kaur College of Nursing (RAKCON), Delhi was sent to Columbia University to earn her Doctorate in Education (DEd) through WHO fellowship.

1954: Government of India constituted committee to review conditions of services, emoluments, etc. of nursing profession (Shetty committee). Shetty Committee Report was published, recommended nursing staff norms of hospital community and other improvements in nursing.

1955: Establishment of child guidance clinic at Rajkumari Amrit Kaur College of Nursing. (RAKCON) for providing services and strengthening community health nursing and pediatric nursing. Ms Margaretta Craig, Principal, College of Nursing, Delhi attended ICN meeting in France, to present a paper on the need for nursing research in India.

1959: Dr Edith M Buchanan, succeeded in establishing the long cherished Master of Nursing (MN) degree program at RAKCON, New Delhi under University of Delhi (October 1959). Healthy Survey and Planning Committee (Dr LN Mudaliar) was constituted by Government of India to review the progress made in health since, Bhore committee recommendation.

1961: Mudaliar Committee report published made some recommendations to improve nursing profession.

1963: A WHO assisted technical project was undertaken at the INC to revise the General Nursing and Midwifery (GNM) course. Dr Buchanan, succeeded in sending Mrs Sulochara Krishnan, one of the first graduate of this newly established, MN degree program, to earn the DEd degree from Columbia University.

1964: Dr Marie Furguson, a public health nurse came to the College of Nursing, Delhi was able to create greater appreciation and understanding of the need and value of research in planning nursing administration and education with senior leaders of the country conducted 'activity studies to define the nursing and non-nursing functions of nursing personnel'.

1965: A WHO publication on 'Guide for School of Nursing' in India was published.

1966: The TNAI established research section under the Chairmanship of Ms Margarata Craig. TNAI conducted 'Time study' with the co-operation of Ms Anna Gupta, Principal, RAKCON, under the supervision of Dr Sulochana Krishnan.

1969-1971: TNAI and Voluntary Health Agencies in India (VHAI), conducted study on survey on the socioeconomic status of nurses in India.

1973: Kartar Singh Committee report on multipurpose workers and Health and Family Planning department published and recommended auxiliary nurse midwife (ANM) and lady health visitors (LHVs) were redesignated and health workers (F) and health assistant (F) to cover the required population at rural area for providing proper health services.

1975: Shrivastava Committee report on three tier-plan of health care delivery system to rural area was recommended.

1976: Dr Marie Farell and Dr Aparna Bhaduri of Rajkumari Amrit Kaur College of Nursing, New Delhi, conducted seminars on nursing research for educationists at Delhi, Mussoorie (Uttarakhand) and Yercaud to strength the nursing research in India.

1978: Government Nurses Association of Karnataka established.

1981: Dr Farrel and Dr Bhaduri's book 'Health Research': A Community-based Approach' published by World Health Organization.

1986: The Nursing Research Society of India (NRSI) was established to promote research within and around nursing environment. Dr (Mrs) Inderjit Walia was founder President. Mrs Uma Hunda was its Secretary. MPhil in nursing program started at RAKCON, under Delhi University.

1987: Reports of the expert committee on health and manpower planning, production and management (Bajaj Committee) published. This committee also dealt with nursing service conditions norms and nurse's emoluments, etc.

1988: The RAKCON, New Delhi was designated as World Health Collaboration Center for Nursing. Developments reports of the high power committee on nursing and nursing profession published. Dr Ruth Hurner book 'Nursing Education in India' published on the basis of survey.

1992: PhD in nursing program started at RAKCON, under Delhi University. Mrs Asha Sharma got registered for the Doctoral course.

SCOPE OF NURSING

There was a time when professional nurses had very little choice of service because nursing was centered in the hospital and bedside nursing. Career opportunities are more varied now for a numbers of reasons. The list of opportunities available are:

1. Staff nurse provides direct patient care to one patient or a group of patients, assists ward management and supervision. Staff nurse is directly responsible to the ward supervisor.
2. Ward Sister or Nursing Supervisor is responsible to the nursing superintendent for the nursing care management of a ward or unit. Takes full charge of the ward. Assigns work to nursing and non-nursing personnel working in the ward. Responsible for safety and comfort of patients in the ward. Provides teaching sessions if it is a teaching hospital.
3. Department Supervisor/Assistant Nursing Superintendent is responsible to the Nursing Superintendent and Deputy Nursing Superintendent for the nursing care and management of more than one ward or unit, e.g. surgical department, outpatient department.
4. Deputy Nursing Superintendent is responsible to the Nursing Superintendent and assists in the nursing administration of the hospital.
5. Nursing Superintendent is responsible to the Medical Superintendent for safe and efficient management of hospital nursing services.
6. Director of Nursing is responsible for both nursing service and nursing educations within a teaching hospital.

7. Community Health Nurse (CHN) services rendered mainly focusing Reproductive and Child Health Program.
8. Teaching in nursing. The functions and responsibilities of the teacher in nursing are planning, teaching and supervising the learning experiences for the students.

   Positions in nursing education are clinical instructor, tutor, senior tutor, lecturer, associate professor, Reader in nursing and Professor in nursing.
9. Industrial nurses are providing first aid, care during illness, health educations about industrial hazards and prevention of accidents.
10. Military Nurse: Military Nursing service became a part of the Indian Army by which means nurses became commissioned officers who are given rank from Lieutenant to Major General.
11. Nursing service in abroad: Attractive salaries and promising professional opportunities, which cause a major increase for nursing service in abroad.
12. Nursing service administrative positions: At the state level, the Deputy Director of Nursing, and the State Health Directorate. The highest administrative position on a national level is the Nursing Advisor to the Government of India.

NURSING AS A PROFESSION

The Code points out very clearly the role of the nurse as a leader and an active participator in professional activities by setting up and carrying out desirable standards of nursing practice and nursing education.

QUALITIES OF A PROFESSIONAL NURSE

For an efficient discharging of nursing duties and for a satisfactory fulfillment of all the aims and aspirations that nursing profession stands for, the following qualities in a nurse are inevitable:

1. **Love:** With all other attendant qualities like mercy, kindness, gentleness, patience and understanding, love is must in a successful nurse. All services for the sick and disabled are sponsored by these qualities. Without these essential characteristics the nurse becomes only a mechanical aid.
2. **Willingness and self-sacrifice:** These two qualities are complimentary to each other. Because nurses are willing to serve under any trying situation, they sacrifice their time, comfort and even material benefits, e.g. Florence Nightingale at Scutari.
3. **Reliability:** A nurse is one who can be depended upon for a faithful discharging of her/his duties, the patients under her/his care, their families, doctors and members of the 'health team' depend on her/him, for she/he is trustworthy and competent.

4. **Resourcefulness:** In critical circumstances nurse uses her/his wisdom and knowledge and performs her/his duties to the best of her/his ability with whatever means that are at her/his disposal. She/he tackles situations with alacrity.
5. **Courage:** In times of confusion, calamity or catastrophe, the nurse manages her/his work with compassion and is ready to meet any problem with courage. She/he is cool and level-headed and does not get agitated easily.
6. **Loyalty and honesty:** Nurses' relationship with the patient, the doctor and associates are marked by utmost loyalty and honesty.
7. **Observant:** A good nurse is always vigilant. She/he keeps a close and constant watch on the patients, their progress, their changes and reactions to treatment, etc. and gives timely reports to doctor. A nurse should anticipate and meet the patients' needs.
8. **Willingness to learn**: A nurse must keep in touch with the latest discoveries and developments in medicine and treatment and must "maintain her/his knowledge and skill at a consistently high level".
9. **Cooperative and considerate**: A nurse learns to live in harmony with patients, doctors and other members of the health team and tries to help them in times of need.
10. **Cleanliness**: A nurse is always neat and clean personally and in her/his work. She/he must be tidy and demand high standards of cleanliness from those whom she/he is associated within her/his profession.
11. **Spirituality**: A nurse must learn to create a spiritual atmosphere for the patient and must try and help the patients to put their confidence and trust in a 'Power' that is higher than any other power in the world.

NEW PERSPECTIVES OF NURSING PROFESSION

Historically, only medicine, law and the ministry were accepted as profession. Criteria of a profession:
Genevieve and Roy Bixler first wrote about the status of nursing as a profession in 1945. These criteria include the following:

1. The services provided are vital to humanity and the welfare of the society. Nursing is the service that is essential to the well-being of the people and to the society. Nursing promotes, maintains and restores the health of individuals, groups and communities. Assisting others to attain the highest level of wellness is the goal of nursing. Caring, meaning nurturing and helping others are the basic components of professional nursing.
2. There is a special body of knowledge that is continually enlarged through research. In the past, nursing was based on principles borrowed

from the physical and social sciences and other disciplines. Today there is a unique body of knowledge to nursing.

3. The services involve intellectual activities. Individual responsibilities (accountability) are a strong feature. Nursing has developed and refined its own unique approach to practice. Nursing process is a cognitive activity that requires both critical and creative thinking and serves as the basis of providing nursing care.

   Individual accountability in nursing has become the hallmark of practice. Accountability is being answerable to someone for something one has done.

   Through legal opinion and court cases, society has demonstrated that nurses are individually responsible for their actions as well as for those of personnel under their supervision.

4. Practitioners are educated in institution of higher learning. There are Basic Nursing Program, Baccalaureate Program, Master's and Doctoral Program in nursing
5. Practitioners are relatively independent and control their own policies and activities (autonomy). Autonomy or control over one's practice is another controversial area for nursing. Although many nursing actions are independent, most nurses are employed in hospitals, where authority resides in one's position.
6. Practitioners are motivated by service (altruism) and considered their work an important component of their lives. Nurses are dedicated to the ideal of service to others, which is known as altruism.
7. There is a Code of Ethics to guide the decisions and conduct of practitioners. The International Council of Nurses (ICN) has established Code of Nursing Ethics through which standards of practice are established, promoted and refined.
8. There is an organization (association) that encourages and supports high standards of practice. Nursing has a number of professional associations that were formed to promote the improvement of the profession. Foremost among these is the Trained Nurses Association of India (TNAI). The purposes of TNAI are to foster high standards of nursing practice, promote professional and educational advancement of nurses and promote the welfare of the nurses.

CONCEPT OF PROFESSIONALISM IN NURSING

ART OF NURSING

Professional nursing practice is grounded in the art of nursing, described as taking a holistic, client-centered focus; being caring and ethical in interactions with patients, families and colleagues; having above average interpersonal skills; and making sound judgments based on experience and knowledge, thus averting potential problems.

COMPETENCE

Professional practice demands competence in relation to knowledge and technical skills. This requires not only a broad base of knowledge, but also depth of knowledge in a chosen area of practice, a desire and ability to continue developing that knowledge base and to share it with others and critical thinking in decision making.

ATTRIBUTES OF PRACTICE

Professional practice reflects a particular approach to one's work with collaboration by far most salient characteristic. Professional nursing practice means working in partnership with other nurses and health professionals in providing client care, being highly organized in managing activities and time, having the ability to manage many complex tasks simultaneously, working autonomously as appropriate and having an open mind and non-judgmental manner.

PERSONAL COMMITMENT

In describing this element of professional practice, respondents referred to the importance of having confidence in one's abilities and taking responsibility for one's actions, including having a sound understanding of the boundaries and limitations of nursing practice. Having a balanced lifestyle and supporting the advancement of the profession were also considered important characteristics of a professional nurse.

VALUES OF A PROFESSIONAL NURSE

To be successful, nurses must be equipped with certain tools and abilities. These skills are developed over time as a nurse gains experience and confidence. These are as follows:

1. **Confidentiality and autonomy:** Nurses should have an awareness of legislation on patient confidentiality and the policies of their own organization. Nurses should not breach confidentiality, unless the circumstances are exceptional. For instance, if the patient is threatening harm to himself/herself or others. Nurses must not discuss patients' details outside of the care setting, and must take care of notes, paper and computer files. Nurses should make all efforts to promote the patient's rights to make his/her own decision whenever possible.
2. **Protection from harm:** The nurse's conduct must protect the patient from harm. Nurse must not undertake something he/she thinks might cause harm to the patient even if he/she has been told or asked to

do so by another person. The nurse is accountable for his/her own actions and might be asked to explain these in later proceedings. If the nurse sees anything he/she fears may endanger the patient, he/she must immediately report this to management.

3. **Professional development:** The nurse has a duty to keep up-to-date with all developments that may have an impact on his/her job. He/she must attend professional development and training activities. Part of his/her duty may involve training and mentoring new and junior staff. Nurses must meet training requirements and pay any fees needed to maintain licensing.
4. **Dedication:** Professional nursing is a difficult profession with many stressful scenarios. Nurses must work long shifts and deal with many vastly different issues on a daily basis. The combination of long work hours, constant care of patients and the stress of seeing death can cause nurses to unravel. Thus, professional nurses need to be calm and level-headed, able to quickly handle a multitude of problems effectively. Nurses are responsible for patient quality of care and the execution of the health care plan. A dedication to the job is essential for a nurse to fulfill the nursing duties.
5. **Systems thinking:** A nurse is faced with a plenty of situations throughout each workday. Each patient has individual problems and requires a different approach. Nurses are expected to develop individualized decisions of care depending on the patient and the specific circumstances.
6. **Caring:** Nurses are required to take care of the patient throughout the entire healthcare process. Their goal is to make the healing process painless and comfortable as possible, without inflicting any unnecessary grief for the patient. In the case of imminent death, nurses must console the patients and the families in order to ease the transition. According to the American Association of Critical Care Nurses, duties of caring include 'vigilance, engagement, and responsiveness of caregivers, including family and healthcare personnel.'
7. **Ethnic and religious sensitivity:** Nurses take care of patients from a variety of ethnic and religious backgrounds. Professional nurses must be sensitive to the specific requirements of various cultures and religions in order to facilitate the patient's health care. Nurses must demonstrate a desire to respect various practices while continuing to adhere to professional standards.

ROLES AND RESPONSIBLITIES OF PROFESSIONAL NURSE

ROLES

The professional nurse occupying the position by accepting responsibility and accountability in:

1. Provide quality nursing to the clients in their care, placing emphasis on the medical psychosocial, spiritual needs of the clients and be mindful of the needs of the relatives or attendants.
2. Cooperating with the nursing units and all other departments within the hospital.
3. Understanding all activities in relaxation to patient care and other assigned duties.
4. Actively participating in the nursing team.
5. Actively pursuing and continuing self education.
6. Actively providing appropriate health education to the individuals, families and groups and community at large in various settings.

FUNCTIONS AND RESPONSIBLITIES

Client Care

Providing safe and effective nursing care within a healthcare setup or community. It includes participating in the delivery of nursing care based on the best practice principles stated by statutory body, maintaining nursing standards, observing and participating in quality improvement programs, fostering congeniality between all members of the healthcare team, assisting with cost containment by utilizing resources effectively, participating in appropriate meetings, workshops or committees related to improving nursing care.

Professional Practice

In professional practice the aspects included are maintaining confidentiality, taking reasonable care in health and safety of persons on the unit, being familiar with the resources to be used in case of any emergency or disaster, adhering to all infection control policies and safety rules, cooperating with management for health, safety and welfare provisions, actively seeking knowledge of the diagnosis and treatment given, actively participating with a zeal as a member of multidisciplinary team, complying with the professional Code of Ethics, demonstrating accountability and responsibility for the professional conduct, practicing with limits of own abilities and qualification, initiating and maintaining effective communication with others.

Management

There are three kinds of management roles, i.e. in planning and in organizing, in implementation and in evaluation. These are the following:

1. In planning, the management roles are to describe the planning process in the assigned clinical area, to assess client's needs, work environment and available resources, to set appropriate priorities for day's work, to anticipate and plan for potential problems or unpredictable events.

2. In organizing, the management roles are to organize work activities, to delegate tasks and share responsibilities, to adhere to organizational policies and procedures, to describe instances of the incorporation of risk management concepts in the assigned clinical setting.
3. In implementation, the management roles are to perform nursing procedures safely, accurately and scientific knowledge based, to describe the decision-making process, to assure continuity of care, to communicate effectively with patients, families and other health personnel, to show sensitivity to the patients' needs, to bring change in the status quo of the organization as required.
4. In evaluation, the management roles are to analyze the flow of communication in the unit and within the organization, to describe the Nurse Manager's role as evaluator of personnel performance, to assess patient care evaluation activities that are done in clinical setting.

CONCLUSION

Nursing has been called the oldest of the art, and the youngest of the profession. As such, it has gone through many stages and has been an integral part of social movements. Nursing has been involved in the existing culture, shaped by it and yet being to develop it. Nursing is known as one of the noblest among all the professions based on spirit and devotion to the services to humanity at large. Nursing is a unique blend of art and science of skill and knowledge. It is a science because it needs vast specialized knowledge in science for its background and it adopts the scientific methods in its application. Nursing is an art as it implies skillful application of this specialized knowledge in approaching the patient as an individual considering his emotions, feelings and environment. Therefore, the primary responsibility of the nurse to help the individual in his daily pattern of living with those activities that are ordinarily performed without assistance.

CHAPTER

2

Philosophies and Objectives of Graduate Nurse

INTRODUCTION

Philosophy, it sets the ideas, principles, goals, standards, values thus it is in reality and truth. Philosophy and education are closely connected that one without the other is meaningless. The term philosophy has been derived from two Greek words, 'Philos' means love and 'Sophia' means wisdom. Thus philosophy means love of wisdom. Philosophy of education may be defined as the application of the fundamental principles of a philosophy of life to the work of education. Philosophy of education offers a definite set of principles and establishes a definite set of aims and objectives. It offers criteria for intelligent interpretation of educational ends and means.

MEANING OF PHILOSOPHY

The following meanings of philosophy have been useful for systematic understanding of education:

1. Philosophy is the science of knowledge.
2. Philosophy is the science of all sciences.
3. Philosophy is the mother of all arts.
4. Philosophy as an activity.
5. Philosophy as a comprehensive picture of the universe.
6. Philosophy as a guide to a way of life.
7. Philosophy and science.

PHILOSOPHY AND BONDS OF EDUCATION

Philosophy and education are closely connected that one without the other is meaningless. Many bonds unite education with philosophy. They are:

1. **Natural bonds:** This bond signifies an association between two or more things or processes that is rooted in their nature. There is a natural association between the spiritual life and education, as well as between the ideals and the cultural standards of the adult generation.

2. **Logical bonds:** The core or heart of any given system of education is found in the ideals, it sets out to attain. These ideals are determined through the philosophy. Once ideals have been established, it may be said to follow logically that a system of education must be set up in order to perpetuate them.
3. **Social bonds:** Education aims at the perpetuation of social institutions, which are based on a philosophy of life and the progress of society.
4. **Cultural bonds:** Culture embraces not only the sum total of people's accomplishments but the ideas and the virtues after which they strive. Therefore, there is a cultural bond between philosophy and education.
5. **Human bonds:** Psychology or the dealing in human relationship is the basis for education. A recognized aim of education is to develop the personality of the student. This is done by knowing the individual student and the ideal that will best serve as a model for the education.

PHILOSOPHY OF NURSING

Nursing philosophies are:

1. I accept responsibility for my accuracy and honesty in all nursing functions and procedures.
2. I believe an individual is a social being with social needs.
3. I believe the private and professional lives of a nurse cannot be completely separated because society, as a whole, sees the profession in the lives of its members.
4. I believe health professional other than nursing are needed to meet the health needs of the public.
5. I believe the nursing profession should be self-governing and directed by nurse.

OBJECTIVES OF GRADUATE NURSES

Nursing is based on values of caring, and aims to help individuals to attain independence in self-care. It necessitates development of compassion and understanding of human behavior among its practitioners to provide care with respect and dignity and protect the rights of individuals and groups. A graduate nursing program is broad based education within an academic framework, specifically directed to the development of critical thinking skills, competencies and standards required for practice of professional nursing and midwifery as envisaged in National Health Policy 2002.

On completion of the four year BSc Nursing program the graduates will be able to:

1. Apply knowledge from physical, biological and behavioral sciences, medicine, including alternative systems and nursing in providing nursing care to individuals, families and communities.

2. Demonstrate understanding of lifestyle and other factors, which affect health of individuals and groups.
3. Provide nursing care based on steps of nursing process in collaboration with the individuals and group.
4. Demonstrate critical thinking skill in making decisions in all situations in order to provide quality care.
5. Utilize the latest trends and technology in providing health care.
6. Provide promotive, preventive and restorative health services in line with the national health policies and programs.
7. Practice within the framework of code of ethics and professional conduct and acceptable standards of practice within the legal boundaries.
8. Communicate effectively with individuals and groups and members of the health team in order to promote effective interpersonal relationships and teamwork.
9. Demonstrate skills in teaching to individuals and groups in clinical/ community health settings.
10. Participate effectively as members of the health team in health care delivery system.
11. Demonstrate leadership and managerial skills in clinical / community health settings.
12. Conduct need based research studies in various settings and utilize the research findings to improve the quality of care.
13. Demonstrate awareness, interest and contribute towards advancement of self and of the profession.

PERSON

In nursing theory, human beings are considered in terms of their physiological, psychological, social, spiritual and cultural selves. People are evaluated in terms of their individual place in society as well as their relationships to their family, community and society as a whole.

Additionally, human beings are viewed in terms of their individual needs and how nursing practice is applied to meet these needs. The purpose of nursing and nursing theory is to identify how a particular individuals needs are either met or not met, to predict future needs and to prioritize those needs in order of importance.

ENVIRONMENT

The environment concept of nursing comprises all the internal and external factors that act on human beings and affect their behavior and development. This includes psychological, spiritual, social, physical and cultural forces as well as the environment in which nursing care is provided. The idea behind this concept is that the environment influences individual and collective health and that individuals who experience a positive, comfortable nursing environment are more likely to demonstrate good health versus those who receive a level of care that is lacking.

HEALTH

The concept of health refers to an individual's physical, mental and social well-being and at what point they are on the health spectrum, which ranges from good health to poor health or death. Health is considered to be affected by genetic factors, environmental factors, lifestyle factors and external mechanisms such as bacteria. A person's place on the health spectrum is constantly changing and in a nursing context, it is the responsibility of nursing professionals to identify the patient's place on the spectrum and to take steps to help that person's health improvement.

NURSING

Nursing refers to the process of caring for the health of human beings and assisting individuals in meeting their needs while also teaching them the basics of caring for themselves. The responsibilities of the nursing profession are to promote good health, to prevent disease when possible, to promote healing in those who are ill and to ease the suffering of dying patients. The concept of nursing extends beyond the healthcare facility to the community and society as a whole, and views individual health and the environment as closely related. Nursing is defined as care that is tailored to the needs of individuals and that is provided in an efficient and effective manner.

BACHELOR OF NURSING COURSE

PHILOSOPHY AND AIMS OF THE ACADEMIC PROGRAM

The faculty believes that nursing is an integral part of the healthcare delivery system and share responsibility by working in collaboration with other allied professions for the attainment of optimal health for all members of society. As an essential health service, nursing includes the prevention of disease, promotion, restoration and maintenance of optimum health for individual and families in hospital and community setting. Professional nursing is broad in scope. It considers all aspects of patient-centered care achieved by a multidisciplined approach. Inherent in the practice of nursing is the teaching and counseling of patient and families. A concurrent study of the arts and science is a necessary requirement for effective professional education and practice.

The faculty conceives education as a lifelong learning process. It seeks to engender appropriate behavioral changes in students in order to facilitate their development, which assists them to live personally satisfying and socially useful lives. Education, social and behavioral sciences and humanities are required for the modification of behavior. The faculty recognizes that the practice of nursing includes the application of knowledge derived from these disciplines.

The faculty acknowledges responsibility for moulding program of studies for students which provides for the development of specialized knowledge, skills and desirable attitudes relevant to nursing and basic to professional duties to be performed; affords practice in independent decision making, stressing the necessity for a systematic approach in solving patient's health care problems; prepares the nurse practitioner to engage in the primary, acute and long-term care of patients of all ages in a variety of settings; stimulates the desire to augment knowledge, skills, abilities and interests through continuing education and creates an atmosphere for the student to become self-directive and a responsible citizen.

OBJECTIVES

The goal of the post certificate degree program leading to a Bachelor of Science in Nursing is the preparation of the trained nurse as a generalist, who accepts responsibility for enhancing the effectiveness of nursing care. The graduate in BSc degree in Nursing demonstrates the ability of:

1. Administer high quality nursing care to all people of all ages in homes, hospitals and other community agencies in urban and rural areas.
2. Apply knowledge from the physical, social and behavioral sciences in assessing the health status of individuals and make critical judgment in planning, directing and evaluating primary, acute and long-term care given by themselves and others working with them.
3. Investigate healthcare problems systematically.
4. Work collaboratively with members of others allied disciplines toward attaining optimum health for all citizens of society.
5. Teach and counsel individuals, families and other groups about health and illness.
6. Understands human behavior and establish effective interpersonal relationships with individuals, families and groups.
7. Recognize the various forces affecting the community's social, health and welfare programs and participate in identifying planning and carrying out community health programs, which meet the community's expectation.
8. Teach in clinical nursing situations and beginning ability in administrative skills and in the teaching of nursing in nursing education programs.
9. Identify underlying principles from the social and natural sciences and utilize them in adapting or initiating changes in relation to those factors.

10. Assume responsibility for continuing learning and for increasing competence in nursing practice.
11. Recognize social and ethical obligations to society.

DEGREE OF MASTER OF NURSING

PHILOSOPHY

Nursing faculty presents the following statement of beliefs about Master of Nursing program. The Master of Nursing program is offered by institution of higher education and is built upon a recognized (by Indian Nursing Council) Bachelor's curriculum in Nursing.

The program prepares nurses for leadership position in nursing and health fields, who can function as specialist nurse practitioners, consultants, educators, administrators and investigators in a wide variety of professional setting in meeting the national priorities and the changing needs of the society.

The program prepares nursing graduates who are professionally equipped, creative, self-directed and socially motivated to effectively deal with day-to-day problems within the existing constraints and this act as an agent of social change. Further the program encourages accountability and commitment to lifelong learning, which fosters improvement of quality care.

OBJECTIVES

Graduates of Master of Nursing program demonstrates:

1. Increased cognitive, affective and psychomotor competencies and the ability to utilize the potentialities for efficient nursing performance.
2. Expertise in the utilization of concepts and theories for the assessment, planning and intervention in meeting the self-care needs of an individual for the attainment of his/her fullest potential in his/her (graduate) field of specialty.
3. Ability to function effectively as educators and administrators.
4. Ability to interpret health related research and develop initial competencies in conducting research.
5. Ability to plan and initiate change in the healthcare system as practice and in the delivery of health care.
6. Leadership qualities for the advancement of the practice of professional nursing.
7. Ability to establish collaborative relationship with members of other disciplines for maintaining and improving health care.
8. Interest in lifelong learning for personal and professional advancement.

MASTER OF PHILOSOPHY PROGRAM IN NURSING

PHILOSOPHY

Nursing shares with the whole university a main focus of preparing its students for service and assisting them to achieve a meaningful philosophy of life. The student is encouraged to develop judgment and wisdom in handling knowledge and skills and achieve mastery of problem solving and creative thinking.

Commitment to lifelong learning is the mark of truly professional person. In order to maintain clinical competencies and enhance professional practice, the students must stay abreast of the new developments and contribute to the advancement of nursing knowledge.

OBJECTIVES

The objectives of the MPhil degree course in nursing are:

1. To strengthen the research foundations of the nurses for encouraging research attitudes and problem-solving capabilities.
2. To provide basic training required for research in undertaking doctoral work.

CONCLUSION

Profession nurse is a graduate of a recognized nursing school who has fulfilled the requirements for a registered nurse in a state in which she is licensed to practice. Candidate who satisfy the basic requirements are selected by the authority to undergo the training in a recognized school or college of nursing. They complete the basic course of study according to the prescribed syllabus approved by the Indian Nursing Council and by the state council. The length of the period of training varies with the type of program. After the successful completion of the course, the candidate receives a diploma or a bachelor's degree in nursing.

CHAPTER

3

Trends and Issues in Nursing

INTRODUCTION

Trends denote general directions and tendencies especially of events and of opinion. Nursing trends refer to direction toward which the different nursing events have moved or are moving, as well as the opinions in and around nursing and tendencies that are found in and about nursing profession. Trends in nursing mean changes currently taking place in any area of nursing, which influence the profession as a whole. These do not occur independently, but each one has a basis of related changes in other fields. These are: If we are aware of current trends it will help us plan for developments in nursing education and nursing services as well as controlling the direction in which the profession moves. A global perception will enable nurses to rise to higher levels in their knowledge, skills and improved performance both in India and around the globe.

FACTORS INFLUENCING TRENDS

The factors influencing the trends in nursing:

1. **Changes in society:** For the past 5 decades, five social factors have greatly influenced present trends in nursing. These are:
   a. Intensive efforts of government to meet the health needs of people.
   b. Gradual improved literacy level of the people with the growing awareness of health needs.
   c. Advanced scientific technology.
   d. The changing role of women.
   e. the continuing growth of population.
2. **Changes in other professions:** Trends in the nursing profession have always been closely related to those in the medical profession. Growing specialization in medical field is resulting in a trend toward increased specialization in nursing. The development of new diagnostic procedure and equipments make specialization even more necessary.

3. **Patient's Bill of Rights:** After the development of the 'Patient's Bill of Rights', the nurses are also accountable for patient's care and have legal responsibilities for the patient.
4. **Developments in other discipline:** These other than medicine also influence trends in nursing profession. Nursing is moving toward more specific nursing functions as other members of health team like dieticians, social workers and physiotherapists are more available and more highly specialized.
5. **Leadership within the profession:** It also influences the trends in nursing. Nursing is moving towards professionalism due to the untiring efforts of nurses who have been dedicated to achieve the aim.
6. **Working and studying in abroad:** This is influenced by many factors within India and in other countries. Shortage of nurses in other countries, higher salary paid in abroad is the main causes for the working of Indian nurses in abroad.
7. **Greater specialization in nursing education and practice:** This is a trend related to that in the medical profession and the growing amount of scientific knowledge available.
8. **Working conditions:** Working conditions for nurses are also changing. There is a gradual change toward, shorter and more convenient hours of duty, better accommodations and higher salaries.
9. **Trends in other countries:** These also influence the trends in the nursing profession in India. The rapid development of the degree program has promoted the same emphasis and development here for professional nursing.

ISSUES RELATED TO NURSING PROFESSION

Issues refer to the items for consideration or questions for discussion. Various issues in nursing profession may be related to profession, education, practice and nurses themselves.

Various issues related to nursing profession are:

1. Status of nursing in society in healthcare delivery system.
2. Values reflected in our nursing performances.
3. Attitudes, humane approach and concern shown in the behavior patterns of nurses.
4. Quality in nursing hand in hand between education and practice.
5. Unique functions of nursing.
6. Different levels of nurses required in the country.
7. Emphasis from traditional to primary healthcare approach.
8. Evidence based nursing research. Nurses in administration.
9. Expanded and extended roles of nurses.
10. Globalization in the profession.

11. Nursing leadership in bringing changes in health scenario according of community demands.

FUTURE CONCERN FOR NURSES

In the near future the issues of concern for the nursing practice involve autonomy and independent practice among nurses, quality of care in community setting and homes, and development of nurse as leaders in the healthcare field. Various challenging healthcare issues are patients refusal toward healthcare, euthanasia, patient advocacy by nurses, cost effective quality nursing care, competency in nursing practice Nurses need to look at these issues, professional values and expectations they face and decide. Once these issues are identified, strategies for promoting the quality care nursing can be delineated.

EXTENDED ROLE OF NURSE

The nurses in India are also prepared and more privileged to face the changes and ready to accept the challenging roles and functions of the nurse as perceived in the globe because of the development in the education and training system. The following roles and positions perceived as in the globe are given below:

1. **Nurse educator** works in schools of nursing, staff development departments. They provide the educational program for student nurses, and nurses teach clients about the self-care and home care.
2. **Clinical nurse specialist** specializes in managing specific diseases and they function as clinicians, educators, managers, consultants and researchers.
3. **Nurse practitioners** are certified to provide healthcare to clients in outpatient or community settings.
4. **Certified nurse-midwife** is certified by the American College of Nurse-Midwives to provide independent care for women during normal pregnancy, labor and delivery.
5. **Nurse anesthetist** having advance training in anesthesiology, provides surgical anesthesia to the client under the supervision of an anesthesiologist during minor surgery with Baccalaureate degrees or Master's degree.
6. **Nurse administrators** manage client care within the healthcare agencies in a middle level or upper level management position.
7. **Nurse researcher** with Doctoral degree investigate nursing problem to improve care and to define and expand the scope of nursing practice.

Advancements in science increase health needs of the society and thereby expect changes in the role of nurses and thus increases the scope for nurses.

TRENDS IN NURSING EDUCATION

The form of teaching has remained unchanged for centuries. The needs of society. The practical side of the matter has been left to chance, whereas specific features of the situation of each country are changing more rapidly. Unfortunately, little or no account has been taken in to consideration for the training of health personnel, but following traditional systems in teaching. What is required now is to make sure that the educational program is relevant? No educational system can be effective unless its purposes are clearly defined.

The members of health team must be trained specially for the task they will have to perform taking into account the circumstances under which they will work, so defining the professional task of health personnel to be trained is the very basis of the educational objectives of training centers/ institutions and must be shaped selectively in terms of the goal to be achieved. If the goal is modified in the course of time the program also to be modified accordingly.

Definition of professional task must proceed from a study of needs, availability of resources, various category of personnel be called upon to do their professional career in a given type of health services. In nursing education, depending upon the needs of the country we need to deicide whom we would like to prepare, the type of health services to be provided and to achieve the institutional goal and educational objectives. For example, generalist or specialist such as graduate midwives, lactation consultants, birth spacing consultants, etc. Depending on this professional task to be identified and prepare the suitable educational objectives and educational programmers as preregistration nursing courses for diploma level and postregistration courses for the higher education framework with the pathways leading towards, an Honors degree or Master's and Doctoral degree.

TRENDS IN NURSING PRACTICE

Definition of professional task becomes precondition for ensuring that the training program is really designed to meet the population health needs. The training programs, professional profile and educational program objectives should provide basis for nursing practice in all three levels of healthcare, such as primary, secondary and tertiary healthcare. The advancement to adopted and develop professional skill as specialist is essential. So that the nurses can be prepared as clinical consultants, administrators and as researches in the various fields of nursing practice in order to make both nursing education and practice identical three principles are fundamental importance.

It must be oriented toward the community as well as the individuals taking account of the needs of each particular activity, i.e. education must be community oriented.

The education must be learner centered. If educational objectives are based on faulty principles, then the 'best system' of training may give 'bad results'.

The support system which should support health systems are:

1. The political system.
2. The structure and authorities of the administrative system.
3. The general system/general infrastructure.
4. The education system.

Unfortunately, most of the time these systems act as obstacles rather than support. Based upon these trends the following issues need to be looked into before developing curriculum.

CONCLUSION

The trend analysis and future scenarios provide a basis for sound decision making through mapping of possible futures and aiming to create preferred futures. The future will see great advantages in prevention, diagnosis and treatment of illness and diseases with increasing demand for heath care and health information. As large hospital are replaced by high tech and small hospitals, health care will be provided in homes and outreach facilities and the focus will be on provider skill, outcomes and user preference and satisfaction. Nurses will be the preferred care providers and entry points for diverse services. On the other hand, there will be challenges related to ethics, rising costs, access to care and quality of care. The multifaceted components in this unfolding will be—the revolutionary advances that we continue to witness in modern medical practice as a result of technological advances from the fields of physics, electronics, instrumentation, chemical and material sciences. The advent of molecular medicine, with work at the frontiers of modern biology particularly on the human genome, and its relevance to the generic basis of disease; the importance of recent advances relating to the human brain the wide range of opportunities becoming available through advances in information technology; the great importance of community and social medicine, of hygiene and epidemiological studies in understanding and preventing disease.

CHAPTER

4

Expanded Role of the Nurse

INTRODUCTION

Contemporary nursing requires that the nurse possess knowledge and skills in a variety of areas. In the past the principal role of nurses was to provide care and comfort as they carried out specific nursing functions, but changes in nursing have expanded the role to include increased emphasis on health promotion and illness prevention, as well as concern for the client as a whole. The contemporary nurse functions in the interrelated roles of caregiver, clinical and ethical decision maker, protector and client advocate case manager, rehabilitator, comforter, communicator and teacher.

EXPANDED ROLES OF NURSE

CAREGIVER

As caregiver, the nurse helps the client regain health through the healing process. Healing is more than just curing a specific disease, although treatment skills that promote physical healing are important to caregivers. The nurse addresses the holistic health care needs of the client, including measures to restore emotional, spiritual and social well-being. The caregiver helps the client and family, set goals and meet those goals with a minimal cost of time and energy.

CLINICAL AND ETHICAL DECISION MAKER

The nurse uses critical thinking skills throughout the nursing process to provide effective care. Before undertaking any nursing action, whether it is assessing the client's condition, giving care or evaluating the results of care, the nurse plans the action by deciding the best approach for each client. The nurse makes these decisions alone or in collaboration with the client and family. In each of these situations, the nurse collaborates and consults with other healthcare professionals.

PROTECTOR AND CLIENT ADVOCATE

As protector the nurse helps maintain a safe environment for the client and takes steps to prevent injury and protect the client from possible adverse effects of diagnostic or treatment measures. Confirming that a client does not have an allergy to a medication and providing immunization against disease in a community-based practice are examples of the nurse's protective role.

In the role of client advocate, the nurse protects the client's human and legal rights and provides assistance in asserting those rights if the need arises. For example, the nurse may provide additional information for a client who is trying to decide whether to accept treatment. The nurse may also defend clients' rights in a general way by speaking out against policies or actions that might endanger client's well-being or conflict with their rights.

CASE MANAGER

As case manager, the nurse coordinates the activities of other members of the healthcare team, such as nutritionists and physical therapists, when managing a group of clients' care. In addition, nurses must also manage the own time and the resources of the practice settings. Differentiated practice models offer nurses opportunities to make decisions about their career paths.

REHABILITATOR

Rehabilitation is the process by which individual's maximal levels of functioning after illness, other disabling events. Frequently clients experience physical or emotional impairments that change their lives and the nurse helps them adapt as fully as possible. Rehabilitative and restorative care activities range from teaching clients to walk with crutches to helping clients cope with lifestyle changes often associated with chronic illness.

COMFORTER

The role of comforter, caring for the client as a person, is a traditional and historical one in nursing and has continued to be important as nurses have assumed new roles. Because nursing care must be directed to the whole person rather than simply the body, comfort and emotional support often help give the client strength to recover. While carrying out nursing activities, nurses can provide comfort by demonstrating care for the client as an individual with unique feelings and needs. As comforter, nurses should help the client reach therapeutic goals rather than encourage emotional or physical dependence.

COMMUNICATOR

The role of communication is central to all effective nursing roles. Nursing involves communication with clients and families, other nurses and health care professionals, resource persons and the community. The quality of communication is a critical factor in meeting the needs of individuals, families, and communities.

TEACHER

As teacher, the nurse explains to clients concepts and facts about health, demonstrates procedures such as self-care activities, determines that the client fully understands, reinforces learning or client behavior and evaluates progress in learning. Some teaching can be unplanned and informal, such as when a nurse responds to a question about a health issue in casual conversation. Other teaching activities may be planned and more formal, such as when the nurse teaches a client with diabetes to self-administer insulin injections. The nurse uses teaching methods that match the client's capabilities and needs, and incorporates other resources, such as the family, in teaching plans.

CAREER ROLES OF NURSE

The proceeding roles and functions apply to all nurses in most practice settings. Career roles, on the other hand, are specific employment positions. Because of increasing educational opportunities for nurses, the growth of nursing as a profession and greater concern for job enrichment, the nursing profession offers expanded roles and different kinds of career opportunities. Examples of career roles include nurse educators and advanced practice nurses, such as clinical nurse specialists, nurse practitioners, certified nurse-midwives, anesthetists, administrators and researchers. Additional no clinical roles include risk managers, quality improvement nurses, and product consultants.

NURSE EDUCATOR

A nurse educator works primarily in schools of nursing, stall development departments (health care agencies and client education departments). Nursing educators generally have a background in clinical nursing, which provides them with practical skills and theoretical knowledge. A faculty member in a school of nursing prepares students to function as nurses.

Nursing faculty members are responsible for teaching current nursing practice theory and necessary skills in laboratories or clinical settings. Nurse educators in nursing schools are usually required to have graduate degrees in nursing education. In addition, they generally have a specific clinical specialty and advanced clinical experience.

Nurse educators in staff development departments of healthcare institutions provide educational programs for nurses within their institution. These programs include orientation of new personnel, critical care nursing courses and instruction about new equipment or procedures. The primary focus of the nurse educator in an agency's department of client education is to teach or disabled clients and families to provide care in the home. In most of the healthcare agencies, however, time budget does not permit a separate client education department. Therefore staff nurses usually incorporate education into a client's plan of care.

ADVANCED PRACTICE NURSE

The advanced practice nurse (APN) has a Master's degree in nursing, advanced education in pharmacology and physical assessment, and certification and expertise in a specialized area of practice (ANA, 1995). An APN usually works in primary, acute, restorative or community healthcare agency. In addition, an APN may specialize in the management of a disease such as cancer, diabetes, cardiovascular, pulmonary disease or in a specific field such as pediatrics or gerontology.

CLINICAL NURSE SPECIALIST

The clinical nurse specialist (CNS) has a Master's degree in nursing and expertise in a specialized area of practice. A CNS may work in primary care, acute care, restorative care and community-based settings. In addition, the CNS may specialize in specific diseases such as diabetes mellitus, cancer, congestive heart failure or in a specific field such as pediatrics or gerontology. The CNS functions as an expert clinician, educator, case in manager, consultant and researcher to plan or improve the quality of care provided to the client and family.

NURSE PRACTITIONER

The nurse practitioner provides health care to clients, usually in an outpatient, ambulatory care or community-based setting and comprehensiveness of care. A significant percentage of primary care encounters extend beyond the boundaries of medicine and demand the expertise of the nurse. The nurse practitioner is able to establish a collaborative provider-client relationship. The major nurse practitioner categories are adult, family, pediatric, obstetrics, gynecology and geriatric nurse practitioner. A nurse practitioner has the knowledge and skills necessary to detect and manage limited acute and chronic stable conditions. The nurse practitioner's educational preparation includes a practitioner program or a Master's degree in nursing.

ADULT NURSE PRACTITIONER

Adult nurse practitioner (ANP) provides primary, ambulatory care to adults with a non-emergency acute or chronic illness, and in some settings tertiary care. ANPs are usually employed in ambulatory care centers or outpatient clinics and work in collaboration with a primary physician.

FAMILY NURSE PRACTITIONER

A family nurse practitioner (FNP) provides primary ambulatory care for families, usually in collaboration with a family care physician. The FNP meets the family's general healthcare needs, manages some illnesses by providing direct care, and guides or counsels the family as needed.

PEDIATRIC NURSE PRACTITIONER

A pediatric nurse practitioner (PNP) provides health care to infants and children, An obstetric-gynecologic nurse practitioner (OGNP) provides primary ambulatory care to women seeking obstetrical or gynecological health care. The nurse practitioner who is also a certified nurse-midwife may independently deliver infants. Gerontologic nurse practitioner (GNP) provides ambulatory or inpatient care to older adults. The GNP's activities include interventions for health maintenance, illness prevention or health restoration.

CERTIFIED NURSE MIDWIFE

A certified nurse-midwife (CNM) is a registered nurse who is also educated in midwifery and is certified by the American College of Nurse-Midwives. The practice of nurse-midwifery involves providing independent care for women during normal pregnancy, labor and delivery, as well as care for the newborn; it may include some gynecological services such as routine Papanicolaou (Pap) smears, family planning, and treatment for minor vaginal infections. A CNM practices with a health care agency that provides medical consultation, collaborative management and referral.

NURSE ANESTHETIST

A nurse anesthetist is an RN who has received advanced training in an accredited program in anesthesiology. Nurse anesthetists provide surgical anesthesia under the guidance and supervision of an anesthesiologist, who is a physician with advanced knowledge of surgical anesthesia.

NURSE ADMINISTRATOR

A nurse administrator manages client care and the delivery of specific nursing services within a health care agency. This administrator may hold a middle-management position, such as head nurse or supervisor, or an upper-level management position, such as assistant or associate director or director of nursing services. Functions of administrators include budgeting, staffing, strategic planning of programs and services, employee evaluation and employee development. Middle-management position usually requires at least a Baccalaureate degree in nursing, and upper-level positions generally require a Master's degree.

NURSE RESEARCHER

The nurse researcher investigates problems to improve nursing care and to further define and expand the scope of nursing practice. The nurse researcher may be employed in an academic setting, hospital, or independent professional or community-service agency. The minimum educational requirement is now a Doctoral degree, with at least a Master's degree in nursing.

CONCLUSION

Nurses will have an essential public health role and patients will become more demanding. Healthier lifestyles, continuum of care, health environments and evidence based practice will be emphasized and in the forefront of nursing agenda. Globalization wills enhance free movement, standardization, and wider opportunities and challenges. The changing work environment will be driven by cost effectiveness and quality of care for which nursing is well positioned.

CHAPTER

5

Development and Trends in Nursing Education

INTRODUCTION

The Nursing Council Act came into existence in 1948 to constitute a council of nurses, which would safeguard the quality of nursing education in the country. The mandate was to establish and maintain uniform standards of nursing education. Today, the Indian Nursing Council is a statutory body that regulates nursing education in the country through prescription, inspection, examination, certification and maintaining its stand for a uniform syllabus at each level of nursing education. They have also ensured easier measures for equivalence, exchange and practice for nurses in any part of the country. On the other hand, the strive for maintenance of a uniform standard and pattern of nursing education has curbed creative development and experiments for expansion of nursing into newer horizons of caring and function.

LEVELS OF NURSING EDUCATION

There are six levels of nursing education in India today. These are:

1. Multipurpose health worker (MPHW) female training (ANM or MPHW-F).
2. Female health supervisor training health visitor (HV) or multipurpose health supervisor-female (MPHS-F).
3. General nursing and midwifery (GNM).
4. BSc (N).
5. MSc (N).
6. MPhil and PhD.

The first three MPHW (F) training, female health supervisor training and general nursing are conducted in schools of nursing. The last three are university level courses and examinations are conducted by the respective universities. Besides, there are several certificate and diploma courses in specialties.

TRAINING SCHOOL

The first midwives school was started at the government hospital in 1871. The formal schools of nursing was started for conducting diploma in general nursing and midwifery programs for a duration of 3½ years in Madras and in other parts of Tamil Nadu. Schools of nursing offering diploma program increased slowly (there were 9 schools of nursing and 4 midwifery schools till 2001) conducted by government of Tamil Nadu.

The number of schools conducted by government of Tamil Nadu is now increased to 17 in 2003 and now the government executed to start one school of nursing in every district hospitals. The numbers of private schools have also increased. Multipurpose health worker schools are also functioning many places in Tamil Nadu conducted by government and private bodies.

COLLEGE OF NURSING

A teachers training program running for a duration of 1 year was functioning in government hospital. In 1967 an integrated 2½ years Bachelor Science degree nursing program attached to Madras Medical College (for trained nurses) commenced replacing the existing diploma program.

In 1980, diploma in community nursing program was started.

In 1983, Bachelor of Science Nursing, 4-year program was started in College of Nursing, attached to Madras Medical College.

In 1995, Master of Science (Nursing) program was started in the College of Nursing, attached to Madras Medical College.

In 2001, a post of Principal for the College of Nursing was sanctioned and started functioning. Dr Sumathi Kumarswamy was appointed as the first Principal. Many candidates have completed Doctoral degree in nursing.

In 2003, a College of Nursing at Madurai started functioning by the government services.

The cadre strength of nursing increased slowly and many categories in nursing services prompted up.

In 1962, a post of Assistant to Director of Medical Services was created and filled at the state level. A post of Deputy Director of Nursing at the state level was created in 1986 and Dr Sumathi Kumaraswamy was appointed as the first Deputy Director of Medical Education in Nursing in 1992.

AUXILIARY NURSE MIDWIFE

DEVELOPMENT OF AUXILIARY NURSE MIDWIFE TRAINING (RURAL HEALTH SERVICES)

During the Second World War, there was a great demand for nursing personnel in the military hospitals as well as in the civil hospitals. So, auxiliary nurses midwife (ANM) services was founded in 1942.

This course was simple and the duration of training period was shorter than the nursing course. The nurses under this course were posted to do useful work under supervision in the hospital or in the health center and to give domiciliary care. ANMs were prepared to meet the demands of the health personnel in the community development programs. After the independence and in the Second 5-year Plan, it was decided to prepare 6,000 ANMs. The private hospitals also were requested to cooperate with the government to start such training institution. The government hospitals were given facilities to train the ANM since 1955.

Today the ANM has a vital role in the health services of the rural health centers such as primary health center, family welfare center, and maternity and child health centers. They can work as a midwife and a health worker in the community. They are also given opportunity to be trained as health visitors or as nurses if they have the basic educational requirements.

The practice of the ANM in the rural center had helped to improve the health status of the people, by health teaching, domiciliary care and regular follow-up of patients and families. ANM in the present healthcare delivery system functions as a multipurpose female health worker. With the present introduction of vocational courses such as nursing in the academic stream as one of the options, it is believed that it will contribute toward the basic nursing care of individuals, families and community for health and happiness. It will also be a foundation course for future diploma and degree programs in nursing.

MULTIPURPOSE HEALTH WORKER (FEMALE) TRAINING

The training grew out of the earlier ANM course. The ANM training was for 2 years and mainly covered maternal, child care and family welfare. In keeping with the policies of the Government of India to have multipurpose health workers, the Indian Nursing Council revised the ANMs syllabus in 1977 and reduced the duration to 18 months. The focus of training is on community health nursing. At the end of the course candidates are eligible for working in health subcenters. There are nearly 500 schools offering this course in India at present. The MPHA-M training course is also conducted in some states with duration of 18 months to render healthcare services at community.

FEMALE HEALTH SUPERVISOR TRAINING

Female health supervisor training was initially meant as a health visitor training course. It went through several modifications and finally became metamorphosed into the current 6 months promotional training. The female health supervisor or MPHA-F course is being conducted in 21 centers in the country. Besides this basics course, several states have their own promotional training courses as requirement for ANMs to be qualified for promotion to supervisors.

GENERAL NURSING AND MIDWIFERY

The general nursing and midwifery course is conducted in 477 centers in the country. The syllabus has undergone many revisions according to the changes in health plans and policies of the government and changing trends and advancements in education, nursing, health sciences and medical technology. The latest revision of the general nursing syllabus by the INC in 1988 has reduced the duration of the course from 3½ years to 3 years. The basic entrance qualification has become intermediate or class XII instead of the earlier class X. Both science and arts students are eligible. The focus of general nursing education is care of the sick in the hospital. Schools of nursing are therefore usually attached to teaching hospital. Three Board examinations are conducted, one at the end of each year. On passing, the candidates are registered as nurses [Registered Nurses (RN)] and as midwives [Registered Midwife (RM)] by the respective state nursing councils.

GRADUATE NURSING EDUCATION

There are two types of graduate nursing education in India, one is of 4-year basic course for fresh entrants and the second is a condensed post basic course for those who have undergone the GNM course.

1. **Four-year BSc (N):** Graduate nursing education started in India in the year 1946 in Christian Medical College (CMC), Vellore and in the Rajkumari Amrit Kaur (RAK) College of Nursing at Delhi University. At present several universities in India offer the course. The entry qualification is intermediate with biological sciences, physics and chemistry. Some universities also give admission to those who have arts background.

   The course focuses on preparation of professional nurses for working at the bedside and for taking up leadership roles in public health nursing. Besides nursing and medical subjects the syllabus includes humanities, arts and allied sciences. The course also includes managerial and teaching subjects to prepare graduates to take up first level teaching and administrative jobs in the hospital. An introductory course in research is also given. Overall, the graduate nursing course in the country offers a broad base in both arts and sciences and lays the foundation for a holistic perspective to health and caring.
2. **Two-year post basic BSc (N):** A 2-year degree course in nursing is offered in several universities in India. This course was specially designed to provide higher educational opportunities for practicing nurses. The entry requirement is that they should have completed the general nursing course and class XII (usually with science). Most places also ask for at least 2 years experience after completing the diploma (GNM) course. Two examinations are conducted by the

university—one at the end of the year, and the other at the end of the 2nd year.

3. **Degree in nursing through distance education:** Distance education in post basic nursing has also been started by Indira Gandhi National Open University (IGNOU) in 1994. This has provided an opening for diploma nurses all over the country to undertake higher education. The IGNOU offers courses through its study centers throughout the country.

POSTGRADUATE NURSING EDUCATION

Presently MSc (N) course is being offered in about 10 universities in the country. The 2-year course is designed to prepare clinical and community health nursing specialists. Besides clinical specialization the students are also taught to conduct research in nursing. A thesis is submitted by each student in partial fulfillment of the requirements for the degree. Courses in education and administration are given to prepare the students to take up responsible administrative and teaching jobs in nursing and allied health areas. The entrance requirement is BSc (N) and 2 years experience as nurses. The candidates also have to pass an entrance test. University examinations are conducted at the -end of the first and second years or at the end of each semester.

MPhiL AND PhD IN NURSING

Till a few years ago nurses had to travel abroad to study PhD course or seek admission in allied disciplines. In the 1980s RAK College of Nursing started an MPhil program as a regular and part-time course. Since then several universities started registering candidates for PhD in nursing. Prominent among these are MGR Medical University, Chennai; Rajiv Gandhi University of Health Sciences, Bengaluru; SNDT University, Mumbai and Delhi University. The Manipal Academy of Higher Education (MAHE) has started both MPhil and PhD programs in nursing. The Indian Nursing Council (INC) has recently initiated a project on starting PhD program in nursing through support from the WHO.

However, nurses keen to obtain Doctorate degrees continue to seek admission into universities and departments with related disciplines such as community health, nutrition, social sciences. The Jawaharlal Nehru University at New Delhi, the Padmavathi Mahila University, Tirupathi and the Centre for Development Studies, Thiruvananthapuram and the Centre for Economic and Social Sciences, Hydcrabad arc somc of thc universities and institutes, where nurses seek to obtain higher degrees.

VOCATIONAL NURSING (AT 10+2 LEVEL)

Since independence India has assumed wide economic and social responsibilities in attempting to provide the security of an adequate standard of living for its people. Investment in education is necessarily a long term on begins to yield results after a generation and in some cases even after a long period. In developing countries like India, due to financial constraints and low gross national product levels, it is difficult to finance universal university education.

Gandhiji had rightly visualized the magnitude of the problem and recommended village upliftment through basic education and development of basic craft in consonance with national growth, most of the youth out of school are workers. The base through which they can earn their livelihood and extend support to their families at grass root level. JP Naik in his paper on new policies, priorities and programs stated that in addition to the existing full time courses of vocational education, it should be possible for a person to transfer himself from general vocational courses and vice versa and carry on credits with him.

To meet the health needs of the population especially at grass root level, multipurpose health worker program was introduced in 1978, to carry on various tasks relevant to promotion of health and prevention of disorders with special emphasis on maternal and child health services. This course of 2 years duration is designed for the candidate with class X certificate (SSC).

CONCLUSION

Nursing has a tremendous capacity to change people. The demands associated with nursing practice require a broad knowledge base and critical thinking abilities along with competent skills. The focus of nursing is shifting towards viewing patients as collaborative beneficiaries rather than passive recipients of care. Nursing requires psychological, social and physical skills and certain attitudes, which are rooted in knowledge. The demands associated with nursing practice require a broad knowledge base for decision-making. Critical thinking abilities and skills in the technological aspects of care. The function of the professional nurse in the hospital is more comprehensive. She will be actively involved in direct nursing care, health teaching, planning for care in home, rehabilitation and service to the outpatients. She may have to teach the students also. The world health organization (WHO) has been considering the future and by 2000 the world experienced major growth in the elderly population, decline in birthrate, especially in Western countries, increases in chronic illness, continuing social unrest, AIDS a major problem, many infectious diseases under control, mental health a key issue and poverty continuing to plague much of the world. Exposure to human ill, sick child and baby, dying patients, cancer patients, renal failure patients, stillbirth etc., closer nurse patient relationship, helplessness, feeling of incompetence in emergency situation, lack of support system, lack of resources, often high unrealistic expectations, high technology equipments, communication breakdown, and heavy workload are the causes of stress among nurses. Nurses are responsible for public anger because—nurses stay 24 hours with client, nurses have to give answers fault made by professionals of other discipline, workload very high, less time for counseling and guidance to patients, unable to explain their own role in clients care and poor orientation to clients.

CHAPTER

6

Professional Organizations

INTRODUCTION

Organizations provide a means through which united efforts are made to elevate standards of nursing education and practice. It also offers a means of voicing and opinions, developing our abilities and keeping informed of new trends. Nursing regulatory bodies are also known as 'professional associations' which are responsible for the licensing of nurses within their respective province or territory. These regulatory bodies set the enforced standards of nursing practice, monitor and enforce standards for nursing education, monitor and enforce standards for nursing practice and set the requirements for registration of nursing professionals. The professional nurse must be aware of these associations, so as to participate in various nursing professional activities of these organizations. To be a part of these associations, the nurse must have lifetime membership with these organizations through proper registration which is must.

FUNCTIONS OF PROFESSIONAL BODIES

Functions of professional bodies include the following:

1. These associations provide a means through which the professional development of a nurse can be channeled with the authority because of its representative character.
2. These associations also provide the nurses with the opportunities for expression of their viewpoints, development of their leadership qualities and abilities.
3. These associations keep the nurses informed of professional news and trends throughout the country and worldwide.

INDIAN NURSING COUNCIL

The Indian Nursing Council (INC) was authorized by the Indian Nursing Council Act of 1947. It was established in 1949 to provide uniform standards in nursing education and reciprocity in nursing registration throughout the country. The Indian Nursing Council is an autonomous body under the Government of India,

Ministry of Health and Family Welfare was constituted by the Central Government under section 3 (1) of the Indian Nursing Council Act, 1947 of parliament. Trained Nurses Association of India (TNAI) members felt that there should be a body to guide and protect nurses in their profession. Before the constitution of INC, the nurses registered in one state were not necessarily recognized for registration in other state, which is must today. The condition of mutual recognition by the State Nurses Registration Councils, called reciprocity, was possible only if uniform standards of nursing education were maintained. Therefore, INC was given authority to prescribe curricula for nursing education in all the states. It was at the same time given authority to recognize programs of nursing education or refuse recognition to the schools and colleges of nursing.

AIMS AND OBJECTIVES

Aims and objectives of Indian Nursing Council are as follows:

1. To establish and monitor uniform standards of nursing education for nurses midwives, auxiliary nurse-midwives and health visitors by doing inspection of the institutions.
2. To recognize the qualifications under section 10(2)(4) of the Indian Nursing Council Act, 1947 for the purpose of registration and employment in India and abroad.
3. To give approval for registration of Indian and Foreign Nurses possessing foreign qualification under section 11(2)(a) of the Indian Nursing Council Act, 1947.
4. To prescribe the syllabus and regulations for nursing programs.
5. Power to withdraw the recognition of qualification under section 14 of the Act in case the institution fails to maintain its standards under Section 14(1)(b) that an institution recognized by State Council for the training of nurses, midwives, auxiliary nurse midwives or health visitors does not satisfy the requirements of the Council.
6. To advise the State Nursing Councils, Examining Boards, State Governments and Central Government in various important items regarding Nursing Education in the Country.

MEMBER REPRESENTS

The council is composed of:

1. State Registration Councils
2. Central and state health departments
3. Military nursing service
4. Indian Red Cross Society
5. University schools of nursing
6. Health schools
7. Post certificate schools

8. TNAI members
9. Medical Council of India
10. Indian Medical Association
11. Members of Parliament.

COMMITTEES

1. **Executive Committee** of the Council to implement on the issues related to maintenance of standards of nursing programs
2. **Nursing Education Committee** of the council is constituted to implement on the issues concerned mainly with nursing education and policy matters concerning the nursing education.
3. **Equivalence Committee** to implement on the issues of recognition of foreign qualifications which is essential for the purpose of registration under section 11(2) (a) or (b) of the Indian Nursing Council Act, 1947, as ammended.

ACTIVITIES OF INC

1. Making the code of nurses.
2. The worldwide accepted definition of a nurse.
3. A book of ethics 'The Nurses Dilemma'.
4. Policy statement on health and social issues.
5. Arrange exchange program for study and employment.
6. Maintain a register on professional qualification of people.
7. Conducting seminars around the world to maintain relationship.

FUNCTIONS

1. It provides uniform standards in nursing education and reciprocity in nursing registration.
2. It has authority to prescribe curriculum for nursing education in all states.
3. It has authority to recognize program of nursing education or to refuse recognition of a program if it did not meet the standards required by the council.
4. It is registering the foreign nurses.
5. It also maintains the Indian Nurses Register.
6. The INC authorizes State Nurses Registration Council and examining boards to issue qualifying certificates.

INTERNATIONAL COUNCIL OF NURSES

The International Council of Nurses (ICN) was founded in 1899 by Mrs Bedford Fenwick in cooperation with nursing leaders from many countries. In 1900, the councils constitution was adopted and the first meeting was held at the World Exposition in Buffalo, New York. Their headquarter is established at Geneva in Switzerland. It is federation of non-political and self-governing national nurses association. The ICN is the global voice of nursing. The main purpose of the ICN is to provide the means through which the national associations can share their interests in the promotion of health and care of the sick.

OBJECTIVES

Objectives of ICN are:
1. To promote the development of the Strong National Nurses Association.
2. To assist National Nurses Association to improve the standards of nursing education and practice.
3. To assist National Nurses Association to improve the status of nurses within their countries.
4. To serve as the authoritative voice for nurses and nursing internationally.

ACTIVITIES

Activities of ICN are as follows:
1. The ICN has published the Code for Nurses.
2. It makes the policy statement on health and social issues.
3. It also maintains and improves the status of nurses and standard of nursing around the world.
4. The council works to improve the nursing education and practice by publishing the guidelines for National Nurses Association.

GOVERNING BODY

The council of national representatives which consists of INC honorary officers and President of the National Member Association. International exchange privileges for nurses have been provided through the INC. This gives the individual nurse the opportunity to observe and obtain employment in other countries and also contributes to improvement of standards.

The ICN publishes the International Nursing Review and the News Letter, which give the news of the ICN and the National Member Association.

INTERNATIONAL RELATIONSHIPS

The International council of nursing has close relationship with many of the world's major international organizations such as World Health Organization (WHO), International Labor Organisation (ILO), United Nations Educational, Scientific and Cultural Organization (UNESCO), United Nations International Childrens Education Fund (UNICEF), Red Cross and its allied leagues. This relationship helps ICN to have related concerns in the healthcare field and allows keeping abreast of trends affecting the future of nursing.

FUNCTIONS

Functions of ICN are:
1. The division of nursing education
2. The division of nursing service
3. The division of social and economic welfare.

TRAINED NURSES ASSOCIATION OF INDIA

The Trained Nurses Association of India (TNAI) is a national professional association of nurses. The present name and organization of nurses were established in 1922, but its history of development goes back to 1905. The TNAI had its beginning in the Association of Nursing Superintendent, which was founded for all nurses to participate at same level.

The level of organization moves to the district, state and national levels. Members of the TNAI are usually most active on the level of the local unit. Activities and conferences, however, are planned regularly by the state branches and provide opportunities for valuable professional participation and development of the individual member.

GOVERNING BODY

The governing body of the TNAI is the council which is assisted by standing committees for economic welfare, nursing research and finance. A full time salaried secretary was first appointed in 1935. A salaried assistant secretary, who also serves as the advisor to the Student Nurses Association was appointed in 1983.

AIMS

The aims of TNAI center upon needs of the individual member and problems in the nursing profession as a whole, such aims include upgrading, development and standardization of nursing education, improvement of living and working conditions for nurses in India and registration for qualified nurses.

Various activities of the TNAI implement its aims. It was active in helping to formulate basic nursing curricula when it first organized. More recently, it has promoted the development of courses in higher education for nurse. It gives scholarship for nurses who wish to go for advanced study either in India or abroad.

The TNAI also stimulates action to organize the state nurses and midwives registration councils. It also helps to remove discrimination against male nurses and initiates study and improvement of economic condition for nurses.

MEMBERSHIP

The TNAI membership is obtained by application and submission of a copy of state registration certificate. Transfer membership from the Student Nurses

Association (SNA) by having a certificate sent from the institution in which the student studied within 6 months after completing the course. A reduced fee is offered to those who transfer membership directly from SNA.

PUBLICATIONS

The publishes TNAI 'The Nursing Journal of India', monthly. Another impressive publication is the 'Indian Nursing Year book'. This contains important reports, trends and statistics about nursing profession in India.

STATE NURSING COUNCIL

State Nurses Registration Council is independent and recognized as a body that can make statues and prescribe by laws for trained nurses and prospective nurses who are undergoing various nursing programs. Although it is an independent body but it has to obtain approval from state government for all the laws passed by it and decision taking. This council helps to maintain a register of names of professional nurses. The names of these nurses are also put into Indian Nurses Registration Council. Registration is must for the diploma and degree courses in nursing. Registration system helps to maintain the high standard amongst the professional nurses. Registration serves a legal protection to the nurse and also to the public as it prevents disqualified and incompetent persons to practice nursing.

The training of nurses, midwives, health visitors and ANMs is to a large extent controlled by the Nurses Registration Councils in the states. Registration in state nursing council is very necessary to be registered in order to practice officially as a professional nurse. Registration councils are functional in all the states of India and they are affiliated to INC.

FUNCTIONS

1. To accredit and inspect schools of nursing in their state.
2. To conduct examinations for General Nursing and Auxillary Nursing courses.
3. To prescribe rules of conduct, take disciplinary actions.
4. Registration of nurses and midwives in their state.
5. Maintenance of register of nurses, midwives and others.
6. To renew registration and upgrade registration.

The state nursing council is an autonomous statutory registration body for registering qualified nurses, midwives, ANMs, MPHWs and health visitors. A council has president/vice president, registrar and staff of the council. The functions of the council includes the registration of qualified nursing professionals, regulation of training programs by conducting inspection, checking malpractice and maintaining professional ethics, foreign verification, coordinating with the INC and with various other government departments and universities. The council conducts inspection for the institution, who are conducting the programs such as ANM, MPHW, DGNM, BSc (N), Post basic BSc (N), MSc (N) and Diploma in nursing education and administration. The council ensures that all facilities are available for conducting any of the nursing program before granting permission. It also conducts the surprise and periodical inspection to identify the deficiencies in that institution. If necessary, it also conducts reinspection to ensure that the deficiencies are rectified. It periodically sends communication to all the educational institutions to inform the issues of importance to nursing and health.

ACTIVITIES

Activities of council are the following:

1. To look after the various nursing educational programs run under its territory.
2. To conduct examinations of GNM and ANM in its areas.
3. To issue certificates of registered nurse and registered midwife to the qualified nurses.
4. Maintenance of various records such as the names and addresses of all registered nurses, registered health visitors, registered midwives, registered nurse dais, registered trained dais in Punjab.

RENEWAL OF REGISTRATION

The registration once done has to be renewed after a specific period of time or after attainment of higher education in nursing. It is done in respect to keep a control on registered persons practicing the profession in the state. The renewal process includes sending a duly filled form certified by the training institution with the copies of all the academic certificates and the required process fees. It is important to renew the registration in order to upgrade the status of the nurse within the state register.

STUDENT NURSES ASSOCIATION

The foundation of the National Student Nurses Association (NSNA) was created in 1969 to honor Frances Tompkins, the association's first executive director, organized exclusively for charitable and educational purposes.' This association was organized 24 years ago, helps to bring students from all over India together for educational, professional, and recreational activities.

The Student Nurses Association (SNA) organized in 1929 is associated under the jurisdiction of the TNAI, in addition to providing a means of personnel and professional development for the nursing students. It serves as a source of membership for the parent organization. In addition the TNAI serves as the advisor for the SNA.

FUNCTIONS

Functions of SNA are:

1. Project undertaking.
2. Sociocultural activities.
3. Exhibitions, public speaking and writing.
4. Organization of conferences.
5. Maintenance of SNA register.
6. Propagation of profession.
7. Improvement of nursing education to improve health care.
8. Aid in the development of the nursing student.
9. Encourage optimal achievement in the professional role of the nurse.
10. Fund raising.

CHRISTIAN MEDICAL ASSOCIATION OF INDIA

The Nurses' League of the Christian Medical Association was founded in 1930.

Christian Medical Association of India (CMAI) is a registered, non-profit, charitable organization. CMAI is the health arm of National Council of Churches in India (NCCI). They undertake programs in training, researcher community service, institutional consultancy, policy advocacy, interface of theology and medicine, information dissemination and others.

OBJECTIVES

Objectives of CMAI are:

1. Prevention and relief of human suffering irrespective of caste, creed, community, religion and economic status.
2. Promotion of knowledge of the factors governing health.
3. Coordination of activities for training doctors, nurses, allied health professionals and others involved in the ministry of healing.
4. Implementation of schemes for comprehensive health care, family planning and community welfare.
5. Rendering health in calamities and disasters of all kinds.

Current Objectives

Current objectives are:

1. To promote cooperation and encouragement among Christian nurses.
2. To promote efficiency in nursing education and services.
3. To secure the highest standard possible in Christian Nursing Education through the Christian Schools of Nursing.

4. To consider the special work and problems of Christian nurses working. Nursing considered to be an occupation now attains the status of profession.

FUNCTIONS OF THE NURSING EXAMINATION BOARD

Functions of the Nursing Examination Board are:

1. To coordinate and bring a uniform standard of nursing education, in accordance with the requirements of the Indian Nursing Council and State Nursing Council.
2. To verify the eligibility requirements of the students before each examination.
3. To arrange to conduct examination and issue diploma certificates to successful candidates.
4. To maintain and enhance the educational standards of Schools of Nursing by arranging continuing education programs/workshops/exhibitions.
5. To prepare the calendar of events at the beginning of each academic year.
6. To decide the disciplinary action against students/concerned staff in case of malpractice in examinations.
7. To nominate members for the panel of examiner's for Ist, IInd and IIIrd year of GNM nursing examinations.
8. To appoint the examiners before annual and supplementary examination.
9. To appoint an auditor to audit the board accounts.

CONCLUSION

Professional organizations provide a means through which your own professional development can be channelized with authority because of their respective character. It provides you an opportunity to express the view-points, develop leadership qualities and abilities and keep well informed of professional trends and news. All qualified nurses must participate in their professional state and national organizations to keep themselves informed of new developments and for upgrading the profession. Philosophy of life, elements of human nature, religious factors, political ideologies, socio-economic factors, cultural factors and expiration of knowledge are the factors determining educational aims. Vocation, knowledge, complete living, harmonious development, mental and emotional development, physical development, moral development, character development, self-realization, cultural development, ideal citizenship and education for leisure are the general aims of education.

CHAPTER

7

Career Opportunities in Nursing

INTRODUCTION

The goal of profession in nursing is to confirm and expand the present body of nursing knowledge, which in turn contribute to improved health care. Establishing a scientific base of nursing knowledge will provide nurses with most current principles of practice, e.g. if it could be demonstrated through research that one method of thermometer disinfections proved to be more effective than another, the better method could be adopted; a comparative study of the different methods of teaching family planning could aid in the selection of the best method for researching family planning; if a study of patient's comfort suggested that a relationship between high level of stress and visiting hours existed, visiting hours could be reduced and the effectiveness of reduced visiting hours could be further evaluated.

NURSING CAREER

Nursing shortages are often a symptom of wider health system or 'nursing shortages are not just a problem for nursing' stated Christine Hancock of Nurses. It is a health system problem, which undermines health social ailments. Nursing in many countries continues to be undervalued as 'Women's work', and nurses are given only limited access to resources to make them effective in their jobs and careers. Health care is labor intensive and demands more nursing service. Policy makes in many countries have already recognized this fact and making necessary changes to attract the best nursing services in numbers and quality. Increases in demand are created due to these policies:

1. Be a serious student with proficiency in the health sciences.
2. Assume legal, moral and ethical accountability for own actions.
3. Use good judgment, be loyal to patients and to the profession.
4. Demonstrate unbiased compassion for all by respecting all people regardless of age, race, social status, sexual orientation and religious beliefs.

5. Show highest degree of motivation to keep up with trends and research in the profession and to value lifelong learning.
6. Learn to handle catastrophe, crisis and everyday challenges, in a confident, efficient and caring way.
7. Have good mental and physical health, plenty of stamina, endurance and sense.

CAREER OPPORTUNITIES IN NURSING

NURSE ANESTHETIST

Provides care to patients before, during and after surgery or delivery. Specific activities include physical assessment, preoperative teaching and preparation, administration and maintenance of anesthesia. Responsible for constantly monitoring every function of the patient's body while the patient is anesthetized. Provides care during the recovery period and as part of follow-up monitoring during the postoperative course.

NURSE EDUCATOR

As the name suggests, the responsibilities include a variety of roles including teaching research and patient care. Central to effective teaching is the solid clinical skills developed from clinical practice. Nurse educator is responsible for lesson planning, instructing, evaluating, learning, counseling, and assisting with solving learning problems. Serves as a primary resource for theory and knowledge development in the discipline of nursing.

STAFF NURSE

The entry-level nurse or nurse without any specialization is called staff nurse, whose responsibilities include making nursing judgments based on scientific knowledge and relies on procedures and standardized care plans. The staff nurse has an incredibly complex job and advances to an intermediate level with experience and become more skilled in developing individual and innovative care plans to meet client needs.

AIDS CARE NURSE

AIDS care nurse is a profession that takes care of a person who is certain to die within a specified time frame. AIDS care nurse responds to the physical, psychological, spiritual and social concerns of patients with AIDS, cares for chronically ill and dying with numerous clinical manifestations.

AMBULATORY CARE NURSE

Ambulatory care nurse provides for the health needs of individuals, families and groups in diverse settings. Emphasis on helping patients, stays well and independent in their home environment as long as possible.

CARDIAC REHABILITATION NURSE

Cardiac rehabilitation nurse meets the need for education and support of patients with coronary heart disease, who are making lifestyle changes to prevent worsening of the disease. Monitors patients during physical workouts to prevent overexertion and/or injury.

CORRECTIONAL NURSE

Correctional nurse provides for the health care of inmates in correctional facilities such as juvenile offender homes, jails, prisons and penitentiaries.

ENDOSCOPY NURSE

Endoscopy nurse provides essential care of patients undergoing procedures for screening, diagnosis and/or treatment of gastrointestinal disorders and may specialize in endoscopy.

GENETIC NURSE

The genetic nurse care for people's genetic health those with genetic problem including screening, early detection, risk identification, treatment and testing.

INFECTION CONTROL NURSE

Specializes in identifying, controlling and preventing outbreaks of infection in healthcare settings and the community in highly contagious situations. Activities include the collection and analysis of infection control data; the planning, implementation and evaluation of infection prevention and control measures; the education of individuals about infection risk, prevention and control; the development and revision of infection control policies and procedures; the investigation of suspected outbreaks of infection and the provision of consultation on infection risk assessment, prevention and control strategies.

INTRAVENOUS THERAPY NURSE

Intravenous therapy nurse initiates, monitors and terminates therapies including medications, antineoplastic agents, investigational drugs, blood products and parenteral nutrition, performs venous and arterial punctures, maintain the intravascular side including tubing and dressings, monitor for infections, initiate emergency therapies, assess patients for adverse reactions and complications and document all patient-directed activities.

NEPHROLOGY NURSE

Nephrology nurse focuses on the prevention of disease and the care of patients with renal problems; works with patients in all stages of chronic renal failure, implementing treatment modalities including efforts to reserve renal function, hemodialysis, peritoneal dialysis or transplant.

NEUROSCIENCE NURSE

Neuroscience nurse care for individuals who have a dysfunction of the nervous system including alterations in consciousness and cognition, communication, mobility, rest and sleep, sensation and sexuality; plans and implements interventions to support bodily functions, promote healing, encourage adoption to persistent neurological difficulties and teaches patients and families about the illness.

OCCUPATIONAL HEALTH NURSE

Occupational health nursing combines concepts of public health and nursing theory in an orientation toward primary prevention or keeping health workers healthy and includes managing workers, compensation records and counseling employees.

ONCOLOGY NURSE

Oncology nurse cares for patients with the diagnosis of cancer in various settings; utilized an empathic and caring approach to patients whose diagnostics and treatment are often painful and life-threatening, administers chemotherapy, conducts patient teaching, and manages illness-treatment-related symptoms.

OPHTHALMIC NURSE

Ophthalmic nurse provides care to persons with disorders of the eyes including blindness or visual impairment; functions range from patient teaching to assistance in surgery.

PERIOPERATIVE NURSE

Provides for the surgical patient's needs by assessing, planning and implementing nursing care patient receive preoperatively, intraoperatively and postoperatively. Nursing activities performed by the preoperative nurse include patient assessment, creating and maintaining a sterile and safe environment.

ORTHOPEDIC NURSE

Orthopedic nurse cares for the actual and potential health problem related to musculoskeletal function; relies on a holistic approach in their assessment of the impact of musculoskeletal conditions on self-care, patient management of the environment, available patient resources, and support systems.

PRENATAL NURSE

Prenatal nurse cares for women, infants and their families from the onset of pregnancy through the 1st month of the newborn's life (prenatal period); monitors the pregnancy, assesses the progression of labor; monitors the status of mother and baby, maintains a sense of clam and comfort during labor; fosters the new mother-infant relationship, teaches parenting skills; assesses and supports the mother in her recovery from childbirth and evaluates the newborn's early adjustment to life.

PSYCHIATRIC NURSE

Psychiatric nurse should possess the art of using one's self in therapeutic ways to assist patients to affect changes in self-understanding and behavior. Views individuals from a holistic perspective, taking into account both physical and mental health needs while focusing on human behavior.

PLASTIC AND RECONSTRUCTIVE SURGICAL NURSE

Cares for patients undergoing cosmetic and maxillofacial surgery, laser and microsurgery and nonsurgical treatments to correct esthetic problems.

REHABILITATION NURSE

The rehabilitation nurse cares for individuals who are experiencing temporary progressive or permanent illness or disabilities that are extensive enough to alter their normal functioning and interrupt their lifestyle.

RESPIRATORY NURSE

Respiratory nurse promotes pulmonary health for individuals, families and communities, and cares for persons with pulmonary dysfunction throughout the lifespan. Respiratory nursing may be preventive, acute, critical or rehabilitative.

TRANSPLANTATION NURSE

Transplantation nurse cares for recipient and living-donor patients throughout the transplantation process from disease state to preoperative-intraoperative experience further to aftercare and long-term follow-up.

TRAUMA NURSE

Trauma nursing involves responding quickly to a wide variety of single and multisystem trauma involving different patient needs, ages, cultures and severity of presenting symptoms. The trauma nurse must respond with decisiveness and clarity to unexpected events by assessing, intervening and stabilizing patients about whom there is minimal information.

FLIGHT NURSE

Flight nurse involves emergency and non-emergency air surface transport of ill and injured patients. This includes interfacility transport and emergency 'scene calls' for trauma and medical emergencies.

FORENSIC NURSE

Forensic nursing combines clinical nursing practice with the law enforcement arena. It involves the investigation and treatment of victims of sexual assault, elder, child and spousal abuse, unexplained or accidental death, trauma and assault as well as perpetrators of these and any criminal activity.

HOLISTIC NURSE

Holistic nurse involves all aspects of wellness and healing of a holistic nature; holism being defined as the mind, body, spirit connection; that it, treating the whole person, not just a disease of symptom.

MEDICAL EDITOR/AUTHOR

Medical editor/author involves all aspects of writing, editing and proofreading technical material for use in biomedical research, education and training, sales and marketing and other communication forms.

MILITARY NURSE

Military nurse provide all aspects of traditional nursing care and practice in both peace and wartime settings through various branches of the military service. Classifications include active duty, reserves and civilian employment.

PEDIATRIC NURSE

Pediatric nurse provides comprehensive care to children, adolescents and their families in various settings. Responds to the physical and psychosocial aspects of health and illness, concern for health promotion and disease prevention, management of physical and mental disabilities and response to acute and chronic illness.

NURSING INFORMATICS

Nursing informatics involves all aspects of computerization as it relates to nursing and healthcare practice.

PERIANESTHESIA NURSE

Perianesthesia nursing provides intensive care to patients as they awaken from anesthesia. The perianesthesia nurse prepares patients for the surgical experience, monitors and supports safe transition from anesthetized state to responsiveness and readies patients for discharge from perianesthesia care unit.

CAREER OF HEALING TOUCH

Nursing encompasses autonomous and collaborative care of individuals of all ages, families, groups and communities, sick or well and in all settings.

Nursing includes the promotion of health, prevention of illness, and the care of ill, disabled and dying people. Advocacy, promotion of a safe environment, research participation in shaping health policy, inpatient and health system management, and education are also vital in nursing roles.

CONCLUSION

Vast opportunities are available for a nurse to develop the career in nursing. There was a time when professional nurses had very little choice of service because nursing was mostly hospital centered and bedside nursing. Today the position is different, wide range of opportunities for nurses for service are available whether married or unmarried, male or female, graduate or a certificate holder with post basic or basic degree or with any specialization or super specialization in various fields. The nurse may choose anyone carrier opportunities here and abroad.

CHAPTER

8

Code of Ethics and Professional Conduct

INTRODUCTION

Ethics in nursing is a particular code of behaviors, characters, conducts and relationship unique only to the nursing personnel. Nursing ethics is 'a system of principles governing the conduct of a nurse, relationship to the patient and family, his/her associates and society at large'. As a guidelines to all those in the nursing profession, the Grand Council of the International Council of Nurses held at Sao Paulo, Brazil on July 10, 1953, adopted, viewed and revised in the year 1964.

DEFINITIONS

1. The Oxford dictionary defines ethics as 'a science of human duty in its widest extent.'
2. The Chambers describes it as 'the science of morals that branch of philosophy which is concerned with human character and conduct.'
3. Webster defines it as 'the morals concerned with or relating to what is right and wrong in matters of human behavior.'
4. A code is needed to educate and orient members of the profession to distinguish desirable from the undesirable behaviors, to regulate relationships with coworkers and clients, and to guide the public in understanding professional conduct.
5. A group of nurses stated, 'ethics is knowledge and attitudes that determine man's relationship to him, to others and to the society.'
6. Ethics is a science that endeavors to interpret the highest standards of written or unwritten principles, doctrines or morals of human duty, human character and conduct of human behavior and human relationships in day-to-day life.

CODE OF ETHICS

In accordance with these requests the Professional Service Committee of the International Council of Nurses (ICN) selected a subcommittee for the revision of the code. The final revised code was submitted to the ICN Council of National Representatives in Mexico in May 1973 at the 15th Quadrennial congress.

The Sub-committee on the Code of Ethics tried to concentrate their attention on the most vital aspects of nursing and built their revised ethical code around five major headings:

1. **Nurses and people:** The nurse's primary responsibility is to those people who require nursing care. The nurse holds in confidence personal information's and use judgment in sharing this information.
2. **Nurses and practice:** The nurse maintains the highest standards of nursing care possible within the reality of a specific situation. The nurse when acting in a professional capacity should at all times maintain standards of personal conduct which credit upon the profession.
3. **Nurses and society:** The nurse shares with other citizens the responsibility for initiating and supporting action to meet the health and social needs of the public.
4. **Nurses and coworker:** The nurse maintains cooperative relationship with coworkers in nursing and other fields. The nurse takes appropriate action to safeguard the individual when care is endangered by a coworker or any other person.
5. **Nurses and the profession:** The nurse acting through the professional organization participates in establishing and maintaining equitable social and economic working conditions in nursing.

APPLICATION OF CODE OF ETHICS IN NURSING

Code of Ethics as applied to nursing are as follows:

1. The nurse provides services with respect for human dignity irrespective of social or economic status, personal attributes, or the nature of health problems.
2. The fundamental responsibility of the nurse is 3-fold; to conserve life, to alleviate suffering and to promote health.
3. The nurse shall maintain at all time the highest standards of nursing care and of professional conduct.
4. The nurse must not only be well prepared to practice but shall maintain knowledge and skills at a consistently high level.
5. The religious beliefs of a patient shall be respected.
6. Nurses hold in confidence all personal information entrusted to them.
7. Nurses recognize not only the responsibilities but the limitations of their professional functions like not to recommend or give medical treatment without medical orders except in emergencies and report such action to a physician as soon as possible.
8. The nurse is under an obligation to carry out the physician's orders intelligently and loyally and can refuse to participate in unethical procedures.

9. The nurse assumes responsibility and accountability for individual nursing judgments and actions.
10. The nurse sustains confidence in the physician and other members of the health team; incompetence or unethical conduct of associates should be exposed but only to the proper authority.
11. The nurse safeguards the patients and the public when health care and safety are affected by the incompetent, unethical or illegal practice of any person.
12. The nurse cooperates with the health team and maintains harmonious relationships with members of other professions and with nursing colleagues.
13. The nurse adheres to standards of personal ethics, which reflect credit upon the profession.
14. In personal conduct nurses should not knowingly disregard the accepted pattern of behaviors of the community in which they live and work.
15. The nurse participates and shares responsibility with other citizens and other health professions in promoting to meet the health needs of the public—local, state, national and international.

Requests poured in from many quarters of the nursing world to review and revise this code against and representation for this purpose was made thorough several national councils.

PROFESSIONAL CONDUCT

NEED OF PROFESSIONAL CONDUCT

Professional conduct is needed for the following purposes:

1. To promote and safeguard the interest and well-being of the patients.
2. To improve and maintain professional knowledge and competence.
3. To acknowledge any limitation in gained knowledge and competence, and declaim any duties or responsibilities unless the nurse is not able to perform in a safe and skilled manner.
4. To work in an open and a cooperative manner with the patients and their families in order to foster their independence and to recognize and respect their involvement in the planning and delivery of care.
5. To recognize and respect the dignity of each patient as a client and respond to the needs of the patients with care, irrespective of their ethnic origin, religious beliefs, personal attributes and the nature of their health problems.
6. To report to the concerned authority at the earliest about any physical, psychological and social problems identified in the patients, which helps to start the treatment at the earliest and prevent the complications of the illness later.

7. To work in a collaborative and cooperative manner with healthcare professionals and others involved in providing care and to recognize and respect their particular contribution within the care team.
8. To avoid any abuse of the privileged relationship with patients in the workplace.

CODE OF PROFESSIONAL CONDUCT (FOR NURSES IN INDIA)

Professional Responsibility and Accountability

To maintain professional responsibility and accountability the nurses:

1. Appreciate a sense of self-worth and nurtures it.
2. Maintains standards of personal conduct, reflecting credit upon the profession.
3. Carriers out responsibility within a frame work of the professional boundaries.
4. In accountable for maintaining practice standards let by the Indian Nursing Council.
5. Are compassionate.
6. Are responsible for the continuous improvement of current practices.
7. Provides adequate information to individuals these allows then to make informed choice
8. Practices healthy behavior.

Nursing Practice

In the course of nursing practice the nurse:

1. Provides care in accordance with set standards of practice.
2. Treats all individuals and families with dignity in providing the physical, psychological, emotional, social and spiritual aspects of care.
3. Respects individuals and families, promoting healthy practices and discouraging harmful practices.
4. Presents realistic pictures truthful in all situations for facilitating autonomous decision making by individuals and families.
5. Endure is safe practice.
6. Consults coordinates, collaborates and follows up approximately when an individual's care needs exceed his/her competence.

Communication and Interpersonal Relationships

Communication and interpersonal relationship plays a key role in the interaction of the nurse with client to effect optimal interaction nurses:

1. Establishment and maintains effective interpersonal relationships with individuals families and communities.
2. Upholds the dignity of team members and maintains effective interpersonal relationship with them.

3. Appreciates and nurtures the professional role of team members.
4. Cooperators with other health professionals to meet the needs of individual's families and communities.

Valuing Human Being

The nurse values human life by:

1. Takes appropriate action to protect individuals from harmful an ethical principles.
2. Considers relevant facts while taking particular decision in the best interest of individuals.
3. Encourages and supports individuals in their, right to speak for themselves on issues affecting health and welfare.
4. Respects and supports choices made by individuals.

Management

Proper management of resources and infrastructure is essential for improving the overall efficiency of the nurse. Hence, the nurse:

1. Ensures appropriate allocation and utilization of available response.
2. Participates in supervision and education of students and other formal provides.
3. Uses judgment in relation to individual competence, while accepting and delegating responsibility.
4. Facilities conducive work culture in order to achieve institutional objective.
5. Participates in performance appraisal.
6. Participates in evaluation of nursing services.
7. Work with individuals to identify the needs and sensitizes policy makers and funding agencies for resource allocation.

Professional Advancement

To escape that he/she is at part with contemporaries in the nursing field the nurse must:

1. Ensure the protection of human rights, while pursing the advancement of knowledge.
2. Participate in determining and implementing quality care.
3. Take responsibility for updating one's own knowledge and competencies. Contribute to the care of professional knowledge and conducting and participating in research.

PROFESSIONAL ETIQUETTE FOR NURSES

Professional etiquette for nurses refers to the ethical manners and moral behavior that a nurse should follow throughout the life of nursing. Maintaining good etiquette reflects good morality in the nurse. The important qualities that make up good professional' etiquette are as follows:

1. Being gentle and polite to all patients, seniors and other health workers in the hospital.
2. Giving respect to the seniors, coworkers and clients.
3. Addressing seniors with proper title such as Sir or Madam.
4. Answering politely and humbly to any questions asked or clarifications sought by the seniors.
5. Giving way to the seniors and standing aside and allowing the senior nurse to pass.
6. Maintaining discipline wherever needed such as in the ward, conference meeting with seniors, classroom and library.
7. Keeping the uniform neat and tidy.
8. Not wearing any jewelry or applying makeup while on duty.
9. Obeying the rules and regulations of the hospital at all times.
10. Getting proper prior permission from colleagues and the sister-in-charge before taking any articles from the ward.

CONCLUSION

Nursing profession uses code for nurses. Ethical concepts are applied to nursing as it guides the professional conduct. This code is adopted and published by the International Council of Nurses. The first code of ethics called the international code of nursing. When a person becomes a member of a profession, he accepts the responsibility of living upon the code of ethics of that profession in nursing, code of ethics provides professional standards for nursing activities which protect the nurse and the patient.

Section II
Health and Nursing Care Delivery

GLOSSARY

1. **Acute illness:** It is characterized by symptoms that are of relatively short duration, usually severe and affect the functioning of the clients in all dimensions.
2. **Adaptation**: Process by which changes occur in any of a person's dimensions in response to stress.
3. **Development**: Increase in capacity or maturation of function. It is related to the maturation and myelination of the nervous system and indicates acquisition of a variety of skills for optimal functioning of individual.
4. **Etiology**: Identification of the cause of a problem. The cause may be direct or a contributing factor in the development of client problem or need.
5. **Growth**: Net increase in size or mass of tissues due to multiplication of cells and increase in the intracellular substances.
6. **Health**: Dynamic state in which an individual adapts to internal and external environments so that there is a state of physical, emotional, intellectual, social and spiritual well being.
7. **Health behavior**: Activities through which a person maintain, attains or regains behavior as an expression of personal health beliefs.
8. **Health-belief model**: Conceptual framework that predicts a person's health behavior as an expression of personal beliefs.
9. **Health-illness continuum**: Scale by means of which a personal's level of health can be described, ranging from high level wellness to severe illness. The scales take in to account the presence of risk factors.
10. **Health promoting behavior:** Considered as third subcategory of health behavior and through assessment, reveal needs for vehicular safety, home safety, domestic violence recognition, recreational safety, occupational safety and health.
11. **Health promotion**: Activities directed toward maintain or enhancing the health and wellbeing of clients.
12. **Holistic health**: A system of compressive or total care that considers the physical, emotional, social, economical and spiritual needs of the person the response to the illness, and the effect of the illness on the person's ability to meet self care needs.

13. **Live born**: This neonate is the product of conception irrespective of weight or gestational age that after separation from mother shows any evidence of life such as breathing, heart rate, pulsation of umbilical cord or definitive movement of voluntary muscles.
14. **Maturation:** It produces an increase in competence, an ability to function at a higher level depending on the child's heredity.
15. **Pathogen:** Microorganism capable of causing disease is a pathogen.
16. **Pediatrics:** Branch of medicine concern with growth, development and care of children and treatment of their diseases.
17. **Therapeutic play:** The process of incorporating play activities in the routine care of pediatric patients to decrease hospital/disease associated stress.

9

Legal and Ethical Issues in Nursing

INTRODUCTION

The law constitutes body of principles recognized or enforced by public and regular tribunals have the administration of justice. The law is the body of principles recognized and applied by the state and the administrations of justice. Law is that portion of the established thought and habit which has gained district and formal recognition, the shape of uniform rules backed by the authority and power of the government.

TYPES OF LAWS

CIVIL LAW

Civil law includes rules and regulations that specify the required course of action to be followed by an individual in business and social relationships with others. It is concerned with relationships among people and the protection of a person's rights.

CRIMINAL LAW

Criminal law defines offences that affect public welfare and security and impose penalties. It includes rules forbidding conduct that is injurious to public order and specifying punishments to be administered to individual who exhibits injurious conduct.

COMMON LEGAL ISSUES

Common legal issues in nursing are:

1. Wrong medications, wrong dosage, wrong route of administration and wrong concentration.
2. Mistaken identity—prepare the wrong patient for an operation, to exchange babies in the labor room, to exchange dead bodies in the mortuary.
3. Failure to communicate.
4. Maintenance of record.

5. Giving explanation and getting the concerned.
6. Bums and false character.
7. Counting sponges and instruments during surgery.
8. Loss or damage to patient's property and fame.
9. Euthanasia or mercy killing: Taking positive step to kill a person in order to end his/her suffering is a murder.

LAW AND NURSE

1. **Responsibility of appointing and assigning:** The nurse administrators have responsibility for staffing and supervising nursing units to ensure safe, effective patient care. Therefore, they have the authority to temporarily reassign a nursing employee to compensate for emergency staff shortages.
2. **Responsibility in quality control:** A nurse manager's legal responsibility for quality control of nursing service imposes a duty to observe report and correct the incompetence of any patient care provider.
3. **Responsibility for equipment:** To protect the patients and employees from injury, a nurse manager must ensure that all patient care equipments are fully functional and the defective equipment is promptly repaired or replaced.
4. **Responsibility for observation and reporting:** Consequently nurses have a legal duty to observe patients frequently and report findings that have diagnostic or treatment value for the patient's physician and other members of the patient's treatment team.
5. **Responsibility to protect public:** The nurse has a legal duty to protect the public from injury by dangerous patients. The manager must ensure that nursing personnel follow the procedures to alert community members to the presence of a potentially dangerous patient in their midst.
6. **Responsibility for record keeping and reporting:** Nurses have legal responsibility for accurately reporting and recording patient's conditions, treatments and response to care. The medical record is an information source document that should be used to plan care, evaluate care, allocate costs, educate personnel, research care measure and substantiate legal claim.
7. **Responsibility for death and dying:** Nurses must be aware of legal definition of death because they must document all events when the patient is in their care.

LEGAL ISSUES IN NURSING

NURSE PRACTICE ACT

Each state has a Nurse Practice Act. The Guidelines and laws outlined in the act pertain to all nurses who are licensed in that particular state.

Nurse limitation is one of those laws. Each nurse has a limitation on what nurse is allowed and trained to do. Nurse must follow the chain of command, especially with the care of a patient. If she/he does not have the authority or knowledge to give a prescription, analyze a laboratory report, or advise the patient on treatment, nurse may not legally do so. Any wrong information or practice she/he commits is punishable by the law and the patient or family may file a suit against the nurse and the health agency or hospital he/she works for.

PATIENT'S ADVOCATE

A nurse has a legal obligation to act as the patient's advocate in case of emergency. The nurse is to act as the liaison between the patient and the healthcare provider, such as physician. The nurse will monitor the patient, ensuring that if any complications or abnormalities arise, a physician notified immediately. The nurse is legally obligated to keep the personal data and information of the patient confidential not doing so is a violation of the Code of Ethics for nurses.

ADMINISTERING MEDICATION

Nurses are responsible for administering the correct doses and medications to patients. If the nurse gives a fatal dosage amount, she/he may face legal malpractice suits. It is also the responsibility to research the patient's records, or ask the patient and family members if there are any allergies or complications that may pose a risk if a certain medication is administered.

INFORMED CONSENT

When a nurse is administering treatment, he/she must explain what the effects and outcomes could be and any other important information. It is the responsibility of the nurse to confirm that the patient or family member who will sign the informed consent form is coherent, and understands all the negative aspects of the treatment. The nurse, patient, or patient family member will sign the informed consent form in front of a witness, a physician or another nurse. Not having this legal document signed and in front of a witness could be a legal issue for the nurse if complications arise during treatment.

NEGLIGENCE

Negligence is the responsibility of the nurse to monitor the patient. If a patient calls for a nurse to come and assist in going to the restroom, for example, the nurse is to assist or if she/he is busy with another patient, have another nurse assist the patient. Ignoring the patient or responding after a lengthy delay could be considered negligence, and if the patient is hurt from trying to move himself/herself, the nurse could face legal suits.

Also, it could be considered negligence if a physician orders the nurse to administer a prescription and the nurse did not do so.

LEGAL ASPECTS RELATED TO NURSING REGISTRATION

A registered nurse (RN) is a nurse who has graduated from a college's nursing program or from a school of nursing and has passed a national licensing examination. A registered nurse helps individuals, families and groups to achieve health and prevent disease. They care for the sick and injured in hospitals and other health care facilities, physicians' offices, private homes, public health agencies, schools, camps and industry. Some registered nurse, are employed in private practice. A registered nurse's scope of practice is determined by each state's Nurse Practice Act. It outlines what is legal practice for registered nurses and what tasks they may or may not perform. Nurse Practice Acts also dictate the scope of practice for nurse practitioners (NPs). An example is prescriptive authority for NPs. In some states, NPs can practice completely autonomously and prescribe any category of medications. In other states, NPs cannot prescribe controlled substances and may only practice with the collaboration of a physician.

CIVIL LAW PENALTIES FOR REGISTERED NURSES

Registered nurses have penalties that are inflicted on them for transgressions such as medical malpractice and breach of confidentiality. These civil law penalties can cause them to be suspended or banned from the nursing practice.

LICENSE REVOCATION OR SUSPENSION PROCEDURE

According to Tennessee law, the reasons for a Tennessee registered nurses license being denied, suspended or revoked are: fraudulent activity with respect to certification, established guilty before a court of law, medical negligence or malpractice, mental dysfunction, unprofessional conduct, drug use and complicity in a crime with another. When these crimes have been committed, the case comes before the Tennessee Department of Health: Board of Nursing, which certifies nurses and eventually makes the judgment as what should be done. The hearing of a case should take place not more than 6 months after the charges have been read.

PATIENT'S BILL OF RIGHT

In 1973, the American Hospital Association adopted Patient's Bill of Rights as national policy statement and distributed it to its members in the health care organizations throughout the nation. There are 12 rights summarized below:

1. The patient has a right to a considerate and respectful care.

2. The patient has a right to obtain complete and concerned information concerning the diagnosis, treatment and prognosis from physician for the patient's expected understanding.
3. The patient has a right to receive the necessary information from physician regarding the treatment and the procedures involved in it.
4. The patient has a right to refuse the treatment to the extent permitted by the law and to be informed about the medical consequences of the action.
5. The patient has a right to privacy concerning own medical care program.
6. The patient has a right to expect all communications and records pertaining to care should be treated as confidential.
7. The patient has a right to expect within the capacity, a hospital must make reasonable response to the request made by the patient for services.
8. The patient has a right to obtain information regarding any of his/her relationship or dealing with hospital or other healthcare institution as his/her care is concerned.
9. The patient has a right to be advised if the hospital proposes to engage or perform human experimentation affecting the treatment.
10. The patient has a right to expect reasonable continuity of care.
11. The patient has a right to examine and receive an explanation of the hospital bills regardless of the source of payment.
12. The patient has a right to know what hospital rules and regulations apply to his/her conduct as a patient.

IMPORTANT PRACTICE STANDARDS FOR BREACH SANCTIONS

The disparity in organizational response to employee malfeasance has a far-reaching impact on the healthcare industry. Consequences include the following:

1. **Confusing message:** An inconsistent organizational response to a breach sends a confusing message to both staff and the public. Healthcare workers moving from one organization to another find differing tolerance levels for enforcing the same directives.
2. **Poor compliance:** Staff in organizations with less stringent enforcement may weigh the level of risk to themselves against the potential advantages. Inequity in sanction application encourages poor compliance by individuals who know they will escape any serious consequence for breaching privacy and security policies.
3. **Public trust erosion:** Public trust is eroded when significant variation is blatantly apparent in how healthcare organizations respond to a privacy or security breach both within and across entities and systems.

The public must feel assured their personal health information has sufficient protections across the healthcare spectrum, particularly in this era of health information exchange.

4. **Weakened position for dispute resolutions:** Inequitable application of sanctions can affect the outcome of personnel actions at arbitration and grievance proceedings. Unequal penalties for similar offenses undermine the organization's ability to prevail in dispute resolutions.
5. **More regulation:** Poor and inconsistent implementation of privacy and security safeguards invites further state and federal intervention. Such laws place an additional administrative and financial burden on facilities. If the industry does not self-correct, then it leaves open the door to state and federal government intervention.
6. **Questionable research:** The validity of research may be in question when patient's privacy or security breaches are not handled consistently and expeditiously.

SAFEGUARDING THE NURSE

1. **Licensure:** All nurses who are in nursing practice have to possess a valid licence, issued by the respective State Nursing Council/Indian Nursing Council
2. **Good Samaritan laws:** In response to health professionals, fear of malpractice claims most states enacted Good Samaritan Laws that exempt doctors and nurses from liability when they render help during emergency. These laws limit liability and offer legal immunity for people helping in an emergency.
3. **Good rapport:** Developing good rapport with the client is very important to prevent malpractice. The ability to develop good rapport with client is dependent on the nurse having good interpersonal communication skills e.g. listening.
4. **Standards of care:** All professional practicing in the medical field are held to certain standards when administering care. It is always better to follow standards of care to avoid malpractice and do not attempt anything beyond the level of competence.
5. **Standing orders:** Nurse may not legally diagnose illness or prescribe treatment, after assessing patient's condition apply standing orders or treatment guideline that have been established by the physician or doctor as appropriate for certain problems and conditions.
6. **Consent for operation and other procedures:** A patient coming in to hospital still retains the rights as a citizen and entry only denotes the willingness to undergo an investigation or a course of treatment. Any investigation treatment of a serious matter or an operation in which an anesthetic is used, requires the written consent of the patient.
7. **Correct identity:** The nurse or the midwife has the great responsibility to make sure that all babies born in the hospital are correctly labeled

at birth and to ensure that never they are placed in the wrong cot or given to the wrong mother.

8. **Counting of sponge, instrument and needles:** Nurses advocate that sponge, instrument and needle counts be performed for all surgical procedures taking place in operation theater. When an instrument left in a patient's body the nurse will probably be liable for any patient injury caused by the presence of foreign body.
9. **Contracts:** This is a written or oral agreement between two people in which goods or services are exchanged.
10. **Documentation:** This is by far the best once a lawsuit field. The medical record is a legal document admissible in court as evidence.

ETHICAL ISSUES IN NURSING

Ethics are the rules or principles that govern right contact. Ethics are designed to protect the rights of human being. Ethics are characteristics of a healthy profession. The Code of Ethics will state what kind of conduct is expected from the members of a profession, what are the responsibilities of its members toward those whom they serve, their coworker, the profession and the society as a whole.

NURSING ETHICS

The nursing ethics provide professional standards for nursing activities which protect the nurse and the patient.

In 1973, the International Council for Nurses (INC) adopted Code of Ethics.

The fundamental responsibility of the nurse is 4-fold to promote health, to prevent illness, to restore health and to alleviate suffering.

The need for nursing is universal. Inherent in nursing is respect for life dignity and rights of men. It unrestricted by considerations of nationality, race, creed, color, age, sex, politics or social status.

Nurses render health services to the individual, the family and the community and coordinate their services with those of related groups.

ETHICAL PRINCIPLES

Ethical principles actually control professionalism nursing practice much more than to ethical theories. Principles encompass basic promises from which rules are developed. Principles are the moral norms that nursing, as a profession, both demands and strives to implement to everyday clinical practice. Ethical principle that the nurse should consider when making decisions are as follows:

1. Respect for persons.
2. Respect for autonomy.
3. Respect for freedom.

4. Respect for beneficence (doing good).
5. Respect for nonmaleficence (avoiding harm to others).
6. Respect for veracity (truth telling).
7. Respect for persons.
8. Respect for justice (fair and equal treatment).
9. Respect for rights.
10. Respect for fidelity (fulfilling promises).
11. Confidentiality (protecting privileged information).

Respect for Persons

Respect for persons not only applies to clinical situations, but also to all life's situations. It directs individuals to treat themselves and other, with a respect inherent to man's humanness. It requires recognition on a sense that all mankind shared a common human destiny. The respect to persons needs to be simplified as it affects nursing practice.

Autonomy

Autonomy that individuals are able to act for themselves to the level of their capacity. It is the right of individual to govern their actions according to their own purpose and reason. Respect for autonomy requires that persons honor another's right to govern him or her. The legal doctrine of informed consent is the direct reflection of autonomy. So it requires that health personnel obtain a patient's informed consent for treatment and for participation in research. The followings are required for a patient to give informed consent for either.

Disclosure

Adequate presentation of relevant information about the proposed treatment or study.

Understanding

Adequate comprehension of the disclosed information.

Voluntary agreement

Free assent, influenced by external controlling factors.

Competence

Adequate decision-making capacity. There are three type of autonomy, i.e. freedom of action, freedom of choice and effective deliberation.

Freedom

The principle of individual freedom decrease that patients be exempt from control by others to select and pursue personal health goals. Nurses as a group believe that patient should have greater freedom of choice within the nation's health-care system. This principle should be observed by staff nurses when planning patient care; by nurse manager when leading subordinates.

Beneficence

The beneficence principle states that the actions one takes should promote good. It dictates that a person is obliged to help others to advance their legitimate and important interests; it requires the balancing of harms and benefits. Benefits promote the clients' welfare and health, whereas harms or risks detract from the client's health and welfare. In other words, providing benefits that enhance the others welfare. Whereas balancing the benefits and harms of intervention made on the others behalf.

Professional education provides awareness that most nursing interventions are capable of producing undesirable, as well as desirable patient outcome. Therefore, the nurse is obliged to ascertain each care measure, likelihood of success, and balance the measures probable benefits and risks in order to select interventions that maximize patient's welfare.

Non-maleficence

The corollary of beneficence, the principle of nonmaleficence states that one should do no harm. The nurse should interpret the term 'harm' to mean emotional and social as well as physical injury. Harm is thwarting, defeating or setting back one person's interest through invasive action by another. Many nurses find it difficult to follow the principle when performing treatment and procedures that bring discomfort and pain to patients. When the principle of sanctity of human life guides healthcare decisions, the principle of nonmaleficence prohibits active and passive enthusive by caregivers of terminally ill patients. As nurse manager performing performance evaluation of subordinates should emphasize their good qualities and give positive direction for growth. Destroying the employees' self-esteem and self-worth would be considered doing harm their principles.

Veracity

Veracity concerns truth telling an incorporates the concept that individuals should always tell the truth. It requires professional caregivers to provide with accurate, reality-based information about their health status and care or treatment prospect. Truth telling is an ethical concern for nurse, because truth is the basis for mutual trust between patient and nurse, and trust is the basis for patient's hope of benefit from nursing services. Nurse managers use this principle when they give all the facts of a situation truthfully and assist their employees to make decisions. However, truth telling may be difficult in a healthcare relationship. Some information that is transmitted from nurse to patient is depressing and/or frightening, e.g. bad news about personal health status.

Justice

Justice concerns the issue that persons should be treated equally and fairly. This principle of justice requires treating others fairly and giving persons their due. When there are resources to distribute in health care, nurses should allocate them in such a way that equal shares go to equal recipients.

The following problems complicate the application of justice:

1. Not everyone is equal in every way; sometimes there are situations in which it seems that one person should receive a greater or lesser share than another.
2. Resources are limited. There is not always enough for each person to receive an equal share.

Questions of justice relate to the fairness with which benefits and burdens are distributed among people. Experience in turn found various principles have to be proposed to guide fair distribution of society's good are as follows:

1. Each person should receive an equal share.
2. The amount given to each person should be proportional to the need.
3. The amount given to each person should be proportional to the amount of work effort.
4. The amount given to each person should reflect the value of work product.
5. The amount given to each person should reflect the value to society.
6. The amount given to each person should be determined by free market exchange. These principles usually arise in times of short supplies or when there is competition for resources of benefits.

Rights

Right is an entitlement to behave in certain way under circumstances, such as nurse's entitlement to freely express personal beliefs and preferences by voting in a political election. Another right is the prerogative to define another's behavior in selected situations, such as manager's prerogative to give assignments to subordinates. A right is also a claim to a specific good, service or prerequisite such as tea break time. Right is also used to mean agreement with justice, law and morality. So right may be mental rights or legal rights related to respective profession. For more details refer Patient's Bill of Rights.

Fidelity

Fidelity is keeping one's promises or commitments. The principle of fidelity holds that a person should faithfully fulfill his duties and obligations. Fidelity is important in a nurse because a patient's hope for relief and recovery rests on evidence of caregiver's conscientiousness. Nurse Managers abide by this principle when they follow through on any promise they have previously made to employees, such as promised leave, a certain shift to be worked or a promotion to perception within the unit.

Confidentiality

Confidentiality is the duty to respect privileged information. The principle of confidentiality provides that caregivers should respect a patient need for privacy and use personal information only to improve care. Nurses should practice confidentiality to decrease patient vulnerability and share from widespread knowledge of personal information divulged during care.

ETHICAL DILEMMAS

A dilemma is defined as situations requiring a choice between two equally desirable or undesirable alternatives. In ethical dilemma, each alternative course of action can be justified by two ways in which a person views the course of action based on his or her value system. Issues in healthcare delivery practices present different alternatives based on whether the issue or course of action is viewed by the patient, the healthcare agency, the legal system or the nurse. Increasingly, staff nurses and nurse managers face difficult decisions caused by tensions between technological capabilities, budgetary structures and quality of life concerns. Nurses in all clinical and functional specialties face the following ethical dilemmas:

1. Need to ration patient care to conserve scarce resources.
2. Need to make treatment and care decisions for terminally ill patients.
3. Need to obtain patients informed consent for care and treatment orders and measures such as:
   a. Do not resuscitate order.
   b. Withholding/withdrawing nutrition and fluids.
   c. Starting/Discontinuing life support system.
4. Response to patient request for assisted suicide.
5. Need to balance the patients need for confidentiality and privacy against society's needs for protection from unreasonable risk.
6. Need to protect autonomy rights of children and incompetent adults concerning consent for research participation.
7. Need to protect justice rights of patients who participate in random trials of experimental treatment.

Usually the dilemma occurs when opposing views are seen for the solution of an issue and a decision must be made. There is no set of procedures or easy answers for how an ethical dilemma should be resolved. Ethical decision making is needed in all steps of the nursing process and all phases of the nursing management process. Ethical reasoning is similar to the nursing process in that it requires critical thinking skills. A nurse can best resolve ethical dilemma by systematically considering all options for solving the dilemma. A ethical dilemma occurs as a result of conflict between moral and principles that support different courses of action.

ETHICAL DECISION MAKING

Nurse's decisions are increasingly constrained by ethical issues. Ethical decision making involves reflection on the following:

1. Who should make the choice.
2. Possible options or courses of action.
3. Available options.
4. Consequences, both good and bad, of all possible options.
5. Rules, obligations and values that should direct choices.
6. Desired outcomes.

When making decisions, nurses need to combine all of these elements using an orderly, systematic, and objective method. There are various models for ethical decision making. Perhaps the easiest ethical decision-making model to remember and to implement in practice is the 'moral model' developed by Thirona and Halloran as follows:

M—Massage the dilemma. Identify and define the issues in the dilemma. Consider the opinions of all major players in the dilemma as well as their value system. This includes patient's family members, nurses, doctors, priest and any other interdisciplinary healthcare team member.

O—Outline the options. Examine all options including those less realistic and conflicting, this stage is designed only for considering options and not for making final decision.

R—Resolve the dilemma. Review the issues and options, applying the basic principles of ethics to each option. Decide the best option based upon the views of all those concerned in the dilemma.

A—Act by applying chosen action this step is usually the most difficult as it requires actual implementation. While the previous steps had only allowed for dialogue or discussion.

L—Look back and evaluate the entire process including the implementation. No process is complete without a thorough evaluation. Ensure that those involved are able to follow through on the final option. If not, a second decision may be required and process must start again at the initial step.

Another exchange of traditional model of ethical decision making are as follows:

1. Identify the problem.
2. Gather data to analyze the causes and consequence of the problem.
3. Explore the optional solutions to the problem.

4. Evaluate the optional solution.
5. Select the appropriate solution from all the options.
6. Implement the selected solution.
7. Evaluate the result.

ETHICAL RESPONSIBILITY

Ethical responsibilities are:

1. Caring demands the provision of helping services that are appropriate to the needs of the client and significant others.
2. Caring recognizes the client's membership in a family and community, and provides for the participation of significant others in his or her care.
3. Caring acknowledges the reality of death in the life of every person and demands that appropriate support provided for the dying person and family to enable, to prepare for, and to cope with death when it is inevitable.
4. Caring acknowledges that the person has the capacity to fact up the health needs and problems in own unique way, and directs nursing action in a manner that will assist the client to develop, maintain or gain personal autonomy, self-respect and self-determination.
5. Caring, as a response to a health need, requires the consent and the participation of the person who is experiencing the need.
6. Caring dictates that the client and significant others have the knowledge and information adequate for free and informed decisions concerning care requirements, alternative and preferences.
7. Caring demands that the needs of the client supersede those of the nurse.
8. Caring acknowledges the vulnerability of a client in certain situations and dictates restraint in actions which might compromise the client's rights and privileges.
9. Caring involving a relationship which is, in itself therapeutic, demands mutual respect and trust.
10. Caring acknowledges that information obtained in the course of the nursing relationship is privileged, and that is requires the full protection of confidentiality unless such information provides evidence of serious impending harm to the client or third party, or is legally required by the courts.
11. Caring requires that the nurse represents the needs of the client and that the nurse takes appropriate measures when fulfillment of these needs is jeopardized by the actions of other persons.
12. Caring acknowledges the dignity of all persons in the practice of educational setting.

13. Caring acknowledges, respects and draws upon the competencies of others.
14. Caring establishes the conditions for the harmonization of efforts of different helping professionals in providing required services to clients.
15. Caring seeks to establish and maintain a climate of respect for the honest conversation needed for effective collaboration.
16. Caring establishes the legitimacy of respectful challenge and/or confrontation when the service required by the client is compromised by incompetency, incapacity or negligence or when the competencies of the nurses are not acknowledged or appropriately utilized.
17. Caring demands the provision of working conditions which enable nurses to carry out their legitimate and responsibilities.
18. Caring demands resourcefulness and restraint accountability for the use of time, resources, equipment and funds, and requires accountability to appropriate individuals and/or bodies.
19. Caring requires that the nurse bring to the work situation in education, practice, administration or research, the knowledge of affective and technical skills, and that competency in these areas be maintained and updated.
20. Caring commands fidelity oneself, and guards the right and privilege of the nurse to act in keeping with an informed moral conscience.

CONCLUSION

Ethics are characteristics of a profession and are called code. The code of ethics will state what kind of conduct is expected from the members of a profession. What are the responsibilities of its members towards those whom, they serve, their co-workers, the profession and the society. The nurse should be aware of some of the legal aspects of nursing, e.g. carelessness or negligence, because of this on the part of nurse may lead to court action against her or the hospital and heavy damages could be awarded against the nurse or her organization.

CHAPTER

10

Health and Illness

INTRODUCTION

Good health is a prerequisite of human productive and developmental process. It is essential to economic and technological development. Health is the condition of being sound by body, mind or spirit, especially free from physical disease or pain. Soundness of body or mind, that condition in which their functions are duly and efficiently discharged (Webster and Oxford dictionary). The concept of health has been defined in a variety of ways. Historically, health and illness were viewed as extremes on a continuum, with the absence of clinically recognizable disease being equated with presence of health. World Health Organization (1974) defined health in terms of well-being and discouraged the conceptualization of health as simply the absence of disease.

DEFINITIONS

1. **Health:** World Health Organization (WHO) defines health as a 'state of complete physical, mental and social well-being, not merely the absence of disease or infirmity.'
2. **Illness:** It is a state in which a person's physical, emotional, intellectual, social, and spiritual functioning is diminished or impaired.

CONCEPT OF HEALTH

Health is a common theme in almost all countries:

- Absence of disease
- Health = Harmony = Being in peace.

Health is the presence of a positive capacity to lead energetic satisfying and productive life. It is a state of optimal physical, mental and social adaptation to one's environment. It is a relative not an absolute concept always involves many levels or degrees.

Other concepts are:

1. **Biomedical concept:** Health is the absence of disease (Germ Theory), normal functioning ability, activities that leads to the survival of the species.

2. **Ecological concept:** Health is a dynamic equilibrium between man and environment. Imbalance results disease. Adaptation to the environment leads to better health and longer life expectancy even in the absence of modern health services.
3. **Psychological concept:** Health is not only a biomedical phenomenon, but one which is influenced by social, psychological, cultural, economical and political factors of the people concerned, mental and emotional fulfillment, self-actualization, absence of neurosis and psychosis.
4. **Holistic concept:** It emphasize on promotion and protection of health. It include all the factors of the other concepts in addition to all human activities such as education, communication, agriculture, industry, housing, recreation, etc.
5. **Spiritual concept:** Profound awareness, appreciation of truth and a sense of bliss.

DIMENSIONS OF HEALTH

1. Health is multidimensional, the WHO definition includes there are specific dimensions like physical, mental and social.
2. Many more may be cited like spiritual, emotional, vocational and political dimensions.
3. These dimensions function and interact with another; each has its own nature and for descriptive purpose will be treated separately.

PHYSICAL DIMENSIONS

1. The state of physical health implies the notion of 'perfect functioning' of the body.
2. Health as a state in which every cell and every organ is functioning at optimal capacity and in perfect harmony with rest of the body.
3. Smooth, easy, coordinate bodily movement.
4. All the senses are intact the resting pulse rate, blood pressure (BP) and exercise tolerance are all within the range of 'normality' of the individuals age.
5. Steady weight gain.

Signs

The signs of physical health in an individual are:

- Good complexion
- Clean skin
- Bright eyes
- Lustrous hair
- Well-clothed with firm flesh
- Not too fat
- Sweet breath

- Good appetite
- Sound sleep
- Regular activity of bowel and bladder.

Evaluations are as follows:

Evaluation

1. Self-assessment
2. Inquiry into symptoms of ill health and risk factors
3. Inquiry into medication
4. Inquiry into levels of activity
5. Inquiry into use of medical services
6. Standardized questionnaires for cardiovascular disease and respiratory disease
7. Clinical examination
8. Dietary assessment
9. Biochemical and laboratory investigations.

MENTAL DIMENSION

1. Mental health is not absences of mental illness, but mental health is the ability to respond to the many varied experiences of life with flexibility and a sense of purpose.
2. A state of balance between the individual and the surrounding world. A state of harmony between one's self and others.
3. A coexistence between the realities of the self, other people and environment.
4. The mind and body were considered independent entities. Later on, it is proved that both are related to mental factor.
5. The mental factor like stress leads to hypertension, peptic ulcer, etc.
6. The mental disorders like depression, schizophrenia have a biological basis.

Mental health is essential component of health, the scientific foundation is not yet clear.

Characteristics of Mentally Healthy Person

1. A mentally healthy person is free from mental conflict, he/she is not at 'war' with himself/herself.
2. The person is well adjusted; and able to get along well with others.
3. Accepts for identity.
4. The person has a strong sense of self-esteem.
5. The person knows himself/herself, his needs, problems and goals (self-actualization).
6. Has good self control, balances with rationally and emotionally.
7. Faces problems and tries to solve them intelligently, i.e. coping with stress and anxiety.

One of the key to good health is a positive mental health; unfortunately our knowledge about mental health is far from complete.

SOCIAL DIMENSION

1. Social dimension has been defined as the "quantity and quality of an individual's interpersonal and the extend of involvement with the community."
2. It includes the level of social skills one possess, social functioning and the ability to see oneself as a member of a large society.
3. It is rooted in positive material environment and positive human environment.

SPRITUAL DIMENSION

1. Spritual dimension is the intangible. Something that transcends physiology and psychology.
2. It includes integrity, principles and ethics, the purpose in life commitment to some higher being and belief in concept that are not subject to the 'state of the art'.

EMOTIONAL DIMENSION

1. Mental health can be seen as 'knowing' or cognition while emotional health relates to feeling, isolating these two separate dimensions is difficult. But some experts in psychology and psychiatry did that one.
2. Now, the mental and emotional aspects of the human may have to be viewed as a separate dimension of human health. Ventilation of emotion is helpful in achieving the health status.

VOCATIONAL DIMENSION

1. Vocational dimension is a new dimension.
2. It is a part of human existences, when work is fully adapted to human goals, capacities and limitations, then the needs will be fulfilled.
3. Work often plays a role in promoting both physical and mental health.
4. Physical work is usually associated with improvement; goal achievement and self-realization in work are a source of satisfaction and enhanced self-esteem.

CONCEPT OF HEALTH AND ILLNESS

1. It is useful for the nurse to be aware of the behavioral components of health, illness and sick.
2. Every person develops a system of health beliefs and attitudes, and these tend to fall within the framework provided by society or cultural heritage.

3. Healthy behavior activities of a person engages in when feeling well to take measures to prevent disease and illness or to detect them before symptom occur.
4. Illness behavior activities of a person edges in when feeling ill that will lead to the defining of the state of health and that will gain help.
5. Sick-role behavior, activities a person engages in believing himself/herself ill. For any individual the level of health behavior is determined by the significance of symptoms—danger value, visibility, ambiguity, fear of unknown, the expectations of those from whom help is sought, feeling about dependence and fear of loss of control, the expectorations of the illness position including past experiences with illness.

STAGES OF ILLNESS BEHAVIOR

Symptom Experience

1. During the initial stage, a person is aware that something is wrong. A person usually recognizes a physical sensation or a limitation in functioning but does not suspect a specific diagnosis.
2. The person's perception of symptoms includes awareness of a physical change such as pain, rash or a lump.

Assumption of the Sick Role

1. The assumption of the sick role results in emotional changes, such as withdrawal or depression, and physical changes.
2. Emotional changes may be simple or complex, depending on the severity of the illness, the degree of disability and anticipated length of the illness.

Medical Care Contact

1. If symptoms persist despite home remedies, become severe or require emergency care, the person is motivated to seek professional health services.
2. In this stage the client seeks expect acknowledgement of the illness, as well as treatment in addition, the client seeks an explanation of the symptoms, cause of the symptoms, course of the illness for future health.
3. Client's illness can be validated at any point on the health illness continuum. A health professional may determine that they do not have an illness or that illnesses are present and may belief threatening.

Dependent Client Role

1. After accepting the illness and seeking treatment, the client enters the fourth stage of illness behavior.
2. In this stage, the client depends on healthcare professionals for relief of symptoms. The client accepts care, sympathy and protection from the demands and stresses of life.

3. It is socially permissible for clients in the dependent role to be relieved of normal obligations and tasks.

Recovery Stage

1. The final stage of illness behavior—recovery and rehabilitation—can arrive suddenly, such as when a fever subsides.
2. The recovery is not prompt, long-term care may be required before the client is able to resume an optimal level of functioning.
3. In the case of chronic illness, the final stage may involve an adjustment to a prolonged reduction in health and functioning.

HEALTH ILLNESS CONTINUUM

Health is a dynamic state that fluctuates as a person adapts to changes in the internal and external environments to maintain a state of well-being. As health and illness are relative qualities existing in varying degrees, it is more accurate to consider health and illness in terms of a scale or continuum, rather than a absolute state.

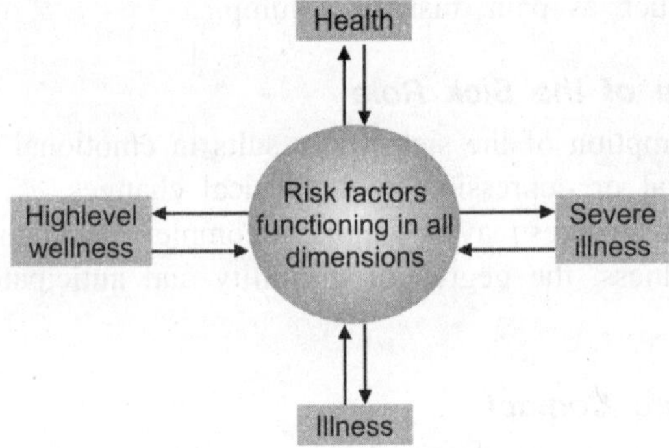

Figure 10.1: Health illness continuum

FACTORS INFLUENCING HEALTH BELIEF AND PRACTICES

Internal Variables

1. **Developmental stage:** A person's thought and behavior patterns change throughout the life.
2. **Intellectual background:** Knowledge about body functions and illness, educational background and past experiences, all influence the health beliefs and practice of patients.
3. **Emotional and spiritual factors:** The patient's degree of calm or stress can influence health beliefs and practices. Spiritual beliefs also influence whether and how a patient seeks or avoids healthy behavior.

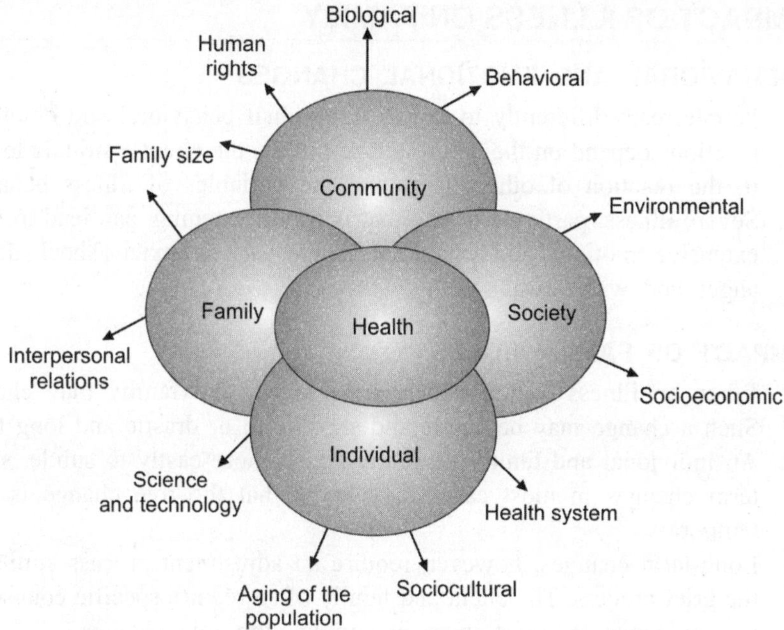

Figure 10.2: Factors influencing health belief practices

External Variables

1. **Family practices:** The way that patient's families use healthcare services, their perceptions of the seriousness of diseases and their preventative care behaviors can influence the health beliefs and practice.
2. **Socioeconomic factors:** Social relationships, economic level and psychosocial factors influence health beliefs and practice.
3. **Cultural background:** It influences beliefs, values and customs. It influences the approach to the healthcare system, personal health practices and nurse-patient relationship.

FACTORS AFFECTING A PATIENT'S HEALTH STATUS

- Smoking
- Nutrition
- Alcohol use
- Habituating drug use
- Driving
- Exercise
- Sexuality and contraceptive use
- Family relationships
- Risk factor modification
- Coping and adaptation.

IMPACT OF ILLNESS ON FAMILY

BEHAVIORAL AND EMOTIONAL CHANGES

1. People react differently to illness. Individual behavioral and emotional reactions depend on the nature of the illness, the client's attitude toward it, the reaction of others to it and the variables of illness behavior.
2. Severe illness, particularly one that is life-threatening, can lead to more extensive emotional and behavioral change, such as anxiety, shock, dental, anger and withdrawal.

IMPACT OF FAMILY ROLES

1. When an illness occurs, the roles of client and family may change. Such a change may be subtle and short term or drastic and long term.
2. An individual and family generally adjust more easily to subtle, short-term changes in most cases they know that the role change is only temporary.
3. Long-term changes, however, require an adjustment process similar to the grief process. The client and family often require specific counseling and guidance to assist them in coping with role changes.

IMPACT ON BODY CHANGES

1. Some illnesses result in changes in physical appearance and clients and families react differently to these changes.
2. When changes in body image occur, such as results from a leg amputation, the client generally adjusts in the following phases—shock, withdrawal, acknowledgment, acceptance and rehabilitation.
3. Withdrawal is an adaptive coping mechanism that can assist the client in making the adjustments.

IMPACT OF SELF-CONCEPTS

1. Self-concept is individual's mental image of themselves, including how they view their strengths and weaknesses in all aspects of their personalities.
2. Self-concepts depends in part of body image and roles but also include other aspects of the psychological and spiritual self.
3. Self-concept changes because of illness may no longer meet the expectations of the family leading to tension or conflict.

IMPACT OF FAMILY DYNAMICS

1. Family dynamics is the process by which the family functions, makes decisions, give support to individual members, and copes with everyday changes and challenges.

2. If a parent in a family becomes ill, family activities and decision making often come to a habit as the other family members, wait for the illness to pass or they delay action, because they are reluctant to assume the ill person's roles or responsibilities.

IMPACT OF ILLNESS ON PATIENT AND FAMILY

1. **Impact of illness on patient:** Short-term and minor illnesses awoke few behavioral changes in the functioning of the patient or family. Severe illness can lead to more extensive emotional and behavioral changes such as anxiety, shock, denial, anger and withdrawal.
2. **Impact on family roles:** When an illness occurs, the role of patients and family may change. This change may be subtle and short-term or drastic and long-term. During illness the patient and family require specific counseling and guidance to assist them in coping with the role changes.

MODELS OF HEALTH AND ILLNESS

HEALTH–WELLNESS MODEL

1. Health-wellness model was developed by Dunn (1997), the high level wellness model is oriented toward maximizing the health potential of an individual.
2. This model requires the individual to maintain a continuum of balance and purposeful direction within the environment.
3. It involves progress toward a higher level of functioning open-ended and expanding challenges to live at the fullest potential.

AGENT-HOST-ENVIRONMENTAL MODEL

1. The agent host-environmental model of health and illness originated in the community health work of level.
2. According to this approach the health or illness of an individual or group depends on the dynamic relationship of the agent, host and environment.
3. The agent is any internal or external factors that its presence or absence can lead to disease or illness.
4. The host is the person or persons who may be susceptible to a particular illness or diseases.
5. The environment consists of all factors outside of the host. It includes physical environment, social environment and biological environment.

HEALTH BELIEF MODEL

1. Rosenstock's (1794) and Beker and Maiman's health belief model addresses the relationship between a person's belief and behavior.

2. It provides a way of understanding and predicating how clients will behave in relation to their health and how they will comply with health care therapies.
3. The first component in this model involves the individual's perception of susceptibility to an illness.
4. The second component is the individual's perception of the seriousness of the illness. This perception is influenced and modified by demographic and sociopsychological variables, perceived threats of the illnesses, and cues to action.
5. The third component is the likelihood that a person will take preventive action which is the person's perception of the benefits of taking action.

HEALTH PROMOTION MODEL

1. The health promotion model proposed by Pender (1996). It was designed to be a complementary counterpart to models of health protection.
2. Health promotion is directed at increasing a client's level of well-being. The model focuses on three functions.
3. The model also organizes cues into a pattern to explain the likelihood of a client's participation in health-promotion behavior.
4. The focus of this model is to explain the reasons that individuals engage in health activities. It is not designed for use with families or communities.

HEALTHCARE DELIVERY SYSTEM IN INDIA

India is a union of 28 states and 7 union territories. States are largely independent in matters relating to the delivery of health care to the people. Each state has developed its own system of healthcare delivery, independent of the Central Government. The Central Government responsibility consists mainly of policy making, planning, guiding, assisting, evaluating and coordinating the work of the State Health Ministries.

The health system in India has three main links:

1. Central
2. State
3. Local or peripheral.

AT THE CENTRAL LEVEL

The official 'organs' of the health system at the national level consist of

- Ministry of Health and Family Welfare
- The Directorate General of Health Services
- The Central Council of Health and Family Welfare.

Ministry of Health and Family Welfare

Functions

Union list

1. International health relations and administration of port quarantine.
2. Administration of Central Institutes such as All India Institute of Hygiene and Public Health, Kolkata.
3. Promotion of research through research centers.
4. Regulation and development of medical, pharmaceutical, dental and nursing professions.
5. Establishment and maintenance of drug standards.
6. Census, collection and publication of other statistical data.
7. Immigration and emigration.
8. Regulation of labor in the working of mines and oil fields.
9. Coordination with states and with other ministries for promotion of health.

Concurrent List

The functions listed under the concurrent list are the responsibility of both the union and state governments are as follows:

1. Prevention and extension of communicable diseases.
2. Prevention of adulteration of food stuffs.
3. Control of drugs and poisons.
4. Vital statistics.
5. Labour welfare.
6. Ports other than major.
7. Economic and social planning.
8. Population control and family planning.

Directorate General of Health Services

Functions

1. International health relations and quarantine of all major ports in country and international airport.
2. Control of drug standards.
3. Maintain medical store depots.
4. Administration of post graduate training programs.
5. Administration of certain medical colleges in India.
6. Conducting medical research through Indian Council of Medical Research (ICMR).

7. Central Government Health Schemes.
8. Implementation of national health programs.
9. Preparation of health education material for creating health awareness through Central Health Education Bureau.
10. Collection, compilation, analysis, evaluation and dissemination of information through the Central Bureau of Health Intelligence.
11. National Medical Library.

Central Council of Health

Functions

1. To consider and recommend broad outlines of policy regard to matters concerning health like environment, hygiene, nutrition and health education.
2. To make proposals for legislation relating to medical and public health matters.
3. To make recommendations to the Central Government regarding distribution of grants-in-aid.

AT THE STATE LEVEL

The health subjects are divided into three groups like federal, concurrent and state. The state list is the responsibility of the state, including provision of medical care, preventive health services and pilgrimage within the state.

State Health Administration

At present there are 28 states in India, each state having its own health administration.

- State Ministry of Health
- State Health Directorate

Four separate major departments, medical and public health are functioning in the state:

1. The Directorate of Health Services or the Director of Medical and Health Services.
2. The Directorate of Health and Family Welfare.
3. The Directorate of Medical Education for the management of medical colleges and hospitals.
4. The Directorate of Public Health Services.

AT THE DISTRICT LEVEL

There are 593 (year 2001) districts in India. Within each district, there are six types of administrative areas.

1. Subdivision
2. Tehsils (taluks)

3. Community Development Blocks
4. Municipalities and Corporations
5. Villages
6. Panchayats:
   a. Most district in India are divided into two or more subdivision, each in charge of an Assistant Collector or Sub-Collector.
   b. Each division is again divided into taluks, in charge of a Tahsildar. A taluk usually comprises between 200 and 600 villages.
   c. The community development block comprises approximately 100 villages and about 80,000 to 1,20,000 population, in charge of a Block Development Officer.
   d. Finally, there are the village panchayats, which are institutions of rural local self-government.
   e. The urban areas of the district are organized into:
      - Town Area Committees (in areas with population ranging between 5,000 and 10,000)
      - Municipal Boards (in areas with population ranging between 10,000 and 2,00,000)
      - Corporations (with population above 2,00,000)
      - The Town Area Committees are like panchayats. They provide sanitary services.
      - The Municipal Boards are headed by Chairmen/President, elected by members.

Functions of Municipal Board

1. Construction and maintenance of roads
2. Sanitation and drainage
3. Street lighting
4. Water supply
5. Maintenance of hospitals and dispensaries
6. Education
7. Registration of births and deaths, etc
8. The Corporations are headed by Mayors, elected by councilors, who are elected from different wards of the city. The executive agency includes the commissioner, the secretary, the engineer and the health officer.

The activities are similar to those of municipalities, on a much wider scale.

1. Panchayat Raj is a 3-tier structure of rural local self-government in India, linking the village to the district.
2. Panchayat (at the village level).
3. Panchayat Samiti (at the block level).
4. Zila Parishad (at the district level).

PANCHAYAT (AT THE VILLAGE LEVEL)

The Panchayat Raj at the village level consists of:

- The Gram Sabha
- The Gram Panchayat

The Gram Sabha considers proposals for taxation and elects members of Gram Panchayat, Panchayat Samiti and Zila Parishad.

Gram Panchayat

The Gram Panchayat covers the civic administration including sanitation and public health and work for the social and economic development of the village.

Panchayat Samiti (at the block level)

The Panchayat Samiti executes the community development program in the block. The Block Development Officer and staff give technical assistance and guidance in development work.

Zila Parishad (at the district level)

The Zila Parishad is the agency of rural local self government at the district level. Its functions and powers vary from state to state.

TYPES OF HEALTHCARE AGENCIES

Health care is provided in various settings.

OUTPATIENT SERVICES

Patients who do not require hospitalization can receive health care in a clinic. An outpatient setting is designed to be convenient and easily accessible to the patient. Hospital settings (to get the material) outpatient services are generally directed at primary and secondary health centers.

CLINICS

Clinics involve a department in a hospital where patients not requiring hospitalization receive medical care.

INSTITUTIONS

Hospital have been the major agency of health care system. Hospitals are classified as:

- Public
- Private
- Military

A public hospital are financed and operated by the government agency at the local, state or national level. Hospitals provide services at free of cost.

Private hospitals are owned and operated by churches, corporations, individuals and charitable organizations. Private hospitals are operated on a for-profit-basis.

Military hospitals provide medical care for the armed forces and their families.

HEALTHCARE SERVICE

1. Health promotion:
   a. Prenatal classes.
   b. Nutrition counseling.
   c. Family planning.
   d. Stress management.
2. Illness prevention:
   a. Screening programs (e.g. hypertension, breast cancer).
   b. Immunization.
   c. Occupational health and safety measures.
   d. Mental health counseling.
   e. AIDS control program.
3. Primary care:
   a. School health units.
   b. Routine physical examination.
   c. Follow-up for chronic illnesses (e.g. diabetes, epilepsy).
4. Diagnosis:
   a. Radiological procedure (e.g. CT scans, X-ray Studies).
   b. Physical examination.
   c. Laboratory investigations.
5. Treatments:
   a. Surgical intervention.
   b. Laser therapies.
   c. Pharmacological therapy.
6. Rehabilitation:
   a. Cardiovascular programs.
   b. Sports medicine.
   c. Mental illness program.

HEALTHCARE TEAM

Nursing is a healthcare profession focused on the care of individuals, families, and communities, so they may attain, maintain or recover optimal health.

PHYSICIAN

A person licensed to practice medicine; a medical doctor to diagnosis and treat the disease.

PHYSIOTHERAPIST

Physical therapists provide services to individuals and populations to develop maintain and restore maximum movements and functional ability throughout the life span. This includes providing services in circumstances where movement and function are threatened by aging, injury, disease or environmental factors. Functional movement is central to what it means to be healthy.

OCCUPATIONAL THERAPIST

An occupational therapist is trained in the practice of occupational therapy. The role of an occupational therapist is to work with a client to help them achieve a fulfilled and satisfied state in life through the use of purposeful activity or interventions designed to achieve functional outcomes which promote health, prevent injury or disability and which develop, improve, sustain or restore the highest possible level of independence.

PODIATRIC

The branch of medicine that deals with the diagnosis, treatment, and prevention of diseases of the human foot. Also called chiropody.

SOCIAL WORKER

Social workers assist people by helping them cope with and solve issues in their everyday lives, such as family and personal problems and dealing with relationships. Some social workers help clients who face a disability, life-threatening disease, social problem, such as inadequate housing, unemployment or substance abuse.

PHARMACISTS

Distribute prescription drugs to individuals. They also advise their patients, physicians and other health practitioners.

DIETICIANS

Dieticians apply the science of human nutrition to help people understand. Workers may be expected to prepare, understand and act on written materials.

DENTIST

Dentist is a part of stomatology (oral or mouth), is the branch of medicine that is involved in the evaluation, diagnosis, prevention and surgical or non-surgical procedures of the teeth.

PARAMEDICAL TECHNOLOGIST

Person helps to do diagnostic test for patient.

RESPIRATORY THERAPY

Respiratory therapy is an allied health field involved in the assessment and treatment of breathing disorders including chronic lung problems.

CONCLUSION

Health is very important for every individual on this earth. Illness is not described in the terms of disease condition, it is the deviation from the normal healthy state and it results in frustration, anxiety, denial, grief and uncertainty. In the illness, all the family members along with the ill person have to adopt towards the direct situation. For providing comprehensive nursing care to the ill person, nurse should have complete knowledge of all kinds of disease, their treatment and also the reaction of patient to illness. Today health and illness process is watched from different angle. The emphasis is now placed on important factors such as health promotion, prevention of illness and rehabilitation of the individuals affected by disturbances in health by various factors in the environment such as socio-cultural, economic and political situations etc. The nurse has to play very important and responsible role in health care team.

CHAPTER

11

Stress and Adaptation

INTRODUCTION

Stress is a universal phenomenon. All people experience it. Parents refer to the stress of missing children, working people talk of the stress of their jobs and students at all levels talk of the stress of school. The concept of stress is important because it provides a way of understanding the person as a unified being, who responds in totality (mind, body and spirit) to a variety of changes that takes place in daily life.

CONCEPTS OF STRESS

Stress can have physical, emotional, intellectual, social and spiritual consequences. Usually, the effects are mixed, because stress affects the whole person. Physically, stress can threaten a person's physiologic homeostasis. Emotionally, stress can produce negative or non-constructive feelings about self. Intellectually, stress can influence a person's perceptual and problem-solving abilities. Socially, stress can alter a person's relationships with others. Spiritually, stress can challenge one's beliefs and values. Many illness have been linked to stress.

Stress is defined in a number of ways:

1. As a stimulus.
2. As a response.
3. As a transaction.

STRESS AS A STIMULUS

Stress may be defined as a stimulus, a life event (sometimes called 'life change') or a set of circumstances causing a disrupted response that increases the individual's vulnerability to illness.

Both positive and negative events are considered stressful. Research has shown that people who have a high level of stress are often more prone to illness and have lowered ability to cope with illness and subsequent stress.

STRESS AS A RESPONSE

Hans Selye defined stress as 'the non-specific response of the body to any kind of demand made upon it'. To differentiate the cause of stress from the response of stress, Selye created the term stressor to denote any factor that produces stress and disturbs the body's equilibrium. Because stress alters the body it can be observed only by the changes it produces in the body. This response of the body, the stress syndrome or the general adaptation syndrome (GAS) occurs with the release of certain adaptive hormones and subsequent changes in the structure and chemical composition of the body.

In addition to adapting globally, the body can also react locally; that is, one organ or a part of the body reacts alone. This is referred to as the local adaptation syndrome (LAS). One example of the LAS is inflammation.

Selye proposed that both the GAS and the LAS had three stages:

1. Alarm reaction.
2. Resistance.
3. Exhaustion.

Alarm Reaction

The initial reaction of the body is the alarm reaction (AR), which alerts the body's defenses against the stressor. Selye divided this stage into two parts:

1. The shock phase
2. The counter shock phase.

During the shock phase, the autonomic nervous system reacts. The person is then ready for fight or flight. The second part of the alarm reaction is called the counter shock phase. During this time, the body changes produced during the shock phase are reversed.

Stage of Resistance

During the second stage in the GAS and the LAS syndrome that the stage of resistance (SR), the body's adaptation takes place. In other words, the body attempts to cope with the stressor and to limit the stressor to the smallest area of the body that can deal with it.

Stage of Exhaustion

During the third stage, the stage of exhaustion (SE), the adaptation that the body made during the second stage cannot be maintained; this means that the ways used to cope with the stressor has been exhausted.

STRESS AS A TRANSACTION

The third stress theory focuses on person- environment-transactions and is referred to as the "transaction or interaction" theory. In this, stress is defined as "transaction". In the transactive model, there is an exchange or transaction between the persons and the environment, which provides feedback to the person-environment- relationship. The proponent of this theory is Richard Lazarus, who emphasized the role of cognitive appraisal in assessing stressful situations and selecting coping options. Lazarus and Folkman (1984) defined psychological stress as a particular relationship between the person and the environment that is appraised by the person as taxing his or her resources and endangering his or her well-being. Lazarus theory focuses on the person- environment transactions and cognitive appraisal of demands and coping options. Appraisal is a judgment process that includes recognizing the degree of demands or stressors, placed on the individual. The appraisal process also involves the recognition of available resources or options that help when dealing with potential or actual demands.

MANIFESTATIONS OF STRESS

Manifestations of the stress experience both physiological and psychological, may be considered coping or mechanisms. Coping is "the cognitive and behavioral effort to manage specific external and/or internal demands that are appraised as taxing or exceeding the resources of the person". Coping can be adaptive or maladaptive. Adaptive coping helps the person to deal effectively with stressful events and minimizes stress. Ineffective coping results in maladaptation.

PHYSIOLOGIC MANIFESTATIONS

Physiologic manifestation may or may not occur in clients experiencing stress, depending on the way the client perceives the stressful event and on the effectiveness of the client's coping strategies. Specific physiologic manifestations are presented below:

1. Pupils dilate to increase visual perception.
2. Sweat production (diaphoresis).
3. The heartbeat increases, which leads to an increased pulse rate to transport of nutrients.
4. Skin is pallid because of peripheral blood vessel constriction, and effect of norepinephrine.
5. Blood pressure increases because of vessel constriction in blood reservoirs.
6. The rate and depth of respirations increase because of dilation of the bronchioles, promoting hyperventilation.
7. Urinary output decreases.
8. The mouth may be dry.

9. Peristalsis of the intestines decreases, resulting in possible constipation and flatus.
10. Muscle tension increase to prepare for rapid motor activity or defense.
11. Blood sugar increases because of gluocorticoids release and gluconeogenesis.
12. Lethargy, mental lassitude and inactivity.
13. There may be decreased physiologic functioning and loss of skeletal muscle tone (parasympathetic dominance).

PSYCHOLOGIC MANIFESTATIONS

Psychologic manifestations of stress include anxiety, fear, anger, depression, cognitive behaviors, verbal and motor responses and unconscious ego defense mechanisms.

COGNITIVE MANIFESTATIONS

Cognitive manifestations of stress are thinking responses that include problem solving, structuring, self-control or self-discipline, suppression, fantasy and prayer. The person assesses the situation or problem, analyzes or defines it, chooses alternatives, carries out the selected alternative and evaluates whether the solution was successful.

VERBAL AND MOTOR MANIFESTATIONS

Verbal or motor manifestations of stress may be the first responses evident. Among these reposes are crying, verbal abuse, laughing, screaming, hitting and kicking, and holding and touching.

NURSING PROCESS FOR STRESS

ASSESSMENT

Determine

1. How would the client rate the stress he/she is experiencing in the following areas?
   - Home
   - Work or school
   - Finance
   - Recent illness or loss of loved one
   - Health
   - Family responsibilities
   - Ethnic or cultural group
   - Religion
   - Relationships with friends
   - Relationships with parents or children

- Relationships with partner
- Recent hospitalization
- Others (specify).

2. How long has the client been dealing with the above stressor(s)?
3. How does the client usually handle stressful situations?
   - Cry
   - Get angry
   - Become verbally abusive
   - Talk to someone (who)?
   - Withdraw from the situation?
   - Structure and control others or situation
   - Go for a walk or physical exercise
   - Try to arrive at a solution
   - Pray for wisdom and courage
   - Meditate or use some other relaxation techniques such as yoga, guided imagery, etc.
   - Others (specify).
4. How does the client's usual coping strategy work? Assess clinical manifestations indication of stress.
   a. Physiologic manifestations:
      - Restlessness
      - Pacing
      - Tremors
      - Muscle tension
      - Rigid posture
      - Purposeless activity
      - Rapid pulse
      - Increased respiratory rate
      - Hyperventilation
      - Heart palpitations
      - Diaphoresis
      - Pallor
      - Clammy hands
      - Dry mouth.

   b. Perceptual changes:
      - Increased awareness and attended or narrowed focus of attention.
      - Inability to focus on what is really happening

   c. Verbalization changes:
      - Increased questioning or information seeking:
      - Seeking help
      - Expressions of concern
      - Feelings of tension

- Apprehension
- Nervousness
- Voice tremors and pitch changes
- Anger.

NURSING DIAGNOSIS

The nursing diagnoses identified by North American Nursing Diagnosis Association (NANDA) (1992), relating specifically to clients experiencing stress include the following:

1. Anxiety related to perceived threat to self-concept, health status and socioeconomic status.
2. Ineffective individual coping related to situational crises, such as natural disasters or loss of loved ones through separation.
3. Fear related to anticipated treatment (e.g. surgery, chemotherapy) or language barrier.
4. Defensive coping.
5. Ineffective family coping, e.g. disabling.
6. Decisional conflict related to conflict with personal values/beliefs or an ethical dilemma.

PLANNING

The nurse develops plans in collaboration with the client and significant support persons when possible, according to the client's state of health. The nurse and client set goals to change the existing client responses to the stressor.

The overall client goals for persons experiencing stress-related responses are to:

1. Decrease anxiety and fear.
2. Increase the ability to manage or cope with stressful events or circumstances.

Suggested outcome criteria are: The client

- Verbalizes a reduced level of anxiety
- Develops realistic goals
- Expresses feelings in a positive way
- Verbalizes feelings to another
- Develops effective coping mechanisms in managing stress.

IMPLEMENTATION

Although stress accompanies every disease and illness, it is also highly individualized; a situation that to one person is a major stressor may not affect another. Some methods help to reduce stress will be effective for one person; other methods will be appropriate for a different person. A nurse who is sensitive to client's needs and reactions can choose methods on intervention that will be most effective for each individual.

MINIMIZING ANXIETY

After clients realize that they are anxious, it is important to discuss all the possible reasons for their anxiety.

When clients can identify the cause of their anxiety, they may find it helpful to explore the cause with the objective of learning better coping strategies.

General Guidelines to Minimize the Client's Anxiety and Stress

1. Support the client and family at the time of illness: By conveying caring and understanding, the nurse can help clients reduce their stress. Feeling that someone else cares is a source of support to stressed people.
2. Orient the client to the hospital or agency: The nurse helps the client adjust to the change from independent wage earner to relatively dependent client. The nurse can help family members by giving information, for instance, about visiting hours and specific unit policies.
3. Give the client in a hospital, some way of maintaining identity: Nurses can help clients to maintain identify by addressing them by the name they prefer and by assisting them to wear their own clothes in a hospital setting, when this is possible.
4. Provide information when the client has insufficient information: Fear of the unknown and incorrect information can frequently cause stress. Additional information or clarification can ally stress.
5. Repeat information when the client has difficulty in remembering: Nurses can assist clients by repeating information when it is requested/required.
6. Encourage the client to participate in the plan of care: Loss of the right to determine their own destiny can be very stressful to some people.
7. Give the client the time to express feelings and thoughts. Allow time for clients to describe their feelings and worries if they wish.
8. Ensure that expectations are within the client's capabilities. Whatever the activity whether an exercise or recreation, the nurse should make sure that it is possible for the client to accomplish it.
9. Be sensitive to specific situations and experiences that increase anxiety and stress for the clients.
10. Assist a client to make a correct appraisal of a situation. Sometimes, through a lack of knowledge people draw incorrect conclusions. Having valid information might relieve the client's stress.

11. Provide an environment in which a person can function independently to some degree without assistance, by adapting eating utensils so that the clients can feed themselves, thereby nurses can lower client's stress levels.
12. Reinforce positive environmental factors and recognize negative ones to help reduce stress.
13. Arrange for other clients with similar experiences to visit the clients, e.g. colostomies or similar conditions.
14. Bring the clients and their support persons into contact with people in community agencies who can help them make valid plans.
15. Communicate with competence, understanding and empathy rather than stress and anxiety.

STRESS MANAGEMENT

Management of stress involves two major changes:
- Change in thinking
- Change in behavior and lifestyle.

COGNITIVE APPROACH

1. Accept death as basic existential condition.
2. Carve out a meaning of life.
3. Realize that stress is inbuilt in life. We are neither the controller of the best nor the future. Present moment is the only reality.
4. Stress inoculation is a psychological and behavioral analogue to immunization on biological level.
5. Cognitive restructuring: Modify negative self-talk to positive self-talk, create willingness to observe own.
6. Dispute irrational beliefs.
7. Positive imagery: Self-visualization.
8. Do not ignore feelings and needs. Suppressing feelings causes' frustration, irritability and stress try to gratify feelings.
9. Accept responsibility because responsibility includes the nation of authorship. Assuming the responsibility is the basic condition for change.
10. Realize we do not control world or events. Attempts to change people and events are self-defecting change attitude from other directness to self-directness.
11. Stop perfectionist attitude and set limit to ambitions and material desires.
12. Do not accept mediocrity in performance but do not entangle in the knots of unrealistic ambitions and overachievement drives. Do not be obsessed with perfection and overambitious ventures.

BEHAVIORAL APPROACH

1. Planning/organizing life, set goals/objectives. Planned and organized life leads to success, goals act as a achievements.

2. Management of habits: Change habits but do not change by sheer will power. It demands change in beliefs and attitudes. It requires process, practice and skill management of time because time is very precious. It is not possible to save time or borrow it. It is possible to make the best and maximum out of it.
3. Time management generates inbuilt discipline in life leading to success and happiness.
4. Do not runaway problems. Avoidance behavior multiplies problems.
5. Avoidance and procrastination leads to more stress. Take every crisis/situation or challenges as an opportunity for growth.
6. Be assertive: Assertion is a form of appropriate behavior in which develops skills of assertiveness.
7. Music can act like a medicine in stress and stress-related disorders. Music can play an effective role in helping and live better.
8. Laughter therapy creates relaxation and reduces stress. Laughter works as an effective muscle exercise.
9. Interpersonal skills enhance self-esteem. These skills make a good communicator. These lead to a better image.
10. Physical appearance reinforces confidence. It strengthens interpersonal skills. Avoid obscene dresses.
11. Engage regularly in leisure/physical exercises. Sublimate energies. Develop and groom hobbies and interests.
12. Develop proper food and sleep habits. Take adequate sleep. Choose and take food thoughtfully.
13. Utilize support system: Supportive relationships are those marked by warmth, empathy and care. Support system helps us to manage stress at least in distinct ways. It gives emotional support.
14. Build on spiritual strength: Spirituality is an essential part of healing process in life. Thinking ourselves as an expression of higher reality. Spiritual intelligence enhance creativity, subsequently helping in setting rules amending the situations.

NURSING INTERVENTION IN STRESS REDUCTION

The first step in managing stress is to become aware of its presence. This includes identifying and expressing stressful feelings (as stated above). The role of the nurse is to facilitate and enhance the coping and adaptation. Nursing interventions depend on the severity of the stress experience and demand. The nurse's efforts are directed to life-supporting interventions and to the inclusion of approaches aimed at the reduction of additional stressors to the client. The importance of cognitive appraisal in the stress experience should prompt the nurse to assess if changes in the way the client perceives and label particular events or situations (cognitive reappraisal) are possible. So, the nurse should also consider the positive effects that result from successfully meeting to stressful demands. Greater emphasis should also be placed on the part of cultural values and beliefs enhancing or constraining various coping options.

An individual personal resource that aids in coping includes health and energy. A health-promoting lifestyle provides these resources and buffers or cushions the impact of stressors. Lifestyle or habits that contributed to the risk of developing illness can be reduced or eliminated. Health risk appraisal is an assessment method designed to promote health by examining the individual personal habits and recommending change where health risk is identified. For example, smoking causes lung cancer and can be prevented by reducing or leaving the habit of smoking.

COPING ENHANCEMENT

Coping enhancement is a nursing intervention and defined as "assisting a patient to adapt, to perceived stressors, changes, or threats which interfere with meeting life demands and roles" (McCloskey, Bulechek 1992). After completing a health risk approach, the nurse could use "coping enhancement to assist the patient in an analysis of the appraisal and to explore methods to improve the person's coping abilities including appraisal of own personal resources.

The activities of coping enhancement are as follows:

1. Appraise the patient's adjustment to change in body image as indicated.
2. Appraise the impact of the patient's life situations on roles and relationships.
3. Encourage the patient to identify a realistic description of change in role.
4. Approve the patient's understanding of the disease process.
5. Approve and discuss alternative responses to situation.
6. Use a calm reassuring approach.
7. Provide an atmosphere of acceptance.
8. Assist patient in developing an objective appraisal of an event.
9. Help the client to identify the information he/ she made interested in obtaining.
10. Provide factual information concerning diagnosis, treatment and prognosis.
11. Provide the patient with realistic choices about certain aspects of care.
12. Encourage an attitude to realistic hope as a way of dealings with feelings of helplessness.
13. Evaluate patient's decision-making ability.
14. Seek to understand the patient's perspective of a stressful situation.
15. Discourage decision-making when patient is under severe stress.
16. Encourage gradual mastery of the situation.
17. Encourage patience in developing relationships.

18. Encourage relationships with persons who have common interests and goals.
19. Encourage social and community activities.
20. Encourage the acceptance of limitation of others.
21. Acknowledge the patient's spiritual/cultural background.
22. Encourage the use of spiritual resources if desired.
23. Explore the patient's previous achievement of success.
24. Explore patient's reason for self-criticism.
25. Confront patient's ambivalent (anger or depression) feelings.
26. Foster constructive outlets of anger and hostility.
27. Arrange situations that encourage patient's autonomy.
28. Assist patient in identifying positive responses from others.
29. Encourage the identification of specific life values.
30. Explore with the patient previous methods of dealing with life problems.
31. Introduce the patient to persons (or group) who have successfully undergone the same experience.
32. Support the use of appropriate defense mechanisms.
33. Encourage verbalization of feelings, perceptions and fears.
34. Discuss consequences not dealing with guilt and shame.
35. Encourage the patient to identify own strength and abilities.
36. Assist patient in identifying appropriate short- and long-term goals.
37. Assist the patient in breaking down complex goals into manageable steps.
38. Assist the patient in examining available resources to meet the goal.
39. Reduce stimuli in the environment that could be misinterpreted as threatening.
40. Appraise patient's needs/desires for social support.
41. Assist the patient to identify available support systems.
42. Determine the risk of the patient's inflicting self-harm.
43. Encourage family involvement as appropriate as possible.
44. Encourage the family verbalize feelings about ill family member.
45. Provide appropriate social skills training.
46. Assist the patient to solve problem in a constructive manner.
47. Instruct the patient about the use of relaxation techniques as needed
48. Assist the patient to grieve, and work through the losses of chronic illness and/or disability if appropriate.
49. Assist the patient to clarify misconceptions. Encourage the patient to evaluate own behavior.

RELAXATION TECHNIQUES

Snyder (1993) and Egan (1993) identified relaxation technique as the major method used to relieve stress, included in nursing interventions. Commonly used techniques cited were progressive muscle relaxation, relaxation with guided imagery and Benson's relaxation response. The goal of relaxation training is to produce response that counter the stress response.

PROGRESSIVE MUSCLE RELAXATION

Progressive muscle relaxation involves tensing and releasing the muscles of the body in sequence and sensing the difference in feeling. It is best if the person lies on a soft cushion on the floor, in a quiet room, breathing easily. Self-taught or instructor-directed exercise that can involve learning to contract and relax muscles in a systematic way beginning with face and ending with feet. This exercise may be combined with breathing exercises that focus on inner self.

RELAXATION WITH GUIDED IMAGERY

Relaxation with guided imagery is the purposeful use of imagination to achieve relaxation and/or direct attention away from undesirable sensations. The nurse helps the person to select a pleasant scene or experience from the past. This image serves as the mental device in this technique. As the person sits comfortably and quietly, the nurse guides to review the scene; trying to feel and relieve the imagery with all of the senses. A tape recording can be made for description of science of experience for the pleasant one.

BENSON'S RELAXATION RESPONSE

Benson and Proctor (1984) describe the following steps for this response which include:

- Step 1: Pick a brief phrase or word that reflects the basic belief systems.
- Step 2: Choose a comfortable position
- Step 3: Close the eyes
- Step 4: Relax the muscle
- Step 5: Become aware of the breathing and start using selected focus word
- Step 6: Maintain a passive attitude
- Step 7: Continue for a set period of time
- Step 8: Practice the technique twice a day.

The response combines meditation with relaxation. The other techniques of stress management will also include the following:

STOPPING THOUGHT

It is a self-directed behavioral approach used to gain control of self-defeating thoughts. When these thoughts occur, the individual stops the thought process and focuses on conscious relaxation.

EXERCISE

Regular exercise, especially, aerobics movement, results in improved circulation, increased release of endorphins on an enhanced sense of well-being.

HUMOR

In the forms of laughter, cartoons, funny movies, riddles, audiocassettes, comic books and joke books, humor can be used for both the nurse and patient.

ASSERTIVE BEHAVIOR

Open, honest, sharing feelings, desires and opinions in a controlled way. The individual who has control over one's own life is less subject to stress.

SOCIAL SUPPORT

Social support may take the form of organized support and self-help groups, relationships with family and friends and professional help.

In addition, meditation, breathing techniques, therapeutic touch, music therapy, and biofeedback can be used as stress management technique.

CONCLUSION

Stress is a state produced by a change in the environment that is perceived as challenging, threatening or damaging to the persons dynamic balance or equilibrium. There is a actual or perceived imbalance in the person's ability to meet the demands of the new situation. The change or stimulus that evokes this state is the stressor. The nature of the stressor is variable, i.e. an event or change that will produce stress in one person will be neutral for another; and even that may produce at one time and place for one person may not do so far the same person at another time and place. A person appraises and copes with changing situations. The desired goal is adaptation or adjustment to the energy and ability to meet new demands. This is stress-coping process, a compensatory process with physiological and psychological components.

CHAPTER

12

Health Care and Nursing Care

INTRODUCTION

Health and health care need to be distinguished from each other for no better reason than that the former is often incorrectly seen as a direct function of the latter. Heath is clearly not the mere absence of disease. Good health confers on a person or group's freedom from illness and the ability to realize one's potential. Health is therefore best understood as the indispensable basis for defining a person's sense of well-being. The health of populations is a distinct key issue in public policy discourse in every mature society often determining the deployment of huge society. They include its cultural understanding of ill health and well-being, extent of socioeconomic disparities, reach of health services, quality and costs of care and current biomedical understanding about health and illness.

IMPORTANCE OF HEALTH CARE

Health care covers not merely medical care but also all aspects of preventive care too. Nor can it be limited to care rendered by or financed out of public expenditure within the government sector alone but must include incentives and disincentives for self-care and care paid for by private citizens to get over ill health. Whereas in India, private out-of-pocket expenditure dominates the cost financing health care, the effects are bound to be regressive. Heath care at its essential core is widely recognized to be a public good. Its demand and supply cannot therefore, be left to be regulated solely by the invisible had of the market. Nor can it be established on considerations of utility maximizing conduct alone.

ORGANIZATION STRUCTURE

1. ***National level***: The organization at the national level consists of the Union Ministry of Health and Family Welfare.

2. ***State level***: The organization at state level is under the State Department of Health and Family Welfare in each state headed by Minister and with a Secretariat under the charge of Secretary/Commissioner (Health and Family Welfare) belonging to the cadre of Indian Administrative Service (IAS).
3. ***Regional level***: Each regional/zonal setup covers three to five districts and acts under authority delegated by the State Directorate of Health Services.
4. ***District level***: This structure of health services is a middle level management organization and it is a link between the state as well as regional structure on one side and the peripheral level structures such as primary health center (PHC) as well as subcenter on the other side.
5. ***Subdivisional/Taluk level***: At the Taluk level, healthcare services are rendered through the office of Assistant District Health and Family Welfare Officer (ADHO).
6. ***Community level***: One Community Health Center (CHC) has been established for every 80,000 to 1,20,000 population, and this center provides the basic specialty services in general medicine, pediatrics, surgery, obstetrics and gynecology.

PRIMARY, SPECIALTY AND HOSPITAL CARE

1. ***Primary***: At present there is one Primary Health Center covering about 30,000 (20,000 in hilly, desert and difficult terrains) or more population. Many rural dispensaries have been upgraded to create these PHCs. Each PHC has one medical officer, two health assistants—one male and one female, health workers and supporting staff.
2. ***Specialty***: This care is available at taluk headquarters hospitals.
3. ***Hospital care***: Varies from secondary care available at taluk district headquarters and tertiary/corporate care at cities.

ROLE OF PRIVATE SECTOR

The Indian Policy welcomes the participation of the private sector in all areas of health activities—primary, secondary or tertiary. However, looking to past experience of the private sector, it can reasonably be expected that its contribution would be substantial in urban primary sector, tertiary sector and moderate in the secondary sector.

The policy also encourages the setting up of private insurance instruments for increasing the scope of the coverage of the secondary and tertiary sector under private health insurance packages.

In the context of the very large number of poor in the country, it would be difficult to conceive of an exclusive government mechanism to provide health services to this category. It has sometimes been felt that a social health insurance scheme, funded by the government, and with service delivery through the private sector, would be the appropriate solution. The administrative and financial implications of such an initiative are still unknown.

It envisages the co-option of the non-governmental practitioners in the national disease control programs so as to ensure that standard treatment protocols are followed in their day-to-day practice.

This policy recognizes the immense potential of information technology applications in the area of telemedicine in the tertiary healthcare sector. The use of this technical aid will greatly enhance the capacity for the professionals to pool their clinical experience.

FOUR BASIC CONCEPTS OF NURSING

The nursing profession is built upon four key concepts such as person, environment, health and nursing. These four concepts encompass the key tenets of nursing philosophy and practice, and define the means by which individuals should be viewed and treated within the nursing profession. The four concepts are interrelated and each is built upon the foundation of the concept that precedes it.

PERSON

In nursing theory, human beings are considered in terms of their physiological, psychological, social, spiritual and cultural selves. People are evaluated in terms of their individual place in society as well as their relationships to their family, community and society as a whole. Additionally, human beings are viewed in terms of their individual needs and how nursing practice is applied to meet these needs. The purpose of nursing and nursing theory is to identify how a particular individual's needs are either met or not met, to predict future needs and to prioritize those needs in order of importance.

ENVIRONMENT

The environment concept of nursing comprises all the internal and external factors that act on human beings and affect their behavior and development. This includes psychological, spiritual, social, physical and cultural forces as well as the environment in which nursing care is provided. The idea behind this concept is that the environment influences individual and collective health and that individuals, who experience a positive, comfortable nursing environment are more likely to demonstrate good health versus those who receive a level of care that is lacking.

HEALTH

The concept of health refers to an individual's physical, mental and social well-being and at what point they are on the health spectrum, which ranges from good health to poor health or death. Health is considered to be affected by genetic factors, environmental factors, lifestyle factors and external mechanisms, such as bacteria. A person's place on the health spectrum is constantly changing and in a nursing context, it's the responsibility of nursing professionals to identify the patient's place on the spectrum and to take steps to help that person's health improvement.

NURSING

Nursing refers to the process of caring for the health of human beings and assisting individuals in meeting their needs while also teaching them the basics of caring for themselves. The responsibilities of the nursing profession are to promote good health, to prevent disease when possible, to promote healing in those who are ill and to ease the suffering of dying patients. The concept of nursing extends beyond the health care facility to the community and society as a whole, and views individual health and the environment as closely related. Nursing is defined as care that is tailored to the needs of individuals and that is provided in an efficient and effective manner.

PATIENT CARE DELIVERY SYSTEM

One important function of the professional nurse at the first-line management position of nursing service department is organizing the activities of the staff into a workable pattern to meet patient needs. She/he should establish effective relationships between the activities to be performed, the workers to perform them.

DEFINITION OF ASSIGNMENT

Assignment refers to 'a written delegation of duties to care for a group of patients by trained personnel assigned to the unit.'

PURPOSES OF ASSIGNMENT

1. To delegate the work to be done to the nursing personnel.
2. To gain the cooperation of the nursing personnel by knowing and accepting the acceptance of the work to be done.

PRINCIPLES OF PERSONNEL ASSIGNMENT

1. Made by the head nurse or nurse in charge for each individual nurse.
2. Based on:
   a. Nursing needs of each patient and approximate time required to care for him/her.
   b. The capabilities, skill level, previous experience and the interest of the staff members.
   c. Job description.

3. Planned weekly and revised daily if necessary to assure continuity of care.
4. Take into account all the direct, indirect and unit activities.
5. Consider the geographical location of the unit and the assigned duties to save nurse's time and effort.
6. Must be balanced among nursing staff.
7. Never to assign the same task to more than one nurse.

PROCESS OF ORGANIZING PATIENT CARE

The head nurse or the nurse in charge should carry out their duties and responsibilities through applying the following steps:

1. **Planning:** Is a process of developing a course of action for meeting the needs of patient. In planning, the head nurse decides what should be done, when, how, where, by whom and to whom.
2. **Assigning:** Assignment of patient and nursing activities are written in the assignment sheet by the head nurse/nurse in charge, based on the principles of assignment.
3. **Leading:** Includes issuing instructions, motivation and coordination of activities, by making rounds, checking performance and conducting conferences.
4. **Evaluating:** By reviewing nursing performance and patient progress to be compared by the assignment and nursing care plan.
5. **Reporting:** The head nurse prepares a nursing unit report, e.g. shift report, which includes patient's needs, special observations, census, bed number, all critically ill and postoperative patients, patients needs special preparation on preoperative stage.

METHODS OF PATIENT CARE DELIVERY (METHODS OF ASSIGNMENT)

1. **Traditional methods**
   - Case method
   - Functional method
   - Team method
   - Modular nursing
   - Primary nursing method.
2. **Advanced method**
   - Case management.

Case Method

Case method is the oldest patient care delivery method. In this method one professional nurse assumes total responsibility of providing complete care for one or more patients (1–6) while he/she is on duty. This method is used frequently in intensive care units and in teaching nursing students.

Advantages

1. High degree of autonomy.
2. Lines of responsibility and accountability are clear.
3. Patient receives holistic, unfragmented care.

Disadvantages

1. Each RN may have a different approach to care.
2. Not cost-effective.
3. Lack of RN availability.

Functional Method

Emerged during 1950s, due to shortage of nurses. This method focuses on getting the greatest amount of tasks in the least time. In this method, the nursing care is divided into tasks and each staff member is assigning to perform one or two tasks for all patients in the unit according to the level of skill required for performance as follows:

Registered professional nurses

Responsible for administering medication to all unit patients, another for changing dressings and administering ordered treatments (such as postural drainage or warm compresses) for all patients.

Technical nurses

Responsible for taking vital signs and recording intake and output for all patients in the unit, while another might be giving baths to all bedridden patients.

Nurse aides

Responsible for making beds for all ambulatory patients and assisting mobility-impaired patients to move in bed or walk in the hall.

Unit clerk

Responsible for answering telephone, delivering messages, recording admissions and discharges, etc.

Advantages

1. Care is provided economically and efficiently.
2. Minimum number of RNs required, so it is efficient when there is a shortage in the staff or there is limited number of professional nurses.
3. Tasks are completed quickly.
4. Useful in emergency situations.

Disadvantages

1. Care may be fragmented.
2. Patient may be confused with many care providers.

3. Caregivers feel unchallenged.
4. Lack of communication among the different persons who care for the patient.
5. Neglecting the humanity of the patient and the individual needs of the patient will be lost in an effort to get the work done.

Team Nursing

Team nursing was developed because of social and technological changes in World War II which drew many nurses away from hospitals, learning aids, services and procedure. Equipment became more expensive and complicated, requiring specialization at every turn. It is an attempt to meet increased demands of nursing services and better use of knowledge and skills of professional nurses.

Definitions

1. Team nursing is based on philosophy in which groups of professional and non-professional personnel work together to identify, plan, implement and evaluate comprehensive client-centered care. The key concept is a group that works together toward a common goal, providing qualitative comprehensive nursing care (Kron, 1978).
2. Team nursing was designed to accommodate several categories of personnel in meeting the comprehensive nursing needs of a group of clients (Donovan, 1975).

Concept of Team Nursing

The concept of team nursing was introduced in the early 1950s. It is a method of nursing assignment that binds professional, technical and nurse aides into small teams. This method allows for efficient utilization of technical and/or nurse aide through the direct supervision, guidance and teaching of professional nurses.

Objectives

The objective of team nursing is to give the best possible quality of patient care by utilizing the abilities of every member of the staff to the fullest extent and by providing close supervision both of patient care and of the individual who give it.

Process of implementing the team method: One registered nurse in the team is appointed by the head nurse to serve as a team leader. The team members commonly consist of at least one professional nurse, one technical nurse, nursing students and nursing aides. All team members may receive reports about their patients' care needs from the team leader or team member on previous shift.

The team leader usually assigns: Professional nurse to care for the most seriously ill patients, to ensure informed observation and skilled interventions.

Often, the team leader assigns the **technical nurse** to bath, feed, move and change dressings for patients.

Aides are assigned to make beds, assist ambulatory patients with bathing and grooming, testing urine and performing simple nursing care procedures.

Team leader usually administers medications and monitors parenteral fluid therapy for all patients assigned to the team. Without team planning and communication through the team conferences, team nursing may become in reality just a variation of the functional method.

Functions of Team Nursing

The two important points of functioning are:

1. The head nurse must know at all times the condition of the patients and the plan for their care and must be assured that assignments and workmanship contribute to quality nursing.
2. The team leader must have freedom to use their initiative and the opportunity to nurse, supervise, and teach unencumbered by the responsibility for administrative detail.

Functions of Registered Nurse

1. In the team nursing RN functions as a team leader and coordinates the small group (not more than four or five) of ancillary personnel to provide care to a small group of patients.
2. As coordinator of the team, the RN must know the condition and needs of all patients assigned to the team and plan for the individualized care for each patient. (Marquis and Huston, 2003).
3. The team leader is also responsible for encouraging a cooperative environment and maintaining clear communication among all team members.
4. The team leader's duties include planning care, assigning duties, directing and assisting team members, giving direct patient care, teaching and coordinating patient activities.
5. The team leader assigns each member specific responsibilities dependent on the role.
6. The members of the team report directly to the team leader, who then reports to the charge nurse or unit manager.
7. Communication is enhanced through the use of written patient assignments, the development of nursing care plans, and the use of regularly scheduled team conferences to discuss the patient status and formulate revisions to the plan of care.
8. However, for team nursing to succeed, the team leader must have strong clinical skills, good communication skills, delegation ability, decision-making ability and the ability to create a cooperative working environment.

Advantages

1. High-quality, comprehensive care with a high proportion of ancillary staff.
2. Team members participate in decision making and contribute their own expertise.

Disadvantages

1. Continuity suffers if daily team assignments vary.
2. Team leader must have good leadership skills.
3. Insufficient time for planning and communication.

Modular Nursing

Modular nursing assignment is used when the nursing staff includes technical and nurse aides, as well as professional nurses. Although two or three persons are assigned to each module, the greatest responsibility for the care of assigned patients falls on the professional nurse. The professional nurse is also responsible for guiding and teaching non-professional nurse.

Definition

Modular nursing is a modification of team nursing and focuses on the patient's geographic location for staff assignments (Magargal 1980).

1. The patient unit is divided into modules or districts, and the same team of caregivers is assigned consistently to the same geographic location.
2. Each location or module, has an RN assigned as the team leader, and the other team members may include licensed practical nurse (LPN)/ licensed vocational nurse (LVN) or unlicensed assistive personnel (UAP). (Yoder-Wise, 2003).
3. Just as in the team nursing, the team leader in the modular nursing is accountable for all patient care and is responsible for providing leadership for team members and creating a cooperative work environment.
4. The concept of modular nursing calls for a smaller group of staff providing care for a smaller group of patients.
5. The goal is to increase the involvement of the RN in planning and coordinating care.
6. Communication is more efficient among a smaller group of team members. (Marquis and Huston, 2003).
7. The success of the modular nursing depends greatly on the leadership abilities of the team leader.

Advantages (Yoder-Wise, 2003)

1. Continuity of care is improved when staff members are consistently assigned to the same module.
2. The RN as team leader is able to be more involved in planning and coordinating care.
3. Geographic closeness and more efficient communication save staff time.

Disadvantages (Yoder-Wise, 2003)

1. Costs may be increased to stock each module with the necessary patient care supplies (medication cart, linens and dressings).
2. Long corridors common in many hospitals, are not conducive to modular nursing.

Note:

1. Modular nursing is similar to team nursing because professional and non-professional employees cooperate in caring for patients under the leadership of a professional nurse.
2. Module nursing is similar to primary nursing because each pair or trio of nursing personnel are responsible for the care of the patients in their caseload from admission to discharge, following discharge and during subsequent admissions to the agency.
3. As with primary nursing, the worker pair or trio arrange or another pair or trio to care for their assigned patients on alternate shifts and days off.

Primary Nursing Method

Primary nursing method is the best in an agency with an all-professional nurse staff. It is a comprehensive, continuous and coordinated nursing process for meeting the total needs of each patient.

Basic concepts in primary nursing

1. **Patient assessment** by a primary nurse, who plans the care to be given by secondary or associate nurse when the primary nurse is off duty. The 24 hours responsibility for care is put into practice through the primary nurse's written directive on a preplanned communication assignment.
2. **Complete communication** of care given in the nursing staff daily reporting method.
3. **Discharge planning** including teaching, family involvement and appropriate references.

Process for Implementing Primary Nursing Method

Head nurse

1. Assigns primary nurse to patients by matching the skills of the nurse to the needs of the patients.
2. Ensures proper scheduling for all shifts, so that if primary nurse is absent in the unit an associate nurse is available for care.
3. Guides, counsels and evaluates care given.
4. May also assign to patients either as a primary nurse or associate nurse.

Professional staff nurse

Primary nurse: Functions of primary nurse include performing the following:

1. Conducting an admission (initial) assessment.
2. Developing, planning, implementing and revising the nursing care plan.

3. Directing care in his/her absence.
4. Collaborating with physicians and families.
5. Making referrals.
6. Teaching health concepts.
7. Making discharge plans.

Associate nurse: May be professional or technical nurse, carries out the nursing care planned by the primary nurse when he/she is not on duty.

Technical nurse: Carry out the nursing tasks assigned by the primary or associate nurses in giving the care.

Nurse aides: Their activities are focusing away from direct contact with the patient and can be utilized as messengers and transporters.

Ward clerk: Responsible for the non-nursing functions of administrative duties.

Advantages

1. High quality, holistic patient care
2. Establish rapport with patient
3. Registered nurse (RN) feels challenged and rewarded.

Disadvantages

1. Primary nurse must be able to practice with a high degree of responsibility and autonomy.
2. Registered nurse must accept 24-hour responsibility.
3. More RNs needed; not cost-effective.

Case Management

Case management is a process of monitoring an individual patient's health care by the case manger, for the purpose of maximizing positive outcomes and containing costs.

The case manger has graduate-level preparation or is at an advanced level of nursing practice. The case manager role requires not only advanced nursing skills but also advanced managerial and communication skills.

The case manager is an individual 'professional nurse' assigned responsibility for this process are as follows:

1. The case manager may follow the patient from the diagnostic phase through hospitalization, rehabilitation and back to home care.
2. Case manager has responsibility and authority for planning, implementing, coordinating and evaluating care for the patient throughout the period of illness, regardless of the patient's movement among various units and services (such as emergency room, surgical unit, recovery unit, etc.).

3. The case manager ensures that plans are made in advance for the next needed step. Through this, the manager assists with decision making and helps to ensure that the patient receives care that will achieve the most positive outcomes in the most efficient manner. This process helps to eliminate costly delays in progress.

Case Manager's Approaches

1. **Case managers employed by the hospitals** follow a patient from the time admission is planned through the time of discharge. This case manager might plan the admitting process to ensure that all preadmission work-ups are completed and that the patient is being admitted at the appropriate time to facilitate follow-up of the problems.
2. **Case managers in private practice** may focus on a particular group of client. For example, the geriatric case manager focuses on managing care for the older client. The private case manger is paid by the client or family usually based on the hours of service provided. The case manager may help the family to identify all the options for care and treatment, ask questions to obtain greater understanding of the overall problem, and work with the family in the decision-making process.

Case Management Tools

The case manager uses two tools, case manager plan (CMP), and critical path diagnosis (CPD) to, design, map, track, monitor, and adjust the patient's course through the care-treatment process.

1. **Case manager plan:** It is a multicolumn plan with accompanying timeline that includes medical and nursing diagnosis, desired care outcomes, intermediate daily goals to supports each outcome, and the daily activities required of nurse, physicians, and other care givers to achieve intermediate goal.
2. **Critical path diagnosis:** It is an abbreviated, one page version of the required physician and nurse action listed in the CMP, together with the exact data on which all key events must occur to achieve the desired outcome by the target date.

The case manager evaluates the patient's progress toward care and treatment goal daily by comparing signs, symptoms and assessment data against information in the CMP and CDP then tracking variances from the expected course of progress.

Advantages

1. **For the patient:**

a. Establishing and achieving a set of 'expected' or standardized patient care outcomes for each patient.

b. Facilitating early patient discharge or discharge within an appropriate length of stay.
c. Using the fewest possible appropriate health care resources to meet expected patient care outcomes.
d. Facilitating the continuity of patient care through collaborative practice of diverse health professionals.

2. For the nurse:

a. Enhancing nurse's professional development and job satisfaction.
b. Facilitating the transfer of knowledge of expert clinical staff of novice staff.

CONCLUSION

Nurses are responsible for determining and planning nursing care. Best nursing care can be given when a written plan for care is made, keep up-to-date and followed by all who participate in patient care. While making a plan, it is necessary to consider and take into account the diagnosis, physical and mental condition, medical care, individual characteristics, nationality, age, weight, education, personal habits and interest, social status, family relationships and handicaps, fear and worries. In addition to this, date of admission, date of operation or deliver, past history of any diseases, etc. should be known for providing the best quality patient care.

CHAPTER

13

Growth and Development

INTRODUCTION

The period of growth and development extends throughout the life cycle. However, the period in which the principal changes occur is from conception to the end of adolescence. The most important period of growth and development is a complex one in which two cells joined as one normally because a thinking, felling person, who eventually takes a responsible place in society.

DEFINITION

Growth: It refers to an increase in physical size of the whole or any of its parts and can be measured in inches or centimeters and pounds or kilometers.

Development: It refers to a progressive increase in skill and capacity to function. It causes a qualitative change in the child's functioning.

MEANING OF GROWTH AND DEVELOPMENT

Growth and development are used interchangeably and taken as synonymous terms. Both related to the measurement of changes occurred in the individual after conception in the womb of the mother. Change is the law of nature. An individual starting from a fertilized egg turns into a fully fledged human adult. **In this turn over process** human undergoes a cycle of change brought about by the process of growth and development in various dimensions such as physical, mental, emotional, social, etc. Therefore in the wider sense both the terms growth and development can be used for any change brought by maturation and learning and essentially is the product of both heredity and development.

CONCEPTS OF GROWTH AND DEVELOPMENT

Different concepts of growth and development are listed below:

1. Growth is one of the parts of developmental process; in strict sense development in its quantitative aspect is termed as growth.

2. Growth may be referred to describe the changes, which take place in particular aspect of the body and behavior of an organism.
3. Growth does not continue throughout life. It stop, when maturity has been attained.
4. The changes produced by growth are the subject of measurement. They may be quantified and are observable in nature.
5. Growth may or may not bring development. A child may grow by becoming fat, but this growth may not bring any functional improvement or development.
6. The term growth refers to an increase in physical size of the whole body or any of its parts.
7. Development refers to progressive increase in physical skill and capacity to function. It cause qualitative change in the child's functioning.
8. Growth is an essential features of life of a child that distinguishes him/her from an adult.
9. The maximum increase in the number of cells occurs in the fetal life as evidenced by an increase in the DNA content of tissues.
10. Children are influenced by genetic factors, home, environment and parental attitudes.
11. Development is closely related to maturation of the nervous system, as primitive reflexes disappear, these are replaced by a voluntary activity.
12. Play is a natural medium for expression, communication and growth in children.
13. Both rate and pattern of growth can be modified most obviously by nutrition.
14. Growth is complex; it is measured both qualitatively and quantitatively over a period of time.

BIOLOGICAL PRINCIPLES OF GROWTH AND DEVELOPMENT

The biological changes brought about in the individual by the process of growth and development tend to follow some well deifined principles. These are known as principles of growth and development. These principles are being described below.

PRINCIPLES OF GROWTH AND DEVELOPMENT

Principles of growth and development includes:

1. **Principle of continuity:** Development follows continuity, it goes from womb to tomb and never ceases. An individual starting life from a tiny cell develops as human body, mind and other aspects of human personality through a continuous stream of development in these various dimensions.

2. **Rate of growth and development is not uniform:** The rate of growth and development is not steady and uniform at all times. It proceeds more rapidly in the early years of life, but shows down in to later years of infancy. Therefore at no stage that rate of growth and development show steadiness.
3. **Principle of individual difference:** According to this principle, there exist wide individual differences among children with respect to their growth and development in various dimensions; each child grows at own unique rate.
4. **Uniformity of pattern:** Although development does not proceed at a uniform rate and show marked individual differences, yet it follows a definite sequence of pattern and somewhat uniform in the offspring. For example, all offsprings of human beings begin to grow from head-wards.
5. **Development proceeds from general to specific responses:** In all the phrases of childs development, general activity proceeds specific activity, the responses are of a general sort before they become specific.
6. **Principle of integration:** The integration refers to the whole and its parts as well as of the specific and general responses that make a child development satisfactory in the various dimentions of growth and development.
7. **Principle of interrelation:** The growth and development in various dimentions like physical, mental, social, etc. are interrelated and interdependent. Growth and development in any one dimension affects the growth and development of the child in other dimensions.
8. **Development is predictable:** With the help of the growth rate and development of a child it is possible to predict the range within which nature of development is going to fall.
9. **Principle of development direction:** By cephalocaudal development proceeds in the direction of the longitudinal axis (head to foot). First the child gains control over his/her head and arm then and his/her legs, so that he/she can stand.
10. **Development is spiral and not linear:** The child does not proceed straightly on the path of development with a constant or a steady pace. Actually child makes advancement during a particular period, but takes rest in the next following period to consolidate his/her development.
11. **Growth and development as a joint product of both heredity and environment:** Child at any stage of influenced growth and development is by a joint product of both heredity and environment. His/her growth and development in any indirectly influenced.
12. **Growth and development proceeds in an orderly sequence:** Growth insight occurs in only one sequence, from smaller to longer. Development also proceeds in a predictable order.

13. **There is an optimum time for initiation of experiences or learning:** A child cannot learn task until his/her nervous system is mature enough to allow that particular learning.
14. **Neonatal reflexes must be lost before development can proceed:** An infant cannot grasp with skill until the grasp reflex has faded, not stand steadily until the walking reflex has faded.
15. **A great deal of skill and behavior is learned by practice:** An infant practices over and over taking a first step before he/she accomplish this securely.
16. **Development involves change:** As the development process, the child undergoes change in all aspects such as physical, psychological, social, spiritual, etc.
17. **Early development is more critical than later development:** In the early stage the child learns all skills from their parents. For example, toilet training is not given properly; child in future will have elimination problems.
18. **Every area of development has potential hazards:** Each stage of growth and development has own risks, which can be avoided if proper care is given.
19. **Happiness varies at different period in development:** Infant will be very happy once it receives all the needs required for toddler. If the child see the toy, which is pleasing, he tries to get in hand by showing the temper tantrum. He/she never adjusts to the situation, but in case of school age child, he/she tries to adjust to the situation.
20. **There are social expectations for every development in mental period:** In every period the society expects certain levels of development for an individual.
21. **Children are competent:** A child wants to be accepted. Each child has its own ability and they always try to achieve their needs.

FACTORS INFLUENCING GROWTH AND DEVELOPMENT

Growth and development depend on not one but combination of many factors, all interdependent. The relatively typical pattern of growth and development is influenced by heredity and environment. Also genetic inheritance and environmental influences are two primary factors in determining a child's pattern of growth and development.

GENETIC FACTORS

Genetic factors, which influence child's growth and development are:

1. **Heredity:** The heredity of a man and women determines that their children. Heredity decides the size and shape of the body, hence family member bear resemblance. The characteristics are transmitted through genes, which are responsible for family illness, e.g. diabetes.

2. **Sex:** Sex is determined at conception, after birth the male infant is both longer and heavier than female infant. Boys maintain this superiority unit about 11 years of age. Girls mature earlier, reach the period of accelerated growth earlier than boys and are than taller on the average.
3. **Race:** Distinguishing characteristics called racial or subracial, developed in prehistoric humans. Similar physical characteristics are seen in people belonging to the same race. As too height, tall and short examples exist among all races and subraces. Among civilized groups, intermarriage has produced mixed racial types.

NUTRITIONAL FACTORS

1. **Poor nutrition:** Nutrition plays a vital role in the body's suscepibity to disease because poor nutrition limits the body ability to resist infection. Poor nutrition also plays a major role in the development of chronic illnesses. Growth and development suffering from protein-energy malnutrition, anemia and vitamin deficiency states are retarded.
2. **Maternal nutrition:** Intrauterine growth retardation and consequently small size of the fetus occur due to nutritional deficiency in mothers, infection and drugs used during pregnancy.

ENVIRONMENTAL FACTORS

1. **Physical environment:** Environment forces act up on the individual. It is the exploding force of an individual potentially to different stimulating forces. The physical environment includes food, temperature, climate, resources, etc.
2. **Mental environment:** It includes the intellectual atmosphere of the school, the libraries, the recreation rooms, laboratories, etc.
3. **Social environment:** It includes social association—the child gets from the beginning. It also includes cultural atmosphere of the society. For example, religion, floklone, literature, art, music, social convertions and political organizations. The rich is the environment, better is the scope for developing an individual in to a healthy human being.
4. **Socioeconomic level:** The child born into a family of low socioeconomic means may not receive adequate health supervision, could leave a child without immunization against measles or other childhood illnesses and thus vulnerable to disease that could cause permanent neurologic damage.
5. **Cultural influences:** Groups of human being create their own cultures, whereas each individual is influenced or shaped by the culture of which he/she is a part. The effects of a particular culture on a child begin before birth because of the manner in which culture views and treat the members of the pregnant women's family.
6. **Internal influences:** There is evidence that all the hormones in the body affect growth in some manner. Deficiency of growth hormone retards growth, while over production results in gigantism.

7. **Characteristics of parents:** Parents with high intelligence quotient are more likely to have children with higher level of inherent intelligence.
8. **Prenatal environment:** Prenatal environment is climate in which the child's develops. The influences of the intrauterine environment on the child's future development are great, particularly since the uterus shields the fetus from the full impact of external adverse condition.
9. **Postnatal environment:** An environment that provides satisfying experiences promote growth. Since growth and development are inter-related, growth in one area influences and in turn is inflienced by growth in all other areas.

CHARACTERISTICS OF GROWTH AND DEVELOPMENT

Growth and development are continuous and orderly processes that have predictable sequences. It is important for the nurse to understand this early period as well as the total life cycle of an individual to better understands the behavior of parents and other adults who provide care for the child.

CHARACTERISTICS

1. **Individual differences:** Each child has an individual rate of growth, but the pattern of growth shows less variability. For example, an infant will be able to sit before standing alone. As noted, the age at which an individual child achieves these skills may occur at any point in a range of time.
2. **Readiness for certain task the critical periods:** During which the learning of certain behaviors occurs are termed critical periods. These are defined as those points at which the maximal capacity for an aspect of development is first present or at which structures to be developed are undergoing rapid growth.
3. **Rate of development:** During the period of growth and development of the total body and its subsystem, growth is sometimes rapid and at times it slows down. Rapid growth occurs during gestation and during infancy. In the preschool years, growth levels off and slows down during the school years.
4. **Sequence of growth and development:** Growth and development proceeds from the head down to the tail or in a cephalocaudal direction. This is particularly evident during the period of gestation and the first year of life. Before birth the head end of the embryo and fetus enlarges and develops before the tail end does. Postnatal, the infant can control the movement of the head before being able to stand and control the feet.
5. **Interrelatedness of growth and development:** Although growth and development—physical, metal, social, emotional, sexual and spiritual proceed at different rates, they are so inter-related in the majority of

children that the result is a progressive development of the whole child, from infancy to adult.

GROWTH OF THE BODY SYSTEM

Circulatory system

1. **Heart rate:** It reduces with increasing age—in infancy, it is 120 beats per minute (bpm), one year: 80–120 bpm, childhood: 70–110 bpm, adolescence to adulthood: 55–90 bpm.
2. **Blood pressure:** Increases with age. The fiftieth percentile ranges from 55–66 mm Hg diastolic to 65–112 mm Hg systolic. These levels increase about 2–3 mm Hg per year starting at age 7 years. Systolic pressure in adolescence higher in males than in females.
3. **Hemoglobin:** Highest at birth 179 per 100 mL of blood. Then decreases to 10–15 g by 1 year. Gradual increase in hemoglobin level to 14.5 g per 100 mL between 1 and 12 years of age. The hemoglobin level higher in males than in females.

Respiratory System

1. **Respiratory rate:** Decreases with increase in age.
   Infancy: 30–40 per minutes.
   Childhood: 20–24 per minute.
   Adolescence and adulthood: 16–18 per minute.
2. **Vital capacity:** Gradual increase throughout childhood and adolescent, with a later life. Capacity in males exceeds than females.
3. **Basal metabolism:** Highest rate is found in the newborn. Rate declines with increase in age, higher in males than in females.

Urinary System

1. Premature and full term newborns have some inability to concentrate urine. Specific gravity (newborn): 0.001 to 1.02
2. Glomerular filtration rate greatly increased by 6 months of age, reaches adult value between 1 and 2 years, gradually decreases after 20 years.

Digestive System

1. Stomach size is small at birth, rapidly increases during infancy and childhood.
2. Peristaltic activity decreases with advancing age.
3. Blood glucose level gradually rises from 75–80 mg per 100 mL blood in infancy to 95–100 mg during adolescence.
4. Premature infants have lower blood glucose levels than do full-term infants.
5. Enzymes are present at birth to digest proteins and moderate amount of fat, but only simple sugars.

6. Secretion of hydrochloric acid and salivary enzymes increases with age until adolescence then decrease with advancing age.

Nervous System

1. Brain reaches 90% of total size by 2 year of age.
2. All brain cells are present by the end of the first year, although their size and complexity will increase.
3. Maturation of the brainstem and spinal cord follows cephalocaudal and proximodistal laws.

PRENATAL DEVELOPMENT

The word 'prenatal' refers to the period before birth. It begins from the time of conception and ends when the baby is born. In the various life stage of man, prenatal period is the earliest and the most important stage because the foundations for future development are laid during this stage.

PRENATAL LIFE

1. Fertilization or conception occurs, when a sperm from the male pierces the cell wall of an ovum or egg from the female.
2. Once the ovum is fertilized, it begins to grow.
3. At first, the fertilized ovum, which is also called zygote consists of only one cell.
4. After few hours, the zygote divided into two new cells.
5. Still later, each of these two cells also divides.

DEVELOPMENT DURING PRENATAL PERIOD

Period of Ovum

1. The first two weeks from the time of conception until the zygote is attached within the uterus is the period of ovum.
2. Conception occurs in the fallopian tube and the zygote travels down to uterus.
3. Zygote starts dividing and multiplying in the beginning of this period.
4. By the time, it reaches the uterus, it is about the size of pinhead.
5. It develops very small tendrils and with the help of these tendrils the ovum attached to the uterine wall is called implantation.
6. Implantation occurs approximately around 10 days after fertilization.

Period of Embryo

1. The period of embryo begins from the time of the zygote attachment to the uterine wall.
2. This period usually lasts from 2 weeks after fertilization to the 8 week by the end of the period of ovum, the eggs has two distinct parts, one inner cell mass and the other an outer layer called trophoblast

3. The inner cell mass differentiates into three clear layers, of the three layers, the outer layer is called ectoderm from which will develop the outer layer of skin, the hair, the nails, parts of teeth, skin glands, sensory cells and the nervous system.
4. The middle layer is called the mesoderm from which will develop the inner skin layers, the muscles, skeleton and the circulatory; and excretory organs.
5. The inner layer is called endoderm from which will develop living of the entire gastrointestinal tract, the trachea, bronchi, lungs, liver, pancreas, salivary gland, thyroid gland and thymus.
6. The outer layer, the trophoblast will develop into accessory tissues, which protect and nourish the embryo.
7. As the embryo grows, additional life supporting structure continues to develop. Among these are the umbilical cord and placenta, which maintain the connection with the mother's body through which the embryo gets nutrients and excrete waste.
8. Umbilical cord is a flexible cord like structure connection the fetus with the placenta.
9. Placenta is a membranous organ into which mother's blood-stream and fetus blood-stream end.
10. Nutrition from the mother blood passes to the fetus through placenta. Also a sac develops, filled with a watery fluid.
11. The embryo, the spontaneous abortion rate is relatively high. Since all organs have their beginning in this stage, development irregularities might occur if the mother takes medicines without medical advice.

Period of Fetus

1. Fetus period extends from the end of the 2nd month of pregnancy until birth.
2. During this time the various body system, which had their origin in the earlier stage become well-developed and begin to function.
3. When the fetus is 3 inches long, muscles are becoming well-developed, and spontaneous development of arms and legs may be observed.
4. The fetal sex can now be distinguished easily by the end of 16 weeks; the mother can feel the movement.
5. By 24 weeks of pregnancy, the fetus is capable of swallowing and sucking. By the time the fetus's eyelids have developed and are functional.
6. The fetal age of 28 weeks is an important one. By this age the fetus's nervous, circulatory and other bodily systems have become sufficiently

well-structured, so that if born prematurely it can survive. As the fetus become older, it becomes more active.

NEWBORN

The birth of an infant is one of the most awe inspiring and emotional events that can occur in one's lifetime. After 9 months of anticipation and preparation, the neonate arrives amid a flurry of excitement. The new human being affects the lives of the parent and also the other family members. The nurse provides family-centered care for neonates and their parents based on an understanding of the effects of heredity and environment; and the newborn infant in the first several days of life.

PHYSICAL GROWTH DURING INFANCY

1. According to medical standards, the period of the newborn extends from birth to the end of the 2nd week or until the navel is healed, this also called the period of neonate.
2. The term neonate is derived from the Greek word 'neo' meaning new and the Latin verb 'nascor' meaning to be born. Hurlock refer to this period as the period of infancy.
3. Before the birth, the baby was inside the mother in a comfortable environment. The entire baby was inside the mother in a comfortable environment. All the needs of the fetus were taken care of by the mother's body.
4. But once the baby is born, the baby has to do such functions as breathing, ingestion, digestion, excretion, etc. by himself/herself.
5. Hence, the newborn baby has to make a number of adjustments.
6. The four most important adjustment—to temperature change, adjustment to breathing, taking in nourishment and adjustment to elimination.
7. Because all babies are not capable of adjustment this period is called a critical period.
8. The most critical time is the 1st day of baby life, full-term baby adjust to those conditions well, but underweight babies and premature babies find difficult to adjust.

APPEARANCE OF THE NEWBORN

1. As soon as the baby is born, he\she cries, this birth cry makes the baby's first breath.
2. All the babies look similar in the newborn stage. A newborn baby's body is coated with a cheese like substance.
3. His/her chinless head seems too big for his/her body. There is hair not only on his head, but at other places of the body also.
4. The genitals are the first large and prominent.
5. Newborn babies have enlarged breasts, which sometimes secrete milk and girl's babies occasionally have a brief menstrual flow.

6. The neonate's scull is not completely formed. There are six soft spots on baby head.

CHARACTERISTICS OF NEWBORN (DURING FIRST WEEK)

Circulatory System

Clamping of cord at birth brings changes in fetal circulation, closure of foramen ovale and ductus arteriosus; and obliteration of umbilical arteries produce an adult like circulation within 1 hour after birth.

1. Regular heart rate 120–160, but variable depending on infants activity; soft hearts murmur common for first month of life.
2. Hemoglobin level high 14–20 g/100 mL of blood.
3. White blood count high, i.e. 6000–22000 mm^3.

Respiratory System

Respirations diaphragmatic, irregular, abdominal, 30–50 per minute, quiet with periods of apnea.

Temperature

Temperature maintained at 97.8°F or 98°F, environmental factors may affect temperature.

Excretory System

1. The first stool is black-green and tenacious, called meconium, by third day, becomes mixed with light-yellow called transitional.
2. Newborn should void during first 24 hours, albumin and urea common during first week because of dehydration.

Integument System

1. Lanugo: Fine, downy, hair growth over the entire body.
2. Milia: Small, whitish, pinpoint spots over the nose caused by retained sebaceous secretions.
3. Mongolian spots: Blue-black discoloration on back, buttocks and sacral region that disappear by first year.

Digestive System

1. The newborn has stores of nutrients from intrauterine existence, therefore needs very little nourishment first few days.
2. Roots and sucks when anything is brought to mouth.
3. Digests simple carbohydrates, fats and proteins readily.
4. Cardiac sphincter of stomach not well-developed, therefore regurgitates if stomach is over fill.
5. Needs to be bubbled frequently to get rid of air bubbles in stomach.
6. Gastric activity remains low for 2–3 months.

Neural

1. Central nervous system (CNS) and brain not well-developed, infant needs constant supply of oxygen.
2. Breathing, sucking and crying are early neural activities necessary for the infant's survival.

Sleep

1. Sleep lowers body metabolism.
2. It helps to restore energy and assimilate nutrition for growth.

Nutrition

1. Initial weight loss of 5–10% of birth weight is normal and usually regained by 10th day of life.
2. Newborn needs to ingest simple proteins, carbohydrates, fats, vitamins and minerals for continued cell growth.

IMMEDIATE NEEDS AT THE TIME OF BIRTH

1. Aspiration of mucus to provide an open airway.
2. Evaluation by use of Apgar score 1–5 minutes following birth score determined by points for heart rate, respiration, muscle tone, reflex irritability and color.
3. Maintenance of body temperature by drying infant and placing next to mother or under radiant warmer.
4. Promotion of interaction between parents and newborn.
5. Constant observation of physical condition.
6. Identification of infant by applying an identification band to infant and mother.
7. Eye care prophylactic installation of ordered medicine (e.g. erythromycin) in each eye to prevent ophthalmia neonatorum.
8. Assessment of behavioral characteristics during transition period—first period of reactivity, period of inactivity, second period of reactivity.

APGAR SCORING

a. Apgar scoring system is developed by Virginia Apgar (USA) in 1952.
b. The core is based on observation of heart rate, respiration, muscle tone, reflex activity and color.
c. Each item is given a score of 0, 1, 2. The assessment of Apgar score is done at 1–5 minutes after birth.
d. Total score of 8–10 indicates ease in adjusting to the extrauterine life. The body's condition is good.
e. Total score of 5–7 indicates moderate difficulty of newborn babies to adjust to the life. The condition is fair.
f. Total score of 0–4 indicates severe distress.

TRANSITIONAL ASSESSMENT

First Stage

First stage of transitional assessment includes:

a. It lasts for about 6 hours after birth. First 30 minutes after birth, the neonate is alert, cries and has stronger sucking.
b. This time is the best for breastfeeding and eye to eye contact.
c. After this 30 minutes of active period the newborn sleeps 5–6 hours.
d. During this reactivity period he may have rapid heart rate, rapid respiration, more secretions and decreased body temperature as extrauterine adjustments adaptation.
e. Exposure needs to be avoided during this period.

Second Period of Reactivity

a. Second period of reactivity is the period from 6 hours to 24 hours after birth, when the neonate awakes after first sleep period.
b. Neonate again becomes active, alert and responsive, gradually baby vital signs stabilize.

NEUROMUSCULAR DEVELOPMENT

1. **Blink reflex:** It may be elicited by shining a strong light such as flashlight or otoscope light on the eye.
2. **Rooting reflex:** If a newborn's cheek is brushed or stroked near the corner of the mouth, the child will turn the head in that direction. The reflex disappears at about the 6th week of life.
3. **Sucking reflex:** When a newborn's lips are touched the baby makes a sucking motion. The sucking reflex begins to diminish at about 6 months of age.
4. **Swallowing reflex:** The swallowing reflex in the newborn is the same as in the adult. Food that reaches the posterior portion of the tongue is automatically swallowed.
6. **Extrusion reflex:** A newborn will extrude any substance that is placed on the anterior portion of the tongue. This protective reflex prevents the swallowing of inedible substance, disappearing at about 4 months of age.
7. **Palmar grasp reflex:** Newborns will grasp on object placed in their palm by closing their fingers in it. It is a primitive reflex, apparently form a time newborns clung to their mother for safety. The reflex disappears at about age 6 weeks to 3 months.
8. **Step (walk):** In place reflex-newborn, who are held in a vertical position with their feet touching a hard surface will take a new quick, alternating steps. This reflex disappears by 3 months of age.
9. **Placing reflex:** The placing reflex is similar to the step in place reflex, except is elicited by touching the anterior surface of newborn's leg against the edge of a bassinet or table.

10. **Plantar grasp reflex:** When an object touches the sole of a newborn's foot at the base of the toes, the toes grasp in the same manner as the finger do. The reflex disappears at about 8–9 months of age in preparation for walking.
12. **Tonic neck reflex:** When newborn lies on these backs, their hands usually turn to one side or the other. The arm and the leg on the side to which the hand turns extend and the opposite arm and leg contract. It is also called a boxer or fencing reflex, because the newborn's position stimulates that of someone preparing to box of fence.
13. **Moro reflex:** A Moro reflex can be initiated by starting the newborn by a loud noise or by jarring the abssinet. The most accurate method of eliciting the reflex is to hold newborns in supine position and allow their heads to drop backward an inch or so.
14. **Babinski reflex:** When the side of the sole of the foot has been firmly stroked, an inverted 'J' curve from the heel upward occurs, the newborn turns the toes. It remains positive (toes fan) until at least 3 months of age, when it is supplanted by the down-turning or flexing adult response.
15. **Magnet reflex:** If pressure is applied to the soles of the feet of newborn laying in a supine position, he/she pushes back against the pressure. This and the two following reflexes are tests of spinal cord integrity.
16. **Crossed extension reflex:** One leg of a newborn laying supine is extended and the sole of that foot is irritated being rubbed with a sharp object such as a thumbnail.
17. **Trunk uncurvated reflex:** When a newborn lies in a prone position and are touched along the pravertebral area by a probing finger, they will flex their trunk and swing their pelvis toward the touch.
18. **Laudau reflex:** A newborn, who is held in a prone position with a hand underneath supporting the trunk, should demonstrate some muscle tone. Babies may not be able to lift their head or arch their back in this position, but neither should they sag into an inverted 'V' position.
19. **Deep tendon reflex:** A patellar reflex can be elicited in a newborn by tapping the patellar tenden with the tip of the finger. The lower leg will move perceptibly if the infant has an intact reflex.

PARENT-CHILD RELATIONSHIPS

Concept of Basic Parent-infant Relationships

1. Early and frequent parent-infant contact is essential for survival (bonding).
2. Child bearing is a development crisis, parenting abilities can be fostered and developed.
3. Biologic changes that occur at puberty and during pregnancy influence the development of nurturance.
4. Interaction between mother and child begins from the moment of conception and can be shared with the father.
5. Love for the infant grows as the patents interact and give cure.

6. As the parent gives to the infant and infant receives the parent in turn receives satisfaction from parenting tasks.
7. Any disturbance in give and take cycle sets up frustrations in parents and infant.
8. Parental behavior is learned and frequent parent infant contact enhances development of parenting abilities; ambivalence is a natural phenomenon as are feeling of resentment.

Infant's Basic Needs

1. Physiologic: Food, clothing, bathing and protection from environment.
2. Emotional: Security, comfort, founding, caressing, rocking being spoken to and contact with one person on a consistent basis.

Mothering and fathering are:

1. Based on biologic inborn desire to reproduce.
2. Role concepts that begin with own childhood experiences.
3. Primitive emotional relationship.
4. Maturing process.
5. Fostered by the parent: Infant interaction that constantly reinforces gratification as needs are met and security develops.
6. Abilities that is learned rather than innate.

Significant phases of maternal adjustments

1. **Taking-in phase:** Mother's needs to be met before she can meet infant's needs, talks about self rather than infant, does not seem interested in infant.
2. **Transition phase:** Characterized by mothers starting to take hold, looking at and reaching for infant, touching with fingertips, talking about infant, etc.
3. **Taking-hold phase:** Kisses, embraces, give care to infant, eye contact, uses whole hand to make contact, calls the infant by name, etc.

Supportive Care to Promote Bonding/Attachment

1. Give parents ample time to inspect and begin to identity with infant, allow the parents to touch, fondle and hold infant.
2. Encourage given and take between parents and infants support these beginning relationships.
3. Teach the parents about their newborn; showing by example helps parents to learn care necessary to meet infants and their own.
4. Evaluate parents and infant's response; and revise plan as necessary, identify beginning of disturbed relationship.

PROBLEMS IN NEWBORN

Preterm or Low Birth Weight Infant

1. Preterm infant born before term (36 weeks or less).
2. Low birth weight infant, weighs 2,500 g or less at birth.
3. Less subcutaneous fat, therefore the skin is wrinkled, blood and bony sutures are visible, lanugo present on birth on face, eyebrows are absent, and ears are poorly supported by cartilages.

Asphyxia Neonatorum

1. Asphyxia neonatorum means non-establishment of satisfactory pulmonary respiration at birth. Clinically it is defined as failure to initiate and maintain spontaneous respiration within 1 minute of birth.
2. The clinical features depend upon the etiology, intensity and duration of oxygen lack, plasma carbon dioxide excess and subsequent acidosis.
3. The basic requirements for initiation and maintenance of pulmonary respiration by airway clearenance, sufficient pulmonary perfusion, oxygen diffusion and dissociation capacity and carbonic anhydrase activity of blood.

Respiratory Distress Syndrome

1. Respiratory distress syndrome is a deficiency in surface- active (detergent like lipoproteins—surfactant), which results in inadequate lung inflation and ventilation.
2. The respiratory distress syndrome occurs commonly in preterm neonates, babies of diabetic mothers and infants delivered by cesarean section or following breech delivery.
3. Clinically manifested by abrupt appearance of dyspnea and cyanosis attack, shortly after birth, X-ray shows ground glass mottling.

Meconium Aspiration Syndrome

1. Meconium aspiration syndrome usually occurs in terms of post-term babies, who are small of gestational age.
2. The meconium stained liquor may be aspirated by the fetus-in-utero or during first breath.
3. The mechanism may block the small air passages or produce chemical pneumonitis.
4. Diagnosis is mainly based on aspiration of meconium from the trachea at birth.
5. The therapeutic interventions are suctioning after head is delivered, oxygenation and ventilation, prophylactic antibiotic therapy and bicarbonate for acidosis.

Cranial Birth Injuries

1. **Caput succedaneum**: Edema with extravasation of serum into scalp tissues caused by molding during the birth process crosses the suture lines of the bony plates of the skull. No treatment is necessary; it subsides in a few days.
2. **Cephalhematoma:** Edema of the scalp with effusion of blood between the bone and periosteum, stops at the suture line, no treatment is necessary. It appears within a few weeks to a few months after birth, resolution of hematoma can lead to hyperbilirubinemia.
3. **Intracranial hemorrhage**: Bleeding into cerebellum, pans, medulla oblongata caused by a tearing of the tentorium cerebelli, occurs in preterm infants and following prolonged labor, difficult forceps birth, precipitate birth, version or breech extraction.

Neuromuscular Birth Injuries

1. **Facial paralysis:** Asymmetry of face caused by damage to facial nerves during difficult forceps birth.
2. **Erb-duchenne paralysis (brachial palsy):** Caused by difficult forceps or breech extraction birth, manifested by a flaccid arm with elbow extended, treatment depends on severity of paralysis.
3. **Dislocation and fracture:** Are diagnosed by crepitation, immobility and variations in range of motion, treatment depend on the site of fracture.

Ophthalmia Neonatorum

1. An eye infection caused by *Neissseria gonorrhoeae* and *Chlamydia trachomatis.*
2. Organism is transmitted from the genital tract of an infected mother during birth or by infected hands.
3. Chlamydial infection can also cause pneumonia.
4. It can be prevented by ophthalmic antibiotic instilled at birth after providing for initial bounding.

NURSING MANAGEMENT IN NEONATE

1. Establish and maintain patent airway by oropharynx suction to clear the respiratory passage.
2. Maintain normal body temperature. Keep the baby away from fan, breeze or air conditioner, maintain the room temperature around 28°–30°C.
3. Protection from infection, handwashing should be practiced before and after caring or touching the baby.
4. Provide adequate nutrition—put the baby to the mother's breast as early as possible after birth. Do not offer artificial feeds when baby has sucking and swallowing reflex.

5. Observe the elimination pattern—the infant passes urine very frequently during early period. If baby does not passes for 10–12 hours, it should be reported to the doctor. The meconium is passed within 24 hours after birth.
6. Providing psychological bonding and supporting cuddling and warmth with close contact with the mother gives the infant feeding of love, affection and security.
7. Parental teaching: Parents should be explained about daily observations, feeding, activity, sleep and elimination.

INFANCY

Infancy is traditionally designed as the period from 1 month to 1 year of age. This year is one of rapid growth and development, with the infant tripling birth weight and increasing length by 50%. During this period, the baby's senses sharpen and with the process of attachment to primary care givers, from his/her first social relationships. Infants are seen at healthcare facilities for health maintenance at least 6 months during the 1st year.

STAGES OF INFANCY

Rapid Growth and Development

1. Infancy is the period of rapid growth and development, inner as well as outer organs developed rapidly at this stage.
2. There is a rapid growth in terms of height and weight; and size.
3. There is rapid development of emotions and almost all the emotions are developed in the child during this stage.
5. Infancy stage is marked by intensive motor activity and restlessness.

Dependence

1. Infant depends upon his/her mother, father and family members for the satisfaction on basic needs.
2. The infant is a helpless creature and can move; and function with the help of others. Even for the emotional satisfaction infant depends upon others.
3. Infant expects that everybody around him/her should love and give entire affection and attention.
4. Infant wants to love and to be loved and in this exchange, totally depends on the mercy of others.
5. In this way the child at this stage is dependent but as the child moves into the later years of infantile behavior, he/she slowly proceeds toward independence.

Self-Assertion

1. The child is helpless and depends upon others for the satisfaction of his/her needs, he/she is quite self-assertive.
2. He/she tries to dominate his/her superior and elder ones, his/her wishes must be fulfilled.
3. He/she thinks, he/she is always right and all round he/she should obey him.
4. He/she is the prince although without crown and tries to assert himself/herself all the time in all situations.

Period of Make-believe and Fantasy

1. Infant live in the world of their own creation, this is a period of rich, but baseless imagination.
2. As on this stage, the infant has limited potentialities and aspires more than, what child can actually get in the actual life.
3. He/she compensates himself/herself in fantasy and makes believe.

Selfish and Unsocial

1. In infancy, the child is almost completely ego-centric and selfish.
2. Child does not want to share his/her toys or give any of his/her possessions to anyone else.
3. Infants want to have all the things even love, admiration and affection reserved for them.
4. Infants do not care for the social and moral codes and principles, and places their self interest at the premium.

Emotionally Unstable

1. Infancy is the period of violent emotional experiences.
2. The emotions at this stage are marked by intensity, frequency and instability.
3. There are spontaneous and the infant is hardly able to exercise control over them.
4. Infants are not able to hide their feelings and in this way, the emotions of the infant is generally in the overt form.

MENTAL DEVELOPMENT DURING INFANCY

Developing Curiosity and Questioning Attitude

1. At this age, the child is very much curious about knowing so many things around him. The world and the environment is new for them.
2. Infants are in the habit of questioning like, what is this? Answers do not interest them as much as asking questions.
3. Their speed of questioning is so rapid that they does not wait the previous answers.

Intellectually not Developed

1. The child at this initial stage is very immature in intelligence.
2. Infants lacks in reasoning and abstract understanding.
3. Infants can think only in concrete terms and is not developed in abstract reasoning and thinking.
4. The powers of observation, perception, concentration, etc. are also not developed.

Rate Memory

1. The child though not developed much intellectually has a very good memory. But this memorization is without reasoning.
2. It is purely a role memory. Infant can cram and reproduce the matter easily.

Creativity

1. The period of infancy is also characterized by the tendency of creative impulse in the child.
2. Infants develops a creative attitude and often engages themselves in making or collecting so many things.
3. He tries to take satisfaction in realizing that he can make, construct and perform the activities as his elders do.

Time Concept is not Developed

For the child at this stage, the divisions of time such as yesterday, today, tomorrow; month, year, etc. are meaningless as he/she not yet developed the concept of time.

Sexual Development

1. Although the sex organs at this stage are not developed, yet the sex tendency is in a continuous stage of development.
2. The findings of psychoanalysis like Freud and others have clearly shown that the sexual life of the infant is an rich as that on an adolescent.
3. An infant passes through the three stages of sexual development—stages of self-love, homosexual and heterosexual.
4. At the initial stage, the child derives pleasure from his/her own body by sucking his/her thumb or touching the sex organs.
5. Later on he/she seeks the satisfaction of his/her sex impulse outside and develops sentiments of love for the mother and father depending upon his/her sex.
6. Finally the child develops heterosexual tendency and in respect the male gets itself attached to the mother and the female child to the father.

PHYSICAL GROWTH

Weight

1. As a rule, most infant double their weight at 4–6 months, they triple it by 1 year.
2. During the first 6 months, infants typically average a weight gain of 2lb/month.
3. During second 6 months, weight gain is approximately 1lb/month.
4. The average 1-year-old male weight 10 kg (22 lb), the average female weight 9.5 kg (2lb).

Height

1. The infant increases in height during the 1st year by 50% or grow from the average birth length of 20 inch to about 30 inch (50.8–76.2 cm)
2. Height, like weight is best assessment, if it is plotted on a standard growth chart.

Head Circumference

1. Head circumference increase rapidly during the infant period, reflecting rapid brain growth.
2. By the end of the first year, the brain has already reached two-thirds of its adult size.

Body Proportion

1. Body proportion changes during the 1st year from that of a newborn to a more typical infant appearance.
2. The mandible becomes more prominent as bone grows.
3. The circumference of the chest is generally less than that of the head at birth by about 2 cm. It is even with the head circumference in some infants as early as 6 months and in most by 12 months.
4. The abdomen remains protuberant until the child has been walking well.

Body Systems

1. In the cardiovascular system, heart rate slows from 120–160 beats per minute (bpm) to 100–120 bpm by the end of the first year.
2. Respiratory rate of the infant slows from 30–60 breaths per minute to 20–30 breaths per minute by the end of the first year.
3. At birth, the gastrointestinal tract is immature in its ability to digest food and mechanically move it along. These functions mature gradually during the infant year.
4. The immune system becomes functional by at least 2 months of age, the infant is able to produce both IgG and IgM antibodies by 1 year of age.

5. Ability to adjust to cold is mature by age 6 months.
6. Kidney, liver and endocrine glands remains immature and not as efficient at eliminating body wastes as in the adult.

Teeth

1. The first baby tooth usually erupts at age 6 months, followed by a new one monthly.
2. Teething pattern can vary greatly among children.

MOTOR DEVELOPMENT

Gross Motor Development

1. **Ventral suspension position:** Refers to the infant's appearance when held in midair on a horizontal plane, supported by the hand under the abdomen. The 3 months old child lifts and maintains the head well above the plane of the rest of the body in ventral suspension.
2. **Landau reflex:** It develops at 3 months. When the infant held in ventral suspension, the infant's head legs and supine extend. When the head is depressed, the hips, knees and elbows flex. This reflex continues to be present in most infants.
3. **Neck righting reflex:** Begins at 4-months-old children. The infant turns, the head to the side, shoulders, trunk and pelvis turn in that direction. This reflex causes the baby to lose his/her balance and roll sideways when lifting up the head.
4. **Sitting position:** A 5-months-old child can be seen to straighten his/her back when held or propped in a sitting position. By 6 months, children sit momentarily without support.
5. **Standing position:** The 9-months-old child can stand holding onto the coffee table, if he/she is placed in that position. At 12 months, a child stands alone at least momentarily.

Fine Motor Development

1. **Thumb position:** It is an ability to bring the thumb and fingers together. It occurs at 4th month.
2. **Pincer grasp:** A major milestone occurs at 9th month, it is a perforce for use of one hand over the other.
3. **At 12th months:** The infant can play pat-a-cake and peek-a-boo, holds a crayon to make a mark on paper. Helps in dressing, such as putting arm through sleeve.

LANGUAGE DEVELOPMENT

1. A child begins to make small, cooing sounds by the end of the 1st month.

2. By 4 months, an infant is very 'talkative', cooing babbling and gurgling when spoken to. He/she definitely laughs loudly.
3. The infant can imitate vowel sounds well, for example, oh-oh, ah-ah and oo-oo at 7 months.
4. By 9 months, the infant usually speaks a first word dd-da or ba-ba.
5. At 12 months, the infant can generally say two words besides ma-ma and dd-da, they use those two words with meaning.

PLAY DURING INFANCY (SOLITARY PLAY)

1. Safety is chief determinant choosing toys (aspirating small objects is one cause of accidental death).
2. The 1 month old children spend a great deal of time watching the parent's face, appearing to enjoy this activity, so much that the face may become their favorite 'toy'.
3. The 3 months old children can handle small blocks or small rattles.
4. A 6-month-old child can sit steadily enough to be ready for bathtub toys such as rubber ducks or plastic boats.
5. Many 9 months old children begin to enjoy toys that go inside one another.
6. The 12 months old child enjoying putting things in and taking things out of container, they like little boxes that fit inside one another or dropping objects such as blocks into cardboard box.

SENSORY DEVELOPMENT

Vision

1. A 1-month-old child regards an object in the midline of vision.
2. Eye movement coordinated most of the time, follows a light to midline. Visual acuity 20/100–20/50 at 1 month.
3. Follows a light to the periphery and has binocular coordination (vertical and horizontal vision) at 3 months.
4. Recognizes familiar object and people at 5 months
5. The 7 months old children pat their image in a mirror. Their depth perception has matured to the extent that they can perform such tasks as transferring toys from hand to hand.
6. By 10 months, the infant looks under a towel or around a corner for a concealed object (beginning of object performance).

Hearing

1. Hearing is demonstrated by the 1-month-old child who quiets momentarily at a distinctive sound such as a bell or a squeaky rubber toy.
2. Many 3 months old children will turn their heads to attempt to locate a sound.

3. At 5 months of age, the infant demonstrate that he/she can localize a sound downward and to the side, by turning the head and looking down.
4. By 10 months, the infant can recognize his/her name and listen acutely when spoken to.
5. By 12 months, the infant can easily locate a sound in any direction and turn toward it.

EMOTIONAL DEVELOPMENT

1. At 1 month, watches face intently while being spoken to.
2. Smiles in response to person or object occur in 3 months.
3. Coos and gurgles when talked to; enjoy social interaction at 5 months.
4. At 6 months, infants are increasingly aware of the difference between people, who regularly care for them and strangers.
5. At 7 months, children show obvious fear of strangers, they may cry, when taken from their parent, attempt to cling to him/her, and reach out to be taken back.
6. Fear of strangers appears to reach its height during the 8th months, thus this phenomenon is often termed eight month anxiety or stranger anxiety.
7. By 12 months, most children have overcome their fear of strangers and are alert, and responsive again when approached. They like to play interactive nursery rhymes and rhythm games and dance with others.

COGNITIVE DEVELOPMENT

1. **Primary circular reaction:** During this time, baby explores objects by grasping them with the hands or by mouthing them. At this stage the infant appears to be unaware of what actions he/she can cause or what actions occur independently. It occurs in 3rd month of life.
2. **Secondary circular reaction:** It occurs at 6 months of age, during this time, the infant is able to realize that his/her actions can initiate pleasurable sensations.
3. **Piaget cognitive process:** It describes congnitive process of infant as sensor motor intelligence for until an individual is about 2 years old, he/she concentrates on regularizing his/her sensation and controlling his/ her motor activity.

NURSING ROLE IN HEALTH PROMOTION OF THE INFANT

1. **Promoting infant safety:** Accidents are the leading cause of death in children. Most accidents in infancy occur because parents either underestimate or over estimate the child's ability. Nursing intervention is to establish sound parent-child relationship and provide anticipatory guidance for the child's safety.

2. **Preventing aspirations:** The accident that leads to the greatest number of infant deaths is aspiration.
3. **Preventing falls:** Falls are the second major cause of infant accidents. No infant, beginning with the newborn, should be left unattended on a raised surface. Normal wiggling can bring a baby to the edge of a bed, couch or table top, resulting in a fall. Teach parents to be prepared for their infant to roll over by 2 months of age.
4. **Nutritional health:** The best food for the infant during the first 12 months of life is breast milk. Breast milk is the most complete diet for the first 6 months but requires supplements of fluoride, iron by 6 months. Iron-fortified commercial formula is an acceptable alternative to breastfeeding. Solids can be introduced by about 6 months.
5. **Activities of daily living:** In the 1st year, caring for the infant—feeding, bathing, dressing and so forth occupies what may seem like nearly all of parents waking hours. All these basic care related activities provide important opportunities for caregivers and infants to get to know one another and to become used to each other's personalities and patterns. Nurses play a key role in teaching parents about these activities, stressing their importance.
6. **Vaccinations**: Diphtheria, pertussis and tetanus (DTP) given at 2,4,6 months, boosters given at 15 months and 5 years of age. Measles, mumps and rubella (MMR), live attenuated vaccine generally given at 12 months of age because of the presence of natural immunity from mother, a second dose should be administered at 4–5 years of age. Infant receive polio, trivalent oral polio vaccine at 2,4,6 months. *Haemophilus influenzae* type B vaccine should be given at 2, 4, 6 and 15 months of age. Chicken pox vaccine (varivax) 1 dose should be given before 12 months.

SOCIAL EMOTIONAL AND BEHAVIOR PROBLEMS OF INFANT

1. **Teething:** Most infants have little difficulty with teething. Generally, gums are sore and tender before a new tooth breaks the surface. Because of this pain, a baby might be resistant to chewing for a day or two.
2. **Thumb sucking**: The need is so intense that many infants begin to suck a thumb or finer at about 3 months of age and continue the habit through the first few years of life.
3. **Head banging**: Some infants rhythmically bang their heads against the bars of crib for a period of time before falling asleep. Excessive head banging done to the exclusion of normal development or activity or head banging past the preschool period, suggests a pathological basis. Such children need a referral for counseling and further evaluation.
4. **Sleeping problems:** Sleeping problems develop in early infancy because of colic or because an otherwise healthy infant takes longer than usual to adjust to sleeping through the night. Breastfed babies tend to wake more often than those who are formula fed because breast milk is more

easily digested. In late infancy, the problem of waking at night the remaining awake for an hour or more becomes common.

TODDLER

The todder period is usually considered from age 1 to 3 years, enormous changes takes place in the child and consequently, in the family. During the toddler period, the child accomplishes a wide array of developmental tasks. Promtiong toddler health and maintaining wellness involves knowledge of normal growth and development processes, an understanding of common significant milestones and the ability to anticipate deviations.

PHYSICAL DEVELOPMENT

1. A child gains only about 5–6 lb (2.5 kg) and 5 inch (12 cm) a year during toddler.
2. Physical growth is slow during toddlerhood; this is because of the toddler's decline in appetite and erratic eating habits.
3. Head circumference equals chest circumferences at 6 months to 1 year of age. At 2 years, chest circumferences are greater than of the head.
4. Toddler tend to have a prominent abdomen—a pooch belly although they are walking, their abdominal muscles are not yet strong enough to support abdominal contents as well as they will later.
5. They also have a forward curve of the spine at the sacral area (lordosis). As they walk longer, this will correct itself naturally.
6. The toddler waddles or walks with a wide stance, this stance seems to increase the lordosis curve, but it keeps the child on his/her feet.

PHYSIOLOGICAL DEVELOPMENT

1. Brain growth continues slowly, corresponding to advancing intellectual skills and fine motor development.
2. Improved coordination and equilibrium parallels the most complete (by 2 years). Myelination of the spinal cord as evidenced by refined walking, jumping and climbing.
3. Respirations slow slightly, but continue to be mainly abdominal.
4. The heart rate slows from 110 to 90 bpm; blood pressure increases to about 99/64 mm Hg.
5. In the respiratory system, the lumen of vessels increases progressively, so that threat of lower respiratory infection is less.
6. Stomach capacity increases to the point that the child can eat three meals a day.
7. Stomach secretions become more acid; therefore, gastrointestinal infections also become less common.

8. Urinary and anal sphincter control becomes possible with complete myelination of the spinal cord.
9. In the immune system, IgG and IgM antibody production become mature at 2 years of age, the passive immunity effects from intrauterine life are no longer operative.
10. The sense of hearing, smell, taste, touch and vision develop, and begin to connect, since toddler utilize all fine senses to explore the world; and exert autonomy and independence.
11. Bladder and bowel control is typically achieving during this time period and children are able to retain urine up to 4 hours before needing to void.

COMMON PROBLEM

1. **Sibling rivalry:** Sibling rivalry defined as intense feeling of jealousy between siblings, often is seen when an infant is born into a family with a toddler.
2. **Temper tantrums:** It is a outward explosive reaction to inward stressful or frustrating situations that are a normal part of toddler life.

PSYCHOSEXUAL DEVELOPMENT

1. According to Freud, toddlers are in the anal stage of development. Fraud first pointed out the tension resolving around toddler, bladder training and viewed toilet training as a possible way of resolving conflict and handling stress.
2. Frued believed, improperly managed toilet training could lead to lifelong psychological trauma with accompanying physical bowel/bladder responses.
3. Toddler is generally able to recognize gender differences by 2 years of age and begin to explore; and recognize body parts during toilet training.

PSYCHOSOCIAL DEVELOPMENT

1. The three major psychosocial tasks of toddlerhood are gaining self-control, developing autonomy and increasing independence.
2. The 15 months old children are still enthusiastic about interacting with people, providing those people are willing to follow the toddlers where they want to go.
3. By 18 months, toddler imitate the things they see a parent doing, such as study or sweep, so they seek out parents to observe and initiate reactions.
4. By 2 or more years, children become aware of gender differences and may point to other children and identify them as 'boy' or 'girl'.

EMOTIONAL DEVELOPMENT

1. Toddler, who does not develop a sense of autonomy may manifest feeling of shame or doubt.
2. Children, who learned to trust themselves and others during the infant year are better prepared to do this than those who cannot trust themselves or others.

COGNITIVE DEVELOPMENT

1. The toddler enters the fifth and sixth stages of sensory motor.
2. During the toddler years, language ability develops rapidly.
3. In tertiary circular reaction stage (12 and 18 months)–describes the toddler as 'a little scientist' because of the child's interest in trying to discover new ways to handle objects or new results different actions can achieve.
4. At the end of the toddler period , children enter a second major period of cognitive development—preoperational thought. During this period, children deal much more constructively with symbols then they did while still in the sensorimotor period of cognition.
5. Cognitively toddler are able to recognize and distinguish between shapes of objects, by they are only beginning to classify objects but they are only beginning to classify objects into categories of use.

PLAY BEHAVIOR

1. The toys toddler enjoys most are those they can play with by themselves and that require action.
2. The 15 months old children are still in a put in, take out stage, so they continue to enjoy stacks of boxes or balls that fit inside each other.
3. They enjoy throwing toys out of a playpen or from a highchair tray as long as someone will pick them up and return them again and again.
4. By age 2, toddler began to spend time, imitating adult action in their play. For example, wrapping a doll and putting into bed, setting the table or driving the car.

SPIRITUAL DEVELOPMENT

1. Fowler defined faith as a relational phenomenon, an active relationship with another, a commitment, belief, love and\or hope, which may be directed toward family, religion, God or friends.
2. Attending religious programs similar to a nursery school that emphasize appropriate behavior and positive self-esteem rather than a lesson is important as well.
3. Children at this stage also know that imitating or confirming to rituals results in approval of others, who are important to the child.

MAJOR LEARNING EVENTS

Toilet Training

1. Physical maturation must be reached and attitude of parents play a vital role.
2. Psychological readiness of a child, such as able to inform the parent of the need to urinate or defecate.
3. Process of training should begin usually with bowel and bladder.
4. Parental response is to choose a specific word for the act.

Need for Independence without Overprotection

1. Parents should be consistent and set realistic limits.
2. Reinforce desired behavior.
3. Be constructive, geared to teach self-control.

HEALTH PROMOTION FOR TODDLERS

Childhood Nutrition

1. Provide adequate nutrient intake to meet continuing growth and development needs.
2. Provide a basis for support of psychosocial development in relation to food patterns, eating behavior and attitudes.
3. Provide sufficient calories for increasing physical activities and energy needs.

Injury Prevention

1. Children under 5 years of age account for over half of all accidental deaths during childhood.
2. More than half of accidental child deaths are related to automobiles and fire.
3. Aspirating small objects and putting foreign bodies in ear or nose.
4. Prevention through parent education and child protection is the goal.

COMMON HEALTH PROBLEMS IN TODDLER

Burns

1. Second and third common causes of death in individuals less than 15 years of age for boys and girls respectively.
2. Causative agents are thermal, chemical, electrical and radiation.
3. The clinical features are edema formation, fluid loss, circulatory stasis, burn shock and decreased cardiac output.

Poisoning

1. Ingestion of a toxic substances or an excessive amount of a substances.
2. More than 90% of poisoning occurs in the home and highest incident occurs in children under 4.
3. Improper storage is the major contributing factor of poisoning.

Fracture

1. In children, bones are more easily injured; fracture can result without major injury to surrounding tissues.
2. Healing occurs rapidly in children, rapidity of healing is inversely related to the age of the child.
3. The clinical features of fracture are generalized swelling, pain or tenderness, diminished function or use of part.

Aspiration of Foreign objects

1. Obstruction of the airway by a foreign object, can occur anywhere from larynx to bronchi.
2. It is most common in children 1–3 years of age leading cause of fatal injury in children less than 1 year of age.
3. Foods that cause asphyxiation include round candy peanuts, grapes and popcorn.
4. The clinical finding of complete obstruction are substernal retractions, inability to cough or speak, increased pulse rate, respiratory rate and cyanosis.
5. Turn the small child upside down (head lower than chest) and deliver up to five quick, sharp back blows with the heel of the hand.
6. Abdominal thrust for children aged 1 year and older [Heimlich maneuver].

Child Maltreat

1. One of the most significant social problem affecting children.
2. Majority of abused children are under 4 years of age about 70–80% of abuse is by parents or other caregivers.
3. It may be intentional physical abuse or neglect, emotional abuse or neglect and sexual abuse of children.
4. Therapeutic intervention includes treat injury and identifies; and protect child from further abuse.

Mental Retardation

1. The Diagnostic and Statistical Manual of Mental Disorders, 4th edition (DSM-IV), defines cognitive impairment on the basis of two criteria; significantly subaverage general intellectual functioning—an intelligence quotient [IQ] of 70 or below.

2. The common causes of cognitive impairment are chromosomal abnormalities, infection in utero and anoxia at birth, fetal alcohol syndrome and head trauma.
3. Assessment done by using standardized tests notably the Wechsler intelligence scale for children [WISC] or the Stanford-Binet.

Cerebral Palsy

1. Non-specific term for a neuromuscular disability or difficulty in controlling voluntary muscles.
2. Major causes are anoxia of the brain, congenital or neonatal infection, trauma or prematururity.
3. Clinical findings are delayed motor, speech development, reflex abnormalities and difficulty in sucking and swallowing.
4. Management includes multidisciplinary approach, mobility devices, surgery to correct spastic muscle imbalance, medication, speech, physio and occupational therapy.

GENERAL NURSING CARE OF TODDLERS

1. **Immunization:** Caregivers should be encouraged to complete the initial immunization series in a timely manner to protect their child from infectious diseases.
2. **Nutrition:** Calorie and nutrient requirements increase with age. So the caretaker should consider for child's appetite, choices and motor skills.
3. **Elimination:** The nurse should educate parents about the signs of readiness for toilet training, which include the ability to demonstrate cognitive awareness of elimination.
4. **Hygiene:** Toddlers are usually bathed either everyday or every other day, depending on their activity and state of cleanliness. It is always important to check the temperature of the bath, water with a thermometer if possible.
5. **Dental health:** An important aspect of the visit is assessment of oral health, education of caretaker regarding correct methods of dental hygiene and counseling on strategies to prevent caries.
6. **Rest and sleep:** Most 2–year-old requires 12–14 hours of sleep each day with one or two naps a day. Nightmare is also common in toddlerhood, since their dreams seem very real.
7. **Safety and injury prevention:** Prevent can be done through parent education and child protection.

PRESCHOOLERS

The preschool years span 3-6. Although physical growth slows, this is a time characterized by reinforcement of the cognitive and social skill begun during the toddler years. The preschooler establishes control of body systems as indicated by the ability to toilet, dress and feed self and is also able to tolerate longer periods of separation from caregivers and interact cooperatively with adult and other children.

CHARACTERISTICS OF PRESCHOOLER

1. **Period of slow and steady growth:** Where the preschooler is the period of rapid and intensive growth the stage of childhood is characterized as the period of slow, steady and uniform growth occurs.
2. **Independence:** Infact at this stage child feels more at home with the world and takes satisfaction by doing his/her work with his/her own efforts. By acquiring experiences and developing physically and socially he/she tries to adjust in the environment.
3. **Emotional stability and control:** The preschoolers exercise control over their emotions and express them in appropriate and socially approved ways. Child emotional behavior is not guided by instinctive causes, but has an appropriate notion behind it.
4. **Developing social tendency:** Children like to play in group and share their toys with others. Feeling of mutual cooperation, team spirit and group loyalties are developed among children of their age.
5. **Realistic attitude:** Child at this stage begins to accept and appreciate the hard realities in place of imaginative idealist. Child begins to take close interest in the world of realities and tries to adapt himself/herself in real environment.
6. **Formation of sentiments and complexes:** The child at this stage is not in the habit of hiding the feelings and checking his/her emotions. Therefore no complexes are formed at this stage of childhood. At this stage of preschooler's emotional behavior get itself structured into sentiments. Various sentiments like religious, moral, patriotic and aesthetic sentiments began to develop at this stage.

PHYSICAL DEVELOPMENT

1. **Biological growth:** Preschooler children grow relatively slow; they become taller and thinner without gaining much weight.
2. **Weight and height:** The preschooler gains approximately 1.8 kg per year. At age of 3 years, the child weighs an average of 14.4 kg and at 5 years, the average weight is 18.3 kg.
3. **Baby proportions:** The typical preschooler looks more like adult than does the toddler because of skeletal maturation. The head and neck continue to decrease in proportion to the size of the rest of the body. The lower extremities grow faster than the head, trunk and arms.
4. **Cardiovascular system:** By age 4 years, heart size is four times of birth size and is now similar to that of the adult heart. Murmurs may be discovered during the late preschooler's period.

5. **Blood values:** During the preschooler's years, fat replaces the red marrow of the long bones. The total leukocyte count is slight higher: 5000–13000 from 4 to 6 years of age.
6. **Respiratory system:** With growth, the length of structures in the respiratory tract has increased and the incidence of infections decreases.
7. **Gastrointestinal system:** The process of digestion is mature at this time, but the gastrointestinal system is vulnerable to stress, which may be manifested by mild to moderate dysfunction.
8. **Genitourinary system:** The urinary system is nearly mature by age 5 years. The urine output in the age group is 600–750 mL/24 h. Daytime bladder control is achieved by the end of the preschooler period, with nightmare control still variable.
9. **Immune system:** Adult level of immunoglobulin A (IgA) are reached during the preschool years. Also children develop antibodies to the agents they are exposed to and to the normal flora in their body.
10. **Nervous system:** By 5 years of age, the nervous system comprises 1/20th of the total body weight. Cerebral dominance is achieved, as demonstrated by the acquisition of handedness.
11. **Motor development:** As children use their muscles, muscle fibers increase in strength and size. Coordination and the ability to voluntary control movements are increased significantly, allowing them to refine their skills.

EMOTIONAL DEVELOPMENT

1. The preschoolers watch adults and attempt to imitate their behavior.
2. Imagination and creativity allow them to fantasize, trying-out roles and behaviors.
3. Preschool children look forward to becoming like their father and mothers. They learn adult roles from their parents, who serve as role models for behavior.
4. A feeling of conflicts may also arise from thoughts, the child realizes actions were not appropriate. Feeling of guilt may also arise from thoughts that the child has different from expected behaviors.
5. The goal of caregivers during period is to assist children to learn about the world and other people. With this help, preschooler gradually modifies their egocentricity.

SEXUAL DEVELOPMENT

1. Sexual energy, generally, at this stage remains dominant, but merges with great forces at the end of the stage.
2. The sexual behavior of the children at this stage is characterized by the development of an attitude of antagonism and indifference toward opposite sex.

3. While this stages the boys and girls play together, they wish to play with the members of their own sex.
4. Due to their varied interests they gradually develop a general attitude of antagonism toward the sexes naturally draws apart. Even when brought together in family gathering boys and girls of this age are barely civil to one another.
5. Sex antagonism more pronounced in boys than in the case of girls, the attitude of antagonism, generally takes the form of indifference.

COGNITIVE DEVELOPMENT

1. During Piaget's preoperational stage, between the ages of 2 and 6 years, the child develops the ability to perform mental operations governed by personal perceptions and linkage to events previously experienced.
2. At this stage the children acquire new experiences and tries to adopt themselves in their environment and prepares themselves to solve the problems.
3. The preschooler gains power of reasoning, thinking observation, concentration, perception, imagination, etc. are developed.
4. Child develops the concept of length, time and distance; and learns to express himself/herself in various ways.
5. The preschooler uses a personal system for organizing objects and events in his/her mind and reasons from one particular to another, often by unrelated events, when in reality the particulars are not linked at all.

MORAL DEVELOPMENT

1. The child's moral development is at the most basic level and right and wrong are determined from rules parents have established.
2. Preschoolers conform to rules strictly for the purpose self-interest, that is to avoid punishment and to have favors returned.
3. According to Kohlberg, moral growth occurs in specific sequences of developmental stages that are preconventional or premoral stage.

SPIRITUAL DEVELOPMENT

1. Preschool children continue in Fowler's stage of intuitive—projective faith.
2. The preschooler has a concrete conception of God, who has physical characteristics and can understand simple religious stories.
3. The preschool children accept the religion of their parents because for them, parents are omnipotent and powerful.
4. Preschool children are old enough to go to Sunday school. Any discussion of religion should be shared experience between parents and their children.

LANGUAGE AND SPEECH DEVELOPMENT

1. Preschool children use language in a symbolic way. They not only imitate sounds at this stage but also use words to represent things.
2. Language is used by preschoolers to communicate their feelings and ideas. They consistently ask questions and learn about the outside world by seeking the meaning of what they experience through sensory stimulates.
3. Preschool children use progressively longer and more complex sentences and their vocabulary grows rapidly.
4. An analysis of child's questions shows a need for information, for relief from anxiety and for attention.
5. Preschoolers delight in trying out a variety of words. They are unconcerned about the consequences of language and are prone to pick up words that parents may prefer, they not to have their vocabulary.

PLAY ACTIVITIES

1. Play facilitates the development of an optional self-identity by establishment of an imaginary friend, which helps a child work through a particular different time.
2. Activities that promote small muscle development encourages a child's creativity and fine motor skills.
3. Preschool children play actively, they climb, run, hammer, open doors with a bang; and slam them shut.
4. The repetitive play of preschool children is an imitation of the life about them. Many play themes stem from a confusion in children's minds about experiences they have had a real life.
5. The children need to be encouraged to express their own creativity rather than fitting them within a mold of adult expectation. They should be allowed and encouraged to play with toys of their choice independent of gender, role, designation.

NURSE'S ROLE IN HEALTH PROMOTION

1. **Nutrition:** Preschooler needs to eat only one-half as much as adult. The daily requirements range from 1,300 to 1,700 calories including 30g proteins. The preschoolers enjoy five meals a day to keep up with energy demand. Food should be selected from the basic four food groups, with a limit of 16 ounces of milk daily.
2. **Accident prevention:** During the preschool years the child begins to explore outside the home and into the neighborhood. It is also important to remember that the preschool aged child is less reckless, will listen more to rules and is aware of potential dangers such as hot objects, sharp instruments or dangerous heights.

3. **Hygiene:** Many preschooler enjoy their bath time, but the parental assistance may be needed for hair washing, and cleaning finger nails and ears.
4. **Dental health:** The number one dental problem during this time is dental caries, which may cause the premature loss of teeth and a consequent alteration of dental arch, compromising development of the permanent teeth. The preschool child should visit a dentist at least 6 months.
5. **Rest and sleep:** The preschooler sleep a total of 12 hours a day. Preschoolers may have difficulty sleeping in a dark, a proper parental support and guidance is essential during time.

SCHOOL CHILD

1. The phase of development from 6 to 12 years, the school-age years, is crucial to establishing positive self-esteems, a sense of belonging and feeling of competence. The school children gain new ideas from adults outside the family, teacher, parents of their friends, policeman and women, television performers, newspaper writers and authors of textbooks with those of their parents.
2. School children learn to think of themselves as person in their own right may resent limits that parents continue to improve on their behavior. Parents need help in understanding the normal growth and development of their child when conflicts areises.Today child can experience the world beyond the classroom with the help of the internet, electronic mail, educational video tapes and cable television.

PHYSICAL GROWTH AND DEVELOPMENT

Biological Growth

1. Weight and height during the school years show a sex related difference. Boys tend to gain slightly more weight through 12 years.
2. The yearly height gain is similar in boys and girls, although boys tend to be taller.

CARDIOVASCULAR SYSTEM

1. The heart assumes a more vertical position in the chest because of left ventricular development and downward placement of the diaphragm.
2. Heart murmur peak during 6–9 years of age.

IMMUNE SYSTEM

1. The immune system continues to develop; response to infection is specific and localized.
2. Normal adult levels of the immunoglobulins are reached during the school years.

3. The increased amount of lymphatic tissue in the nasopharynx continues to cause blockage of the eustachian tube.
4. As the child reaches puberty and the amount of lymphatic tissue decreases, ear infection decreases in direct proportion.

NERVOUS SYSTEM

1. By 10 years of age, the nervous system is essentially mature.
2. The maturity is evident in the sensory and motor functions as well as in the cognitive process.

SENSORY DEVELOPMENT

1. By the time the child reaches the age of 6 years, central visual acuity is established.
2. At age 7 years, visual acuity should be 20/20, which is the adult level.
3. The accommodative and refractive powers of the eye also reach stability.
4. The sense of taste and smell fully mature prior to the school years, allows for greater discrimination.

SKELETOMUSCULAR DEVELOPMENT

1. Skeletal growth is particularly noticeable in the long bones of the extremities. Growing pain, which occur because the long bone grows faster than the attached muscles.
2. Muscle strength and size also increase at a gradual rate during school-age years and six basic gross motor skills such as balancing, catching, throwing, and running, jumping, climbing, continue to be refined.
3. At the same time, improved balance and coordination enable the school-aged child to explore new physical activities such as bike riding and roller lading.
4. Boys have a greater number of muscle cells than girls, so it is common to find they do well gross motor activities such as throwing and running.

MOTOR DEVELOPMENT

1. Motor development progress in a cephalocaudal and proximal to distal direction, with reinforcement of both gross motor and fine motor skills occurring as the central nervous system matures.
2. The developmental theory of Erik Erikson identified the major task of the school-age period as identity versus inferiority.
3. During this time, energy is channeled into activities such as school projects, sports and bobbies. The school–age child also develops the ability to work with others on school projects and athletic terms in preparation for becoming a citizen of the world.
4. School children must grow out of the dependency on their family and must find satisfaction in the company of peer groups and adults outside the home environment.

5. During the school years the child develops whole some attitudes toward set as a person and learns the appropriate masculine or feminine social role.

PSYCHOSEXUAL DEVELOPMENT

1. Freud believed that, starting at age 6 years and throughout school age, the child enters a calm period in the development of their sexuality called latency.
2. Freud theorized the school-aged child identified with the same sex parent by modeling the behaviors and emotional of this parent and learned about sex-role behavior and identify by observing caregiver instructions, the media and friendship with children of the same gender.
3. School-age children become much less ecocentric and direct their energies beyond themselves. During the early latency period children associate with same sex peers and tend to ignore members of the same age and tend to draw apart from them.
4. Boys and girls should be informed about the reproductive cycle and their respective roles as they approach puberty.

SPIRITUAL DEVELOPMENT

1. In school years, Fowler identified school children as being in the mythic-literal faith stage.
2. During these years, children are learning many specifics about their children that will develop into a religious philosophy to be used in their interpretation of the world.
3. As children reach pubescence, they begin to be less mythical in their thinking and their beliefs are more controlled by reason.
4. As the child enters preadolescence, he/she realizes self-centered prayers are not always answered and there is no magic involved in religious beliefs, blind faith that previously existed in the younger child is replaced by reason.

COGNITIVE DEVELOPMENT

1. Piaget suggested that around 6 years of age children start to move from the egocentric view of the preschool age to the more open and flexible thought of the school-aged child.
2. By 7–11 years during concrete operational stage characterized by considerable growth in thinking, imagination and language, which allows school-age children to expand and understand their world.
3. School-age children are increasingly able to classify objects in a more complex manner then they could during the preschool years.
4. The school children mental ability permits them to carry on converse and reverse process. They can solve problems because they can manipulate symbols.

5. During the school age periods, children think not only of the present but also the past and future. Since children can recall events that happened in the past, they become aware that exist over a period of time.

MORAL DEVELOPMENT

1. The school-aged child is at the conventional level of moral development, when the conscience develops an internal set of 'rules' that must be followed in order to 'be good'.
2. During third stage of moral development, the child's morality is based on avoiding the disapproval of others and maintaining a positive relationship with friends, family and teachers.
3. Children at this level can also demonstrate rigid behavior in an effort to obey the law. These children can take into account circumstances surrounding and incident rather than just looking at the result.

LANGUAGE AND SPEECH DEVELOPMENT

1. During this period of development, children show tremendous growth in their ability to use words.
2. They extend their vocabulary by 20,000–30,000 words.
3. Their sentence structure and use of grammar continue to improve and the use if adjectives and pronouns increases.
4. Speech proceeds from egocentric to social. The unique culture of their children is reflects in language acquisition and speech patterns.

PLAY ACTIVITIES

1. Plays activities vary with age, number of play activities decreases, whereas the amount of time spent in one particular activity increases.
2. Likes games with rules because of increased mental abilities.
3. Likes games of athletic competition because of increased motor ability.
4. Play serves as a learning tool for children and their play changes with developmental needs.
5. Play becomes more formal, more organized, more competitive and to a degreeless physical active.
6. Parent can assist their school children with learning the rules of organized sports. Although parents may not attending sports events and others activities in which their children participate.

MENTAL ABILITIES OF SCHOOL CHILDREN

1. Readiness for learning, especially in perceptual organization—names months of year, knows right from left, can tell time; can follow several directions at once.
2. Acquires use of reason and understanding of rules, needs consistency.
3. Trial-and-error problem solving become more conceptual rather than action oriented.
4. Reasoning ability allows greater understanding and use of language.

NURSE'S ROLE IN HEALTH PROMOTION

Nutrition

1. Children aged 7–10 years require 80 calories per kilogram of body weight.
2. After age in years through adolescence, boys require more protein and iron.
3. Careful meal and physical activity are crucial for the physical and emotional health of the school aged child.

Accident Prevention

1. Factors contributing to the high incidence of accidents for this group are their increased independence, desire to have peer approach and increased involvement in physically challenging activities.
2. Most accidents are related to motor vehicles, but firearm injuries continue to increase in incidence. The second most frequent cause of accidental death is drowning.
3. Accidents also occur when children are skating, skateboarding or riding a bicycle or mini-bike.

Elimination

1. School children are old enough to attend school all day, they have learned to control and independently care for their own elimination patterns.
2. Usually stools are well-formed and school-aged children have one to two stools per day. The amount of urine passed is depended on intake of water content, temperature, time of the day and child's emotional state.

Hygiene

1. Children older than 6–7 years of age are capable of caring out their own personal hygiene practices daily and by the time when they are 8 to 9 years can be held responsible for independely bathing, grooming, dressing and properly discarding their sold clothing.
2. As children become more aware of changes in their bodies are they reach late school age, they begin to take more interest in and are more reliable in their own grooming, and cleanliness.

Dental Health

1. Dental caries resulting from poor nutrition is still a significant problem in the school-age population. Raw sugars and candies are common contributors to the development of dental caries.
2. Dental checkups are recommended every 6 months, the school system should incorporate a dental health educational program into the curriculum.

Sleep and Rest

1. A 6-year-old child may need 11–12 hours of sleep, whereas a 12-year-old generally needs only 10 hours.
2. Sleep is essential during the school-age years to foster physical growth and academic performance, and failure to receive adequate rest can lead to irritability and lack of attention span at school.
3. Nightmares and night terrors are less common during the school-age years.

Sex Education

1. Sex education is important and that school–age children be educated about pubertal changes and responsible sexual practices.
2. Sex education should be incorporated into health education throughout the school years in a manner that is appropriate to age and development.

COMMON PROBLEMS ASSOCIATED WITH SCHOOL CHILDREN

School Phobia

1. School phobia is fear of attending school. It is a type of 'social phobia' similar to agoraphobia (fear of going outside the home).
2. Children who resist attending school this way may develop physical signs of illness such as vomiting, diarrhea, headache or abdominal pain on school days.
3. The causes of resistance to school, the child may be over dependent on the parents or may be reluctant to leave home because he/she feels that younger siblings will usurp the parent affection while he/she is at school.
4. Handling school phobia requires coordination among the school, school nurse and healthcare providers, who diagnoses the problem.
5. The nurse is the ideal person to coordinate such efforts and to help the parent allow the child some independence not only in going to school but in other activities.

Stealing

1. During early school age, most children go through a period in which they steal loose change from their mother's purse or father's dresser.
2. This usually happens at around 7 years of age, when they are learning how to make change and discovering the importance of money.
3. Youngsters, who continue to steal, may require counseling, because they should have progressed beyond this normal development step by this age.

Recreational Drug Use

1. Recreational drug use was once considered a college or high school problem, is now a problem of school age. Illegal drugs are available

to children as early as elementary school and certainly by the time they reach the seventh or eight grades.

2. Alcohol is available in so many homes and often can be purchased in small stores without proof of age, it is a commonly abused drug of this age group. Cocaine is becoming increasingly easy for children to obtain.
3. Parents should suspect of recreational drug use if their child regularly appears irritable, inattentive or drowsy. School health personnel should be aware of the increase in this practice among students and look for warning signs.
4. Children need to be counseled against this because the recreational drug use leads to cardiovascular irregularities, uncontrollable aggressiveness and possible cancer in later life.
5. Both nurses and parents should be role models of excellent health behaviors when earning for school-age children.

Obesity

1. Many perteenagers, particularly boys, become overweight. Some have been overweight since infancy their propubertal nutral weight gain makes them obese.
2. Obese children begin to develop many of the same health problems as obsess adults such as hypertension and elevated total cholesterol level with possible atherosclerosis.
3. A weight reduction program for school-age children that emphasis long term life changes such as intake about 1200 calories low in fat and designed to reduce weight, active exercise program and counseling program.

ADOLESCENT

Adolescent is the time period between 13 years and 18–20 years, which serves as a transitional period between childhood and adulthood. It is a time of explosion, excitement and discovery; and sometimes confusion; and despair. Adolescent consist of early, middle and late stages. Each is distinguishing by several aspects of adolescent lives and constitutes the ages 12–14, 15–17 and 18–21years.

PHYSICAL GROWTH AND DEVELOPMENT

weight and Height

Most of the girls are 1–2 inches taller than boys coming in to adolescence and generally stop growing within 3 years from menarche. Thus, those girls who start menstruating at 10 years of age may reach their adult height by age 13 years.

Musculoskeletal Development

1. Significant changes occur in skeletal size, muscle mass, skin and adipose tissue. Full bone length is first reached in the extremities and moves inwards.
2. The skeletal system grows faster than the muscles and muscle mass increases more rapidly than the heart size.

Teeth

1. Adolescent gains their molars (wisdom teeth) between 18 and 21 years of age. The jaw reaches about size only toward the end of adolescence.
2. Adolescent, whose third molars erupt before the lengthening of the jaw is complete may experience pain and may need these molars extracted because they do not fit their jaw line.

Central Nervous System

1. Brain growth continues during adolescence, the cell that support and nourish the nervous proliferate even though the number of neurons does not increase.
2. Continued growth of myelin sheath allows faster neural processing and is reflected in the adolescent's increasing ability to think abstractly and hypothesize.

Cardiorespiratory Development

1. The heart almost doubles in weight and increase in the size by about one-half during adolescence.
2. The lung increases in length and diameter during adolescence and the respiratory rate averages 16–20 breaths per minute.
3. Males have greater capacity, volume and rate because their great shoulder width and chest size.
4. The slower of respiratory system growth relatives to the growth of other body system may be another cause of the inadequate oxygenation and fatigue sometimes experienced by adolescents.

Gastrointestinal System

1. Rapid maturation of the gastrointestinal system occurs during adolescence, and by the 21st birthday, all 32 teeth have erupted.
2. Gastric acidity and capacity increase up to 1,500 mL to accommodate and facilitate digestion of the increased food intake that occurs in response to rapid growth.

Genitourinary System Development

1. Secretion of neurohormonal releasing factors by the hypothalamus stimulates the anterior pituitary gland to release follicle-stimulating hormone (FSH) and luteinizing hormone (LH).

2. In females, FSH stimulates ovarian follicle growth and estrogen production. Estrogen causes breast changes including enlargement and darkening of the reproductive organs such as vagina, uterus, ovaries and growth and darkening of pubic and axillary hair.
3. In males, FSH is responsible for sperm production and maturation of the seminiferous tubules. LH promotes testicular maturation and testosterone production. Testosterone causes the musculoskeletal system and development of the male reproductive system.

Sexual Development

1. Adolescence is the physiologic period between the beginning of puberty and cessation of bodily growth.
2. Puberty is the stage of life at which secondary sex changes begin. Girls begin dramatic development and maturation of reproductive organs at approximately age of 10–13 years; for boys 12–14 years.
3. Androgenic hormones are responsible for muscular development, physical growth and increase in sebaceous gland secretions that cause typical acne in both boys and girls.
4. In girls pubertal changes typically occurs such as growth spurt, increase in the transverse diameter of the pelvis, breast development, growth of pubic hair, onset of maturation, growth of axillary hair and vaginal secretions.
5. The average age at which menarche (the first menstrual period) occurs is 12.5 years. It may occur as early as age as 9 or as late as age 17, however, still be within a normal age range.
6. A menstrual cycle can be defined as periodic uterine bleeding in response to cyclic hormonal changes. It is the process that allows for conception and implantation of a new life.
7. Education regarding menstruation is an important aspect of comprehensive sexuality education.

Psychosexual Development

1. According to Freud, the physical changes of puberty reawaken the sexual and aggressive energies felt toward parents during latency to late childhood.
2. Freud argued many psychological issues adolescents face are attributable to physiological changes.

Psychosocial Development

1. According to Erikson, the development ask of youngsters in early and midadolescence is to form a sense of identity. If the young person's do not achieve a sense of identity, they develop a sense of role confusion.

2. Body image: Adolescents, who developed a strong sense of industry during their school age have learned to solve problems and are best equipped to adjust to their new body image.
3. Value system: Adolescents need to be able to tasks to peers to develop values. They dress identically with other members of the group.
4. An important part of adolescents self-understanding is the value they place on their definition of who they are, which involves self- competency and self-worth.
5. According to Erikson, the youth who is not sure of his/her identity shies away from interpersonal intimacy or throw himself/herself into acts of intimacy, which may involved in intimate relations.

Cognitive Development

1. The final stage of cognitive development, the state of formal operations, begins at age 12–13 years and grows in depth over the adolescent years.
2. This step involves the ability to think in abstract terms and use the scientific method to arrive at conclusions. Problem solving in any situation depends on the ability to think abstractly and logically.
3. They can create a hypothesis and think through the probable consequences. Thinking abstractly is what allows adolescent to project themselves into the minds of others and imagine how others view them or their actions.
4. Another significant change is cognitive development. Adolescence generally becomes more sophisticated in their ability to understand words and their related concepts.
5. Another important aspect of adolescent's cognitive development is their broadening ability to assume another perspective.

Moral Development

1. Kohlberg's conventional level of moral reasoning, which has been shown to emerge during adolescence and to persist as the predominant stage of moral functioning through adulthood.
2. Adolescent male would likely reflect judgment-based reasoning of fourth stage thinking, whereas female adolescents would more likely reflect the relationship based on the third stage.
3. Abstract thinking—new level of social communication and understanding can comprehend satire and double meanings.

Spiritual Development

1. Almost all adolescent's question the existence of God and any religious practices they can taught.
2. This questioning is a part of forming a sense of identity and establishing a value system at a time in life when they draw away from their families.

3. Religious and scientific views are often compared as teens decide what is true more emphasis is placed on internal aspects of religious commitment rather than on attending church.
4. Adolescent's become more oriented toward spiritual and ideological matters and less oriented toward practice, rituals and strictly observing religious costumes.
5. The late adolescent tends to re-examine and re-evaluate the beliefs and values of childhood; and become more personalizes less bound to the traditional religious practices expressed to when younger.

HEALTH PROMOTION DURING ADOLESCENT

Nutrition

1. The nutrional objective is to provide nutritional support for demand of rapid growth and high energy expenditure.
2. Support development of appropriate eating habits through variety of foods, regular pattern and good quality snacks.
3. Nutrition education may be made through association with teenagers concerns about physical appearance, finger control, complexion, physical fitness, athletic ability.

Safety Measures

1. Accidents, most common those involving motor vehicles are the leading cause of death among adolescents.
2. Drowning is one of the chief accident and athletic injuries tend to occur during adolescence because of the vigorous level of competition that occur.
3. Appropriate education regarding sexual maturity, reproduction, sexual behavior, driver education, hazards associated with smoking, alcohol and drug abuse.

Elimination

1. The elimination patterns for adolescents are similar to adults. They should void an average of 700–1400 mL/day urine and have stool everyday.
2. Constipation in adolescents may be due to a physiological disorder, eating disorder or improper nutritional patterns.

Hygiene

1. Skin care is especially important during this age because of the increased activity of the sebaceous gland, which contributes to acne, increased sweat gland activity requires careful cleansing as well as the use of deodorant and body powders.
2. For female, menstrual hygiene is especially important and may require extra attention.

3. It is important to remind parents and other adult as well as the adolescent that these physical changes that may require more attention to hygiene are normal.

Dental Hygiene

1. Adolescents are generally very conscious about toothbrushing because of fear of developing bad breath.
2. During adolescents, malocclusion, gingivitis and dental trauma may occur. Malocclusion occurs due to dental crowding or mandibular/facial bone growth changes.
3. The dental teaching should include brushing the teeth at twice a day using a soft-bristled brush and fluoride toothpaste, flossing daily, eating a well-balanced diet and regular dental visits.

Rest and Sleep

1. Protein synthesis occurs most readily during sleep. Because of this, adolescents need proportionately more sleep than school-age children to support the growth spurt during this time, which demands the formation of so many new cells.
2. Nurses need to educate both parents and adolescents on the importance of adequate rest and sleep; and encourage teens to have realistic activity schedules that do not overextend their time.
3. An adolescent's excessive anxiety and fatigue may also result in sleep disturbances, which can continue into adulthoods since adult sleep cycles and habits are formed during adolescent.

HEALTH PROBLEMS DURING ADOLESCENTS

Alcohol Abuse

1. Alcoholism and alcohol abuse in adolescence are increasing. Many adolescents, who do drink use it as a mind altering device since it allows participation in risk-taking activities, they might otherwise avoid.
2. There are numerous hazards of alcohol ingestion. Some may be seen in adolescents including hepatitis, pancreatitis, gastritis and neuritis and cirrhosis, ulcer of gastrointestinal tract, cerebellar degeneration and delirium termers.
3. Parents and nurses with adolescents who abuse or other mind altering drugs and their family members need to explain about detrimental effects.

Homosexuality

1. Nurses need to recognize that even though many young people explore their own sexual orientation or homosexual attractions, few who engage in homosexual behavior during adolescents, continue the practice into adulthood.

2. Nurses and caregivers recognize that homosexual experimentation is not the same as establishing homosexual orientations, acknowledge same bisexual relationships and attractions, and phrase questions about sexuality and sexual activity carefully.

Suicide

1. The number of adolescents committing suicide has increased dramatically over the last few decades.
2. Stresses related to physiosocial, physiosexual or physiological issues have been identified as cause for the increasing number of adolescent suicides.
3. Risk factors of adolescents are previous history of suicide, family history of psychiatric disorders, living without home, history of physical or sexual abuse, unable to meet scholastic expectations of parents and teachers.
4. Suicide programs for teens should be directed at school staff, community agency personnel and students themselves by providing information relative to warning signs, fact and programs, which can enhance self-esteem and social competence.

ADULTHOOD

The young and middle adulthood is a period of challenges, rewards and crises. Challenges may include the demand of work and raising families, although adult can also be rewarded by successes in their carrier endeavors and in their personal lives. Adult development involves orderly changes in characteristics and attitudes. Developmental changes are based on earlier characteristics help to shape subsequent behavior and characteristics.

CONCEPTS OF YOUNG ADULTHOOD

1. Young adulthood is the period between the late teens and the mid to late 30s.
2. During young adulthood, individuals increasingly separate from their families of origin, establishing carrier goals and decide whether to marry and begin families or remain single.
3. Young adults are active and must adopt to new experiences. The transition into middle age occurs when young persons become aware that changes in reproductive and physical abilities signify the beginning of another stage in life.
4. Middle age is a time of continuing transitions when individuals may reassess their goals in life and add new goals.
5. The adult face such crises as caring for their aging parents, possibilities of job loss in a changing economic environment and dealing with their own developmental needs as well as their family members.

MATURITY DEVELOPMENTAL TASK

1. People are said to have reached maturity when they have reached a balance of growth in physiological, psychological and cognitive areas.
2. Matured individual feels comfortable with abilities, knowledge and responses that they have developed over the years.
3. They look at the world with a broad view, based on a blend of insight, emotion and imagination. They take problems that can be solved but recognize and learn it live with unsolvable problems.
4. Mature people are open to suggestion and can accept constructive criticism without a major loss of self-esteem.
5. They weigh other person's input and recommendations what making decisions, but are not overly influenced or intimated by others, above all, mature people develop by learning from their own and other experiences
6. Other characteristics of maturity are related to interpersonal communication or behavior.
7. Mature person acknowledge accomplishments and shortcoming. The mature adults confront tasks openly, use decision-making techniques to solve problems and are accountable and responsible for their actions.

THEORIES OF YOUNG ADULTHOOD

Levinson's Phases of Young and Middle Adult Development

1. Early adult transition (ages 18–20) when the person separates from the family and desires independence.
2. Entrance into the adult world (ages 21–27) when the persons prepares for and tries out career and lifestyles.
3. Transition (ages 28–32) when the person may greatly modify life activities and thinks about future goals.
4. Setting down (ages 33–39), when the person experiences greater stability.
5. The payoff years (ages 40–65), a time for maximal influence, self direction and appraisal.

Gilligan's (1993) Intellectual and Moral Development

1. Gilligan's theory proposes that intellectual and moral development differ between men and women.
2. Women struggle with the issues of care and responsibility; and in turn their relationships progress toward a maturity of interdependence.
3. As women progress toward adulthood, the moral dilemma changes from how to exercise their right without interfering in the right of others to how to lead a normal life, which includes obligations to themselves and their families; and people in general.

Gordon (1991)

1. As women entered professional areas, they hoped to develop the caring and nurturing roles in their male colleagues.

2. Women have long recognized that, without caring, the perceived quality of life is changed. As a result women maintained caring in the home and educational frustrated in their development.
3. However, women become frustrated in their development because the responsibility of caring was not shared and frequently nurturing become a gender-specific responsibilities,.

Diekelmann's Developmental Tasks

1. Young adults alive independence from parental controls.
2. They begin to develop strong friendship and intimate relationships, and intimate relationships outside the family.
3. They establish personal set values.
4. They develop a sense of personal identity.
5. They prepare for lifework and develop the capacity for intimacy.

PHYSIOLOGICAL DEVELOPMENT

1. The young adult has completed physical growth by the age of 20. The young adult usually quite active, experience severe illnesses less commonly than older adults.
2. A personal life assessment of the young adult includes assessment of general life satisfaction, hobbies and interests.

COGNITIVE DEVELOPMENT

1. Rational thinking habits increase steadily through the young and middle adult years. Fromal and informal educational experiences, general life experiences and occupational opportunities dramatically increase the individual's conceptual, problem-solving and motor skills.
2. Identifying preferred occupational areas is a major task of young adults. When people known their educational preparation, skills, talents and personality characteristics, occupational choceies are easier and they generally more satisfied with their choices.
3. The young adults are continually evolving and adjusting to changes in the home, work place and personal lives their decision-making processes should be flexible.

PSYCHOSOCIAL DEVELOPMENT

1. The young adult is usually caught between wanting to prolong the irresponsibility of adolescence and wanting to assume adult commitments.
2. The years from 35 to 43 are the time of vigorous examination of life goals, relationships; alterations are made in personal, social and occupational lives.
3. During young adults, people generally give more attention to occupational and social pursuits. During this period individuals attempt top improve their socioeconomic status.

4. During young adult, they take major decisions concerning career, marriage and parenthood.

HEALTH PROMOTION DURING YOUNG ADULT

1. Young adult lifestyles may put them at risk for illnesses or disabilities during their middle or older adult tears. Young adults may also be genetically susceptible to certain chronic disease such as diabetes mellitus and familial hyperchostermia.
2. Violence is the greater cause of mortality and morbidity in the young adult population. Death and injury can occur from physical assault, motor vehicle or other accidents, and suicidal attempts.
3. Intoxicated young adults may be severely injured in motor vechiel accidents that may result in death or permanent disability to other young adults as well.
4. Sexually transmitted diseases have immediate effects such as dischare, discomfort and infection. They may also lead to chronic disorders, which can result from genital herpes, infertility, gonorrhea or even death.

OLDER ADULT

Geriatrics, the care of aged, aging is a normal process of time-related change that occurs throughout life. It involves all aspects of the organism and is largely characterized by decline in functional efficiency and decreased capacity to compensate and recover from stress. It does not necessarily occur in an inter-related or synchronous manner, but it does involve physiological, psychological and social changes that interact to influence behavior and adaptation.

CONCEPTS OF OLD AGE

1. Old age is a normal part of human development and is the final phase of the life cycle.
2. Aging is not something that happens to the other person, but is a unique and highly personal experience that affects everyone who lives long enough.
3. Successful adaptation to the aging process probably correlates with the person's previous ability to cope and adopt to change.
4. Other influences include environmental factors, education and socio-cultural determinants as well as the health status of the entire body.
5. Gerontology, the study of the aging process and its effects on older persons, become more important with each passing day.

DEVELOPMENTAL THEORIES OF OLD AGE

1. Certain theoretical models of human development help to point out important turning points during the late years of the cycle.

2. The theories concerning the life cycle incorporate the social, psychological and biological factors of developmental growth and relate them to age to identity milestones and time development.
3. The theories of Buhler, Jung and Erikson, which are considered to be three of the most prominent theories of adult development, have as a common theme, the goal of personal resolution in the second half of life.
4. Buhler's theories perceived that the period from 65 on is one of awareness of the experience of fulfillment or failure and the remaining years are spend in either a continuance of previous activities or a return to the need satisfying orientations of childhood.
5. Jung suggested that in the second half of life the individual direct his/her attention inward, so that through an intensive inner exploration he/she may find a meaning and totality in life that makes the acceptance of death possible.
6. Erikson's theory explains that the years between 40 and 50, challenge those values that a person places on physical power in favor of the value placed on wisdom. People who cling to their waning physical powers becoming more and more depressed, but persons who shift to using their mental abilities as a primary resource appear to age more successfully.
7. The theorists view the first part of life as growth and expansion; and the later part of life as inner withdrawal and contraction.
8. The task of later life involves finding meaning and wholeness in life and considerations about oncoming death.

KINDS OF AGE

Biological Aging

1. Aging occurs with such changes as whitening of the hair, wrinkling of the skin, decline in eye focus and high-register hearing.
2. Biological aging depends on a combination of factors, including genetic inheritance, finances and good health.
3. The most serious change for most people is their heightened vulnerability to and lessened ability to recuperate from various illnesses.

Psychological Aging

1. Psychological aging refers to a role the individual assigns to himself/herself as he/she reaches a certain chronological age.
2. The two major threat felt by the older persons are the deterioration of his/her concept of self, which results in loss of self-esteem and extensive and continual grief over frequently occurring losses.
3. The plight of the aged in the youth-oriented society continues to receive attention and the process of gerontological counseling is now recognized as a specialized form of helping.

4. The older people should encourage seeing themselves as in a dynamic period of growth rather than in a period of rapid deterioration. The older person, for the most part, wishes to be treated as a person on worth and dignity.

Sociogenic Aging

1. Society imposes role on people as they reach a certain chronological age. Older persons are seen by many people in our society as either nonpeople or expendable people, merely because they lived longer.
2. Older people have been told by our society that they are supposed to be physically, socially, sexually and intellectually infirm–slow in comprehending events going on around them and rigid in their ways of thinking and behaving.
3. Society also seems to take the attitude that older people should run away and hide until they die. It is important to note the combination of psychological than biological aging for many people.

PHYSIOLOGICAL CHANGES DURING OLD AGE

Changes in Homeostasis

1. Homeostasis is the body's ability to maintain a stable internal environment. The complex mechanism of homeostasis regulates fluid and electrolyte balance, blood pressure, temperature and food intake.
2. Man is dependent upon the functional integrity of the cell and the stability of the internal environment. If the homeostatic mechanisms are functioning properly, the body is able to adopt or react stress.
3. However, with aging these mechanisms become less efficient and reserve power is lost. This in turn makes the person more vulnerable to disease. Recovery is also affected since more time is required for the body return to normal after illness.

Changes in the Nervous System

1. The nervous system is extremely vulnerable to the aging process, as seen in the progressive loss of cells that occurs with advancing years.
2. There are approximately half as many brain cells in the frontal area at age 80 as at 40, with resulting decrease in brain weight.
3. The steady loss of neurons begins surprisingly early in life and affects both brain and spinal cord. There is also a decrease in the blood flow to the brain.
4. Both physiologic changes in the brain and the reduced blood supply may be related to personality changes sometimes encountered elderly.

Changes in Special Senses

1. The aging process produces varying degree of impairment in hearing, vision, smell, taste and pain perception as well as diminished sensation of touch and slowing reflexes.
2. Decreased in the sense of smell and in the number of taste buds at times contributes to a loss of appetite.
3. Diminished sensitivity to thirst needs can lead to dehydration and confused behavior as a result of fluid balance.
4. Hearing impairment, which usually is first noticed in the higher frequencies, can result in impairment of speech discrimination and loss of the full sense of background noises.
5. Vision is affected by a decrease in visual acuity and accommodation to glare and by a marked diminution of night vision and peripheral field of vision.
6. Perception of some types of pain decreases and referral of pain from one part of the body to another seems to become more common with advancing age.
7. The temperature-regulating mechanisms are less reliable and heat-generating activities are reduced.

Cardiovascular Changes

1. In older people, the heart is able to pump effectively under normal circumstances, but because it lacks much of its physiological reserve, it reaches poorly to sudden stress such as blood loss, excessive parenteral fluids or sudden effort.
2. When normal homeostasis is upset, congestive heart failure, arrhythmias and myocardial ischemia may develop.
3. The signs of arteriosclerosis become clinically recognizable when it has reached advanced stage in the elderly.

Respiratory Changes

1. Most of the changes that occur in pulmonary function in the aged result from loss of elastic tissue surrounding the alveoli and alveolar ducts and from changes in the anteroposterior of the chest owing to rib and vertebral calcification.
2. There is also changes in the tissues of the lungs and decline in its functional capacity, size and structure as well as weakening of the respiratory muscles.
3. Vital capacity becomes reduced while there is a concurrent increase in residual volume. Changes in the pulmonary vasculature also occur.

Changes in the Kidney Function

1. Kidney function decline with age because of a reduction in the number of glomeruli and diminished filtration; and tubular function.

2. The blood flow to the kidney is reduced as a result of decreased cardiac output and increased peripheral resistance.

Metabolic Changes

1. As the body ages, the basal metabolic rate slows and the quantity of oxygen used by the tissue is reduced.
2. As metabolic processes change, the glucose tolerance curve tends toward that of the diabetic. If normal standards for glucose tolerance tests were applied to the aged, 50% of this population would be classified as diabetes.

Musculosketal Changes

1. Generally, there is a slow and steady atrophy of muscles that result in muscle wasting, particularly of the trunk and extremities.
2. With loss of muscle power there is a decrease in strength, endurance and agility.
3. Bones gradually lose calcium and bone porous; and lighter, because bone become more brittle, falls are especially dangerous in the elderly.
4. Ligaments calcify and ossify; and joints become stiffened from erosions of cartilaginous joint surfaces. Changes in the lining of joint cavities can produce degenerative changes.

Skin and Connective Tissue Changes

1. The skin is among the first structures to show the most obvious associated with aging.
2. As the person ages, there is loss of subcutaneous supporting tissue and resultant thinning of the skin. With the loss of subcutaneous fat, the skin assumes the characteristic appearance of aging—folds, lines, wrinkles and slackness.
3. The dermis become relatively dehydrated and loses strength and elasticity. The skin in general is prone to excess dryness and itching.
4. As a preventive measure, older people should avoid overexposure to the sun, which tends to accelerate aging of the skin and increases the tendency to skin cancer.

Reproductive Changes

1. Physiologic changes occurring with menopause can affect sexual function and activity in older women. Atrophy of the vaginal canal and diminished vaginal secretions can lead to local irritation, bleeding and pain with sexual activity.
2. In older male, there may be diminished and delayed ability to achieve a full penile erection and a reduction in the frequency associated with psychological changes.

HEALTH PROMOTION MEASURES FOR ELDERS

Health Appraisal

1. Varied health assessment techniques can be implemented to help detect and identify elderly people at risk.
2. Many authorities believe that a comprehensive physical examination, including blood examinations, urinalysis and stool test should be carried out annually.
3. Assessment of health habits is necessary as a basis for health counseling. Positive measures for maintaining health include weight control, exercise, proper nutrition, avoidance of cigarette smoking and protection of accident prevention.

Nutritional Support

1. Dietary inadequacies in the elderly results from factors such as poor nutritional habits, economic constrains and underlying disease condition.
2. Nutrition can have a tremendous impact on health maintenance and disease prevention as well as on the treatment of disease.
3. Older people are vulnerable to low nutrient intake. Dietary studies show that calcium, thiamine, ascorbic acid and vitamin A are the nutrients, most commonly lacking in the diets of the aged.
4. The addition of moderate amount of fiber to the diet may alleviate constipation and flatulence. The high incidence of osteoporosis in older women seems to be age related.
5. Other factors contributing to nutritional deficiencies are social isolation, lack of interest in cooking and eating, and problems in food shopping.

Exercise

1. Activity is one key to the prevention of premature aging. Many of the health problems of the aged arise from a lack of conditioning and diminished response to stress.
2. Exercise maintains muscular tone throughout the body and is effective in the prevention of premature aging and rehabilitation following cardiovascular diseases.
3. Exercise training improves functional capabilities, increase vitality and has psychological benefits.

Temperature Regulation

1. Older people cannot tolerate a cold environment and are very susceptible to hyperthermia. The nursing approach is to provide extra blankets may be added for warmth.
2. Efforts are directed to maintain heat and humidity at comfortable levels by fans, air conditioning and humidifiers or dehumidifiers during hot weather.

Hygienic Care

1. With aging, the skin becomes thin and inelastic, predisposing the elderly patient to prevent pressure sores.
2. For elderly people, foot care is essential in order to maintain mobility, physical well-being and independence. A common foot disorder of this age group includes calluses, bunions, toenail problems, corns and fungus infections.
3. The components of dental care for the aging patients include eating a proper diet, maintaining oral health and denture-bearing structure, being motivated to speak proper care and having adequate dental services available.
4. Problems of constipation and bowel incontinence often can be reduced through systematic habit training. Constipation occurs because of altered mobility, decreased mucus secretion and changes in muscle tone and elasticity of the colon, as well as changes in diet.

Recreation

Recreation is more than just having fun; it is fundamental to physical and mental well-being. No matter how old or disabled one becomes, the desire for the dignity that comes only through purposeful activity is never lost.

COMMON HEALTH PROBLEMS OF ELDERLY

Disease and Aging

1. The aged are particularly vulnerable to disease because of such factors as it decreased physiological reserve, a less flexible homeostatic mechanism and lessened defensive mechanism of the body.
2. Chronic diseases have been called the companions of the aged and most persons over 65 years are affected by at least on chronic disease.
3. The major disorders of old age include heart disease, malignancy, cerebrovascular disease, influenza and pneumonia.
4. Disease in the aged does not always present with classic signs and symptoms. The usual clinical manifestations may be absent, attenuated or disguised and atypical signs and symptoms may present.

Falls in the Elderly

1. A fall may be a frightening experience that can lead to immobilization and possibly to pneumonia and complete loss of the ability to walk.
2. Falls by the elderly result from age-related physiologic decline in postural control and deterioration of the central nervous system from lightheadedness, postural hypotension, heart block and arrhythmias.
3. Special danger arises from osteoporosis, a condition in which the bones lose calcium and thus become thin and brittle. This condition renders an elderly person susceptible to major fractures.

Depression

1. Depression is the most common emotional disorder in the aged. Depression and grief are common with aged since losses are inevitable.
2. Depression resulting from losses can easily be overlooked and may be mistaken for physical or organic mental illness. The patient may exhibit anger, denial, withdrawal or other maladaptive responses that move him/her further away from reality.
3. Depression in the aged is usually manifested by feelings of apathy, quietness and emptiness, which may be mistaken for senile changes.
4. Treatment in elderly, usually referred to community health resources such as the community mental health services, can be very beneficial.

Chronic Organic Brain Syndrome (Senile Dementia)

1. The term dementia refers to signs and symptoms of intellectual dysfunction owing to differing etiologies and varying pathophysiology mechanisms that can occur alone and in combination.
2. It is believed to result from diffuse impairment of brain tissue. The most common long term disorders are cognitive functions (attention, learning, memory) in the elderly are seen in senile dementia (often called Alzheimer's disease).
3. Senile dementia generally refers to a disturbance of mental status or mental deterioration occurring after the age of 65 years. There are neuro-pathological changes associated with changes in the patient's cognitive function, which may include loss of neurons, neurofibrillary tangles, granulovascular changes and neuritic (senile) plaques in the brain.
4. Senile dementia is devasting to the human personality and is a source of anguish and frustration to the patient and loved ones.
5. Senile dementia and related disorders are associated with a high mortality rate and significantly shortened life expectancy.

Acute Brain Syndrome

1. Acute brain syndrome is a temporary psychiatric state caused by a physiologic or an anatomical insult to brain tissue.
2. The disorder have a relatively sudden onset and potentially reversible. They associated with acute physical illness of physiologic disturbances, cardiac and circulatory problems, neurologic conditions, cerebrovascular disorders, dehydration, electrolyte imbalance, alcohol or drug toxicity and wide variety of infections.
3. In management of acute brain syndrome, the basic disease must be treated or the etiologic toxic agent must be removed.
4. Specific treatment is aimed at alleviating or curing the condition that underlies thc confusion—antimicrobials for infection, removal of drugs, removal of fecal impaction, correction of heart failure, treatment of stroke.

5. Appropriate medications such as the phenothiazines, which exert much of their calming action on the lower brain centers, may be administered.

CONCLUSION

Growth and development are used interchangeably and taken as synonymous terms. Both related to the measurement of changes occurred in the individual after conception in the womb of the mother. Human growth from infancy to maturity involves great changes in body size and appearance, including the development of the sexual characteristics. The growth process is not a steady one—at sometimes growth occurs rapidly, at others slowly. Individual patterns of growth vary widely because of differences in heredity and environment. Children tend to have physiques similar to those of their parents or of earlier forebears; however, environment may modify this tendency. Living conditions, including nutrition and hygiene, have considerable influence on growth. Development is a series of orderly progression towards maturity. It implies overall qualitative changes resulting in the improved functioning of the organism.

Section III
Nursing Theories

GLOSSARY

1. **Client:** An individual, family, group, population or entire community who requires nursing expertise. In some clinical settings, the client may be referred to as a patient or a resident. In research, the client may be referred to as a participant.
2. **Collaboration:** A joint communication and decision-making process with the expressed goal of working together toward identified outcomes while respecting the unique qualities and abilities of each member of the group or team.
3. **Competencies:** Statements about the knowledge, skills, attitudes and judgments required to perform safely and ethically within an individual's nursing practice or in a designated role or setting.
4. **Critical thinking:** A purposeful, disciplined and systematic process of continual questioning, logical reasoning and reflecting through the use of interpretation, inference, analysis, synthesis and evaluation to achieve a desired outcome.
5. **Nursing:** The health profession in which a person provides the following services: (a) health care for the promotion, maintenance and restoration of health; (b) prevention, treatment and palliation of illness and injury, primarily by (i) assessing health status, (ii) planning and implementing interventions, and (iii) coordinating health services.
6. **Nursing diagnosis:** A clinical judgment about an individual's mental or physical condition to determine whether the condition can be improved or resolved by appropriate interventions of the registered nurse to achieve outcomes for which the registered nurse is accountable.
7. **Nursing science:** Knowledge (e.g. concepts, constructs, principles, theories) of nursing derived from systematic observation, study and research.
8. **Critical thinking:** Process of examining one's own thinking and assumptions to arrive at a broader viewpoint.
9. **Deductive reasoning:** Reasoning from the general to the specific.
10. **Environment:** Internal and external surroundings that affect the client.
11. **Health:** Degree of wellness or well-being that the client experiences.
12. **Holistic:** Approach that takes into account the client as a physical, mental, emotional, and spiritual being.
13. **Inductive reasoning:** Forming generalizations from a set of facts or observations.

14. **Objective data:** Signs that are detectable by an observer or can be tested against an accepted standard.
15. **Subjective data:** Symptoms; facts, perceptions, or sensations apparent only to the person affected.
16. **Theories:** Ways of looking at a discipline—such as nursing—in clear, explicit terms that can be communicated to others.

CHAPTER

14

Nursing Practice Theories

INTRODUCTION

As a science, nursing is in its infancy. Professional nurses are aware of this and conscious of the need for both nursing theory development and theory based practice. As nursing comes of age, not only as a practice discipline but also as a scholarly discipline, there will be increasing interest in delineating the theory base of nursing. Some believe that theory development is the most crucial task facing nursing (Chinn and Jacob, 1978). This study of theory helps to develop analytical skills, challenge thinking, clarifies values and assumptions, determines purposes for nursing practice, education and research. The contributions of many theorists outside of nursing profession formed the knowledge based for nursing practice for many years. New disciplines are often slow to develop their own theories and nursing was no exception. Even now, theories from the physical, biological, social, and behavioral sciences in addition to more recent nursing models and theories are used extensively in nursing practice.

MEANING

Theories are general explanations which scholars use to explain, control and understand commonly occurring events. Theories are best understood as preliminary explanations that reflect the current understanding of events. "Theory is defined as a set of propositions used to describe, explain, predict and control events". Here set refers to a group of circumstances, situations and so on, joined and treated as a whole; propositions refers to statements about how two or more concepts are related; concepts refers to an abstract classification of data, temperature; describe means of tell about in details; explain means to offer reasons for; predict means to foretell/forecast; control means to exercise as regulating influence over; and phenomena refer to theory includes the joint functions of theory, i.e. description, explanation, prediction and control.

IMPORTANCE OF NURSING THEORIES

Theory helps in providing knowledge to improve practice by describing, explaining, predicting and controlling phenomena. Nurses power is increased through theoretical knowledge because systematically developed more likely to be successful. In addition, nurses will know why they are doing, what they are doing if challenged. Theory provides professional autonomy by guiding the nursing practice, education and research functions of profession. And also there has been interest in identifying a body of nursing knowledge that is essential to professional nursing practice. Theory development contributes to knowledge building and is seen a means of establishing 'nursing as a profession'.

The commitment to that nursing practice based on sound, reliable knowledge is intrinsically valuable to nursing. That is to say, knowledge is desirable by its nature. The growth and enrichment of theory and of itself is an important goal for nursing as a scholarly discipline, to pursue. Now nursing practice settings are complex and the amount of data available to nurses are virtually endless. Nurses must analyze a tremendous amount of information about each patient and decide what to do. If a theory helps practicing nurses categorize and understand what is going on in nursing practice, if it helps them predict patients responses to nursing care, and if it is helpful in clinical decision making, it is useful as a guide to nursing practice.

DEVELOPMENT OF NURSING THEORIES

The development of nursing science and theory is a scholarly activity. Developing this science involves generating knowledge; although this knowledge can be used with knowledge from other disciplines, it is designed to advance and support nursing practice and health care. As nursing continues to evolve, nurses theorize about the nature of nursing practice, the principles on which practice is based, and the proper goals and functions of nursing in society. Conceptional and theoretical nursing models are used to provide knowledge to improve practice, guide research and curricular and identify domain and goals of nursing practice. Nursing theories provide the nurse with goals of assessment, nursing diagnosis and intervention; common ground for communication; and professional autonomy and accountability. They also guide future directions for nursing research; practice, education and administration.

Theories of nursing can help the nursing student to understand how the roles and actions of nurses fit together in nursing. The brief descriptions of selected nursing theories are as follows.

NIGHTINGALE'S THEORY (ENVIRONMENTAL MODEL)

Florence Nightingale, the matriarch of modern nursing, who is establishing the discipline of nursing, spoke with firm conviction about the 'nature of nursing as a profession that required knowledge distinct from medical knowledge'. The overall goal of this knowledge has been explained the practice of nursing as different and distinct from the practice of medicine, psychology, and social work. Nightingale conceptualized disease as a reparative process and described the nurses' role as manipulating the environment to facilitate this process. Her ideas regarding ventilation, warmth, light, diet, cleanliness, variety and noise are presented in her classic nursing textbook, i.e. Notes on Nursing (1859).

Nightingale believed that every woman at one time or another would be a nurse, in the sense that nursing was to have the responsibility for someone's health. This she proved women with guidelines for nursing care and advice on 'how to think and how to nurse'.

Major Concepts as defined by Nightingale

1. **Patient,** viewed as individual or person, is responsible, creative in control of their lives and health, and desiring good health. However, the patient is regarded as being acted upon by the nurse or affected by the environment.
2. **Health** viewed as a state of being well; using ones power to the fullest.
3. **Illness** defined as the reaction of the nature against the condition in which we have placed ourselves. Disease is a reparative mechanism, an effort of nature of remedy, a process of delay.
4. **Environment** refers to that external to the persons, but affecting the health of both sick and well persons. Environment, one of the chief sources of infection must include fresh air, fresh water, efficient drainage, cleanliness, and light.
5. **Nursing,** defined as a service to people, is intended to relieve pain and suffering. Goal of nursing is to promote the reparative process by manipulating the environment. Client's environment is manipulated to include appropriate noise, nutrition, hygiene, light, comfort, socialization, and hope. Nightingale's descriptive theory provides nurses with a way to think about nursing or a frame of reference that focuses on patients and the environment. Her principles encompass the areas of practice, research and education.

PEPLAU'S THEORY (1952)

Hildegard E Peplau was born on Sept 1909, and graduated from Pottstown, Pennsylvania Hospital, School of Nursing in 1931. The nature of science and nursing refers to the body of verified knowledge found within the discipline of nursing, i.e. mainly knowledge from the biological and behavioral sciences. The synthesis, reorganization or extension of concepts drawn from the basic and applied sciences, which is their reformation tend to become new concepts have led to the growth of nursing science. Then the evolution of Peplau's theory of interpersonal relations resulted. Peplau's theory focuses on the individual nurse and the interaction process; the result is the nurse-client relationship. The major concepts defined/viewed are as follows:

Psychodynamic Nursing

Psychodynamic nursing is being able to understand one's own behavior to help others identify felt difficulties, and to apply principles of human relations to the problems that arise at all levels of experience. She describes the structural concepts of interpersonal process and both the nurse-patient relationship to be based on psychodynamic nursing.

Nurse-patient Relationship

Nurse-patient relationship described by the Peplau in four phases, i.e. orientation, identification, exploitation and resolution:

1. **In orientation phase** the individual has a felt need and seeks professional assistance. The nurse helps the patient recognize and understand his/her problem and determine their need for help.
2. **In identification phase** the patient identifies with those who can help him (relatedness). The nurse permits exploration feelings to aid the patient in undergoing illness as an experience that reorients feelings and strengthens positive forces in the personality and provides needed satisfaction.
3. **In exploitation phase** the patient attempts to derive full value from what is offered him/her through the relationship. Now goals to be achieved through personal efforts can be projected and power shifted from the nurse to the patient as the patient delays gratification to achieve the newly formed goals.
4. **In the phase of resolution,** old goals are gradually put aside and new goals are adopted. This is a process in which the patient frees himself/herself from identification with the nurse.

Nursing Roles

Peplau describes six different nursing roles that emerge in the various phases of the nurse-patient relationship as given below:

Role of the stranger: In this role both nurse and patient are stranger to each other, the patient should be treated as he/she is and with ordinary courtesy. This coincides with the identification phase.

Role of resource person: In this role nurse provides specific answers to questions, especially health information, and interprets to the patient the treatment or medical plan of care. Here the nurse also determines what type of response is appropriate for constructive learning, either straight-forward factual answers or providing counseling.

Teaching role: It is a combination of all roles. Peplau separates teaching into two categories, i.e. instructional which consists largely of giving information and is the form explained in educational literature and practical which is using the experience of the learner as a basis from which learning products are developed.

Leadership role: It involves the democratic process. The nurse helps the patient to meet the tasks at hand through a relationship of cooperation and active participation.

Surrogate role: The patient casts the nurse in the surrogate role. The nurse's attitudes and behaviors create 'feeling tones' in the patient that reactivate feelings generate in a prior relationship. The nurse's function is to assist the patient in recognizing similarities between himself/herself and the person recalled by the patient. Nurse then helps the patient to see the differences in his/her role and that of the recalled person. In this phase, nurse and patient defines areas of dependence, independence and finally interdependence.

Counseling role: Peplau believes the counseling role has the greatest emphasis on psychiatric nursing. Counseling functions in the nurse-patient relationship by the way nurses response to patient demands.

Nursing

Nursing is described by Peplau as a significant, therapeutic, interpersonal process. It functions comparatively with other human processes that make health possible for individuals in communities. When professional health teams offer health services, nurses participate in the organization of conditions that facilitate natural ongoing tendencies in human organism. 'Nursing is an educative instrument, a maturing force that aims to promote forward movement of personality in the direction of creative constructive, productive, personal, and community living'.

Person

Person refers to man. Man is an organism that lives in an unstable equilibrium.

Health

Health is defined by Peplau as 'a word symbol that implies forward movement of personality and other ongoing human processes in the direction of creative, constructive, productive, personal and community living'.

Environment

Environment is defined in terms of 'existing forces outside the organism and in the context of cultures', from which morals, customs, and beliefs are acquired. However, general conditions that are likely to lead the health always include the interpersonal process.

According to this theory the client is an individual with a felt need and nursing is an interpersonal and therapeutic process. Nursing goal is to educate the client and family and to help the client reach mature personality development. Therefore nurse strives to develop a nurse-patient relationship in which the nurse serves as a research person, counselor and surrogate. This theory creates a 'making force' through which interpersonal effectiveness assists in meeting the client needs.

HENDERSON'S THEORY (1955)

Virginia Henderson was born in 1897, a native of Kansas city, Missouri, spent her developmental years in Virginia because her father practiced law in Washington DC. During World War I, she developed an interest in nursing. The major concepts defined by Henderson are as follows.

Nursing

Henderson defines nursing in functional terms, i.e. 'the unique function of the nurse is to assist the individual, sick or well, in the performance of those activities contributing to health or its recovery (or to peaceful death) that he would perform unaided if he had the necessary strength, will or knowledge. And to do this is such a way as to help him gain independence as rapidly as possible'.

Health

Henderson did not define health, but looking into several definitions of health. She views health in terms of patient's ability to perform unaided the 14 components of nursing care. She says it is 'the quality or health rather than life itself, that margin of mental physical vigor that allows a person to work most effectively and to reach his highest potential level of satisfaction of life'.

Environment

By using Webster's definition, Henderson defines 'environment as the aggregate of all the external conditions and influence affecting the life and development of an organism'.

Person (Patient)

Henderson views the patient as an individual who requires assistance to achieve health and independence or peaceful death. The mind and body are inseparable. The patient and his family are viewed as a unit.

Needs

Henderson did not define a need, but she identifies 14 basic needs of the patient, which comprises the components of nursing care. These include the need to:

1. Breathe normally.
2. Eat and drink adequately.
3. Eliminate body wastes by all avenues of elimination.
4. Move and maintain a desirable position.
5. Sleep and rest.
6. Select suitable clothing, i.e. dress and undress.
7. Maintain body temperature within the normal range by adjusting clothing and modifying the environment.
8. Keep the body clean and well groomed and protect the integument,
9. Avoid dangers in the environment and avoid injuring others.
10. Communicate with others in expressing emotions, needs, fears or opinions, worship according to one's faith.
11. Worship according to one's faith
12. Work in such a way that there is a sense of accomplishments.
13. Play or participate in various forms of recreation.
14. Learn, discover or satisfy the curiosity that leads to normal development and health and use the available health facilities.

Henderson viewed nursing as an art and a discipline separate from medicine, and viewed the nurse's role as that of a substitute for the patient, a helper to the patient and a partner with the patient. The 14 basic needs compose Henderson's components of nursing care.

ABDELLAH'S THEORY (1960)

Faye Glenn Abdellah was born in New York City, a 1942 Magna cum Laude graduate of Fitkin Memorial Hospital, School of Nursing, she received BS, MA and DEd from Teachers College at Columbia University. She completed her doctoral work in 1955. The nursing theory developed by Faye Abdellah et al. emphasized delivering nursing care for the whole person to meet the physical, emotional, intellectual, social and spiritual needs of the client and family. The major concepts defined by Abdellah are as follows:

Nursing

Abdellah defined nursing as 'service to individuals and families, therefore to society. It is based upon an art and science which mould the attitudes, intellectual competencies and technical skills of the individual nurse into the desire and ability to help people sick or well to cope with their health needs, and may be carried out under general or specific medical direction.

Abdellah was clearly promoting the image of the nurse who was not only kind and caring but also intelligent, competent and technically well prepared to provide service to the patient/mankind.

Nursing Problem

Nursing problem is a problem that is presented by the patient in a condition faced by the patient or family, which the nurse can assist them to meet through the performance of her professional function. The problem can be either an overt or covert nursing problem:

1. An overt nursing problem is an apparent condition faced by the patients or family which the nurse can assist him or them to meet through the performance of her professional functions.
2. A covert nursing problems is a concealed or hidden condition faced by the patient or family which then nurse can assist him or them to meet through the performance of her professional functions.

The functions of the nurses are to identify and solve the specific problems of clients. This identification and classification of problems was called the 'typology of 21 nursing problems, i.e. Abdellah 21 nursing problems were divided into the following three areas:

1. Physical, sociological and emotional needs of the patient.
2. Type of interpersonal relationships between the nurse and patient.
3. Common elements of patient care.

The 21 nursing problems are as follows:

1. To maintain good hygiene and physical comfort.
2. To promote (achieve) optimal activity, exercise, rest, sleep.
3. To promote safety through prevention of accidents, injury or other trauma and through the prevention of the spread of infection.
4. To maintain good body mechanics and to prevent or correct the deformity.
5. To facilitate the maintenance of oxygen supply to all body cells.
6. To facilitate the maintenance of nutrition of all body cells.
7. To facilitate the maintenance to elimination.
8. To facilitate the maintenance of fluid and electrolyte balance.
9. To recognize the physiological responses of the body to disease conditions—pathological, physiological and compensatory.
10. To facilitate the maintenance of regulatory mechanisms and functions.
11. To facilitate the maintenance of sensory function.
12. To identify and accept positive and negative expressions, feelings, and reactions.
13. To identify and accept interrelatedness of emotions and organic illness.
14. To facilitate the maintenance of effective verbal and non-verbal communications.
15. To promote the development of productive interpersonal relationships.
16. To facilitate progress toward achievement of personal spiritual goals.
17. To create and/or maintain a therapeutic environment.

18. To facilitate awareness of self as an individual with varying physical, emotional and developmental needs.
19. To accept the optimal possible goals in the light of limitations, physical and emotional.
20. To use community resources as an aid in resolving problems arising from illness.
21. To understand the role of social problems as influencing factors in the cause of illness. When using Abdellah's approach, the nurse needs knowledge and skills in interpersonal relations, psychology, growth and development, communication and sociology as well as knowledge of the basic sciences and specific nursing skills.

Problem Solving

Problem solving refers to the process of identifying overt and covert nursing problems and interpreting, analyzing and selecting appropriate causes of action to solve these problems. This process closely resembles the nursing problems.

The nurse is a problem solver and decision maker. The nurse formulates an individualized view of the client's needs, which may occur in the following areas:

- Comfort, hygiene, and safety
- Physiological balance
- Psychological and social factors
- Sociological and community factors.

The specific clients' needs, which are often referred to as Abdellah's 21 nursing problems, that is useful in identifying the needs, plan and implement the nursing intervention, accordingly.

ORLANDO THEORY (1961)

Ida Jean Orlando was born in 12 August 1926. In 1947, she received a diploma in nursing later on received BS (PhD) and MA in mental health consultation. From Machen College, Columbia University, she worked as a staff nurse, nursing supervisor, teacher, research associate.

Orlando describes her model as revolving around five major interrelated concepts:

1. Function of professional nurses.
2. Present behavior of the client.
3. Immediate reaction or internal response to nurse.
4. Nursing process discipline.
5. Improvement.

Major concepts of her model defined are as follows:

1. Nurses responsibility means whatever help the patient may require for the needs to be met.

2. Need situational, defined as requirement of the patient which is supplied, relieves or diminishes immediate distress or improves immediate sense of adequacy or well-being.
3. Personal behavior means any observable, verbal or non-verbal behavior.
4. Immediate reactions include both the nurse and patients' individual perceptional, thoughts and feelings.
5. Nursing process discipline includes the nurse communicating to the client, his or her own immediate reactions, clearly identifying that the item expressed belongs to the nurse, then asking for validation or correction.
6. Improvement means 'to grow better', 'to turn', 'to profit', 'to use', 'to advantage'.
7. Purpose of nursing refers to supply the help a patient requires in order for the needs to be met.
8. Automatic action, i.e. those nursing actions decided upon for research other than the patient immediate need.
9. Deliberate action, i.e. those actions decided upon after ascertaining a need and then meeting this need.
10. Orlando views that nursing should be a distinct profession that functions autonomously. Although nursing has been historically aligned with medicine and continuous to have close relationship with medicine, nursing and practice of medicine are clearly separate profession. She states that function of professional nurse is conceptualized as finding out and meeting the patients immediate need for help. Accordingly the goal of nursing is to respond to client's behavior in terms of immediate needs. To interact with client to meet immediate needs by identifying client behavior, reaction to nurse and nursing action to be taken.

To Orlando, the client is an individual with a need that when met, diminishes distress, increase adequacy or enhances well-being. Her theory focuses on nurses' reactions to client behavior in terms or the client immediate need. This theory contains those main elements like client behavior, nurse reaction and nurse action which compose the nursing situation. After nurses thoroughly assess the client's needs, they recognize the impact that need on the clients level of health and then act automatically or deliberately to meet the need, ultimately reducing client distress.

HALL'S THEORY (1962)

Lydia E Hall began her career in nursing as a graduate of the York Hospital, School of Nursing in York, Pennsylvania. She then earned her BS and MA degrees from Columbia University. Nursing circles of care (body), core (person) and cure (disease) are the central concepts of Hall's theory:

1. Care alludes to the 'hands on' intimate bodily care of the patient and implies a comforting; nurturing relationship (the body—natural and biological sciences intimate bodily care—aspects of nursing 'the cure').

2. Core involves the therapeutic use of self in communicating with the patient. The nurse reflects questions appropriately and helps the patient clarify motives and goals facilitating the process of increasing patient's self awareness (the person—social science therapeutic use of self-aspects of nursing—the core).
3. Cure is the aspects of nursing involved with administration of medications and treatment. The nurse functions in this role as an investigator and potential painer (the disease—pathological and therapeutically sciences—seeing the patient and family through medical care—aspects of nursing 'the cure'). According to this theory the goal of nursing is to provide care and comfort to client during disease process. The client is composed of the following overlapping parts, i.e. person (core) pathological state and treatment (cure), and body (care). Nurse is a caregiver. The professional nurses function most therapeutically when patients have entered the second stage of their hospital stay. This stage is the recuperating or non-acute phase of illness. The first stage of illness is the time of biological crisis, with nursing being an ancillary to medicine. After the crisis period the patient is more able to benefit and learn from the teaching that nurses can offer.

WIEDENBACH THEORY (1964)

Ernestine Wiedenbach's interest in nursing began with her childhood experiences with nurses. She earned master's degree from Columbia University. The major concepts defined by Wiedenbach are as follows:

1. **Patient:** She defines patient as an individual who is receiving help of some kind, be it care, instruction or advice, from member of the health profession or from worker in the field of health.
2. **Need for help:** A need is anything that individual may require maintaining or sustaining himself/herself comfortably or capably in the situation. A need for help is any measure or action required or desired by the individual, which has potential for restoring or extending his/her ability to cope with the demands implicit in the situation.
3. **Nurse** is a functioning human being. For the nurse whose actions are directed toward achievement of a specific purpose, thoughts and feelings, a discipline role to play.
4. **Purpose** that nurse wants to accomplish through what she does—in the overall goal.
5. **Philosophy,** an attitude toward life and reality evolves from each nurse beliefs and code of conduct, motivates the nurse to act, guides the thinking about when he/she is to do and influences the decisions. It stems from both culture and subculture. It is integral part of nurse. It is personal in character, unique to each nurse and expressed in the way of nursing.

6. **Practice:** Overt action, directed by disciplined thoughts and feelings toward meeting the patients need for help. It constitutes the practice of clinical nursing; it is goal direction, deliberately carried out and patient curaterd. Knowledge, judgment skills are necessary for effective practice. Identification, administration, validation are three competence of practice directly related to the patient care.

According to Wiedenbach's theory 'nursing is a practice which is related to the individuals who need help because of behavioral stimulus. The goal of nursing is to assist individuals in overcoming obstacles that interfered with the ability to meet demands or needs brought about by condition, environment, situation or time. Clinical nursing has following component, i.e. philosophy, purpose, practice and art.

Wiedenbach identifies five essential attributes to professional person (nurse). These characteristics are as follows:

1. Clarity of purpose.
2. Mastery of skill and knowledge essential for fulfilling purpose.
3. Ability to establish and sustain purposeful working relationship with others, both professional and non-professional.
4. Interest in advancing knowledge in the area of interest and creating new knowledge.
5. Dedication of furthering the goal of mankind rather than to self aggrandizement. She also stated the following four assumptions related to person:
   a. Each human being is endorsed with unique potential to develop within himself/herself resources which enable to maintain and sustain himself/herself.
   b. The human being basically strives toward self-direction and relative independence, and desires not only to make best use of the capabilities and potentialities but to fulfill his/her responsibilities.
   c. Self-awareness and self-acceptance are essential to the individual sense of integrity and self-worth.
   d. Whatever the individual does represents best judgment at the amount of his/her doing it.

LEVINE'S THEORY (1966)

Myra Estrin Levine obtained diploma from Cook Country, School of Nursing in 1944 and MSN from Wayne State University in 1962. She views the person's sense of identity and client as an integrated being who instructs with and adapts to the environment.

In her view 'nursing is a human interactions'. The essence of Levine's theory is that 'when nursing intervention influence adaption favorably or toward renewed social being, then the nurse is acting in a therapeutic sense, when response is unfavorable, the nurse adds supportive care. The goal of nursing is to promote wholeness. Whole, health, hale is all derived from Anglo-Saxon word 'hal'. Wholeness (holistic) emphasizes a sound, organic, progressive, mutually between diversified functions and parts with an entirety, the boundaries which are open and fluent. 'Holism' means that human beings are more than the different from the sum of their parts. Perceiving the 'wholes' depends upon recognizing the organization and interdependence of observable phenomena.

Conservation Principles of Nursing

Levine believes that nursing intervention is a conservation activity, with conservation of energy as a primary concern. Health is viewed in terms of the conservation of energy in the following areas, i.e. which Levine calls the 'four conservation principles of nursing':

1. Conservation of client energy.
2. Conservation of structural integrity.
3. Conservation of personal integrity.
4. Conservation of social integrity.

Integrity is from Latin integer, meaning 'being control of one's life'. Conservation is also from the Latin word 'conservatio' meaning to keep together. Conservation describes the way by which complex system are able to continue to function even when severally challenged.

The brief description of conservation principle of nursing are as follows:

Conservation of energy: The individual requires a balance of energy and constant renewal of energy to maintain life activities. That energy is challenged by process such as healing and aging. Conservation of energy has long been used and nursing practice even with the most basic procedures.

Conservation of structural integrity: Healing is the process of restoring structural integrity. Nurses should limit the amount of tissue involved in disease by early recognition of functional changes and by nursing interventions.

Conservation of personal integrity: Self worth and a sense of identity are important. Nurses can show respect to the patients calling them by their name, respecting their wishes, valuing personal possessions, providing privacy during procedures, supporting their defenses and teaching them. The nurse goal is always to impart knowledge and strength, so that the individual can resume a private life—no longer patient, no longer dependent.

Conservation of social integrity: Life gains meaning through social communities and health is socially determined. Nurses fulfill professional roles, provide family members, asses with religious needs, use interpersonal relation to conserve social integrity.

Adaptation is a process of change whereby the individual retains integrity within the relation of the environment. In Levine's approach, nursing care involves conservation activities aimed at the optimal use of the client's resources.

JOHNSON'S THEORY (1968)

Dorothy E Johnson was born on 21 Aug, 1919, in Savannah and received BA from Armstrong Junior College and got MPH degree from Harward University in Boston, 1948. Johnson's perceives nursing is an external force aiming to preserve the organization of the patient behavior. While the patient is under stress by means of imposing regulatory mechanism or by providing resources. As an art and science, it supplies external assistance both before and during system or balance disturbance and therefore requires knowledge of order, disorder and control.

She views man as a behavioral system with patterned, repetitive and purposeful ways of behaving that link him to the environment. Person is a system of interdependent parts that requires some regularity and adjustment to maintain balance. She perceives health as an inclusive dynamic state influenced by biological, psychological and social factors. Health is the desired value by health professionals and focuses on the person rather than illness.

Johnson theory of nursing focuses on how the client adapts to illness and how actual or potential stress can affect the ability to adapt. The goal of nursing is to reduce stress, so that the client can move more easily through recovery. This theory focuses on basic needs in terms of the following categories of behavior:

1. Security-seeking behavior.
2. Nurturance-seeking behaviors.
3. Master of oneself and ones environment according to internalize standards of excellence it.
4. Taking nourishment by socially and culturally acceptable ways.
5. Ridding the body of nurse socially and culturally acceptable way.
6. Sexual roles identify behavior.
7. Self-protected behavior.

According to Johnson, nurses assess the client's needs in these categories of behavior, called behavioral subsystem and plan, and provides nursing care to resolve problems in meeting the clients' needs.

ROGERS THEORY (1970)

Martha E Rogers was born on 12 May, 1914 in Dalls, Texas. She has done diploma in nursing in Knoxville General Hospital, School of Nursing (1936), Doctoral in nursing in Johns Hopkins University, Baltimore in 1954.

Roger felt that historically the term 'nursing' most often has been used as a verb simplifying 'to do' when nursing is perceived as a science. The term 'nursing' being a noun, signifies body of knowledge. She describes nursing as a learned profession that is both a science and an art. 'Nursing is a humanistic science dedicated to compassionate concern for maintaining and promoting health, preventing illness and caring for and rehabilitating the sick and disabled'. Nursing seeks to promote symphonic interactions between the environment and man, to strengthen the coherence and integrity of the human beings and do direct and redirect patterns of interaction between man and his environment for the realization of maximum health potential.

Roger considers man (unitary human being) as an energy field co-existence within the universe. An energy field constitutes the fundamental unit of both the living and non-living. Field is unifying concept and energy signifies the dynamic nature of the field. Energy fields are infinite, so she identified only two, i.e. the human field and the environment field:

1. The unitary human being (human field) is defined as an irreducible, indivisible, pandimensional energy field identified by pattern and manifested characteristics that are specific to the whole and which cannot be predicted from knowledge of the parts.
2. The environment field is defined as an irreducible pandimensional energy field identified by pattern and integral with human field. Each environmental field is specific to its given human field. Both change continuously and creatively. Unitary man evolves along life process. Client continuously changes and coexists with environment.

Roger viewed the terms health and illness as value leader, arbitrarily defined but as part of the same continuum, i.e. health occurs when patterns of living are in harmony with environmental change and illness occurs when patterns of living conflicts with environmental change and are deemed unacceptable.

The four dimension used in Rogers theory of energy fields, openness (universe of open system) pattern and organization and to derive principles about how human beings develops. Her views on nursing primarily as a science and is committed to nursing research. Nursing, therefore, corporate knowledge of the basic sciences and physiology, as well as nursing knowledge. The science of nursing aims to provide a body of abstract knowledge growing out, of scientific research and logical analysis and capable of being translated into nursing practice. Nursing body of knowledge is a new product specific to nursing.

According to this theory the goal of nursing is to maintain and promotc health, prevent illness and care for and rehabilitate ill and disabled client through humanistic science of nursing.

OREM'S THEORY

Dorothea Elizabeth Orem, one of the American foremost nursing theorists was born in Baltimore, Maryland. She began her nursing career at Providence Hospital, School of Nursing, Washington DC, where she received diploma in nursing and she also recipient of BSN and MSN of Catholic University America. Orem's self-care deficit theory of nursing as a general theory consists of three related theories:

1. Theory of self-care (describes and explains self-care).
2. Theory of self-care deficit (describes and explains why people can be helped through nursing).
3. Theory of nursing system (describes and explains relationship that must be brought about and maintained for nursing to be produced).

The major concepts defined by Orem's are as follows:

Self-care

Self-care is a learned, good-oriented activity of individuals. It is behavior that exists in concrete life situations directed by persons to self or to the environment to regulate factors that affects their own development and functioning in the interests of life, health or well-being.

Self-care requisites are expression of purposes to be attained, results desired from deliberate engagement in self-care. They are the reasons for doing actions that constitute self-care. There are three categories of self-care requisite as given below:

Universal self-care requisites: These are common to all human beings and include the maintenance of air, water, food, elimination, activity and rest, and solitude and social interaction, prevention of hazards and promotion of human functioning.

Development self-care requisites: These are self-care requisites that they promote processes for life and maturation and prevent conditions deleterious to maturation or mitigate those effects.

Health deviation self-care requisites: These are defined by Orem that disease or injury affects not only specific structures and physiologic or psychological mechanisms but also integrated human functioning. When integrated functioning is seriously affected the individuals' developing or developed powers of agency are seriously inspired either permanently or temporarily — discomfort, frustration resulting from medical care also create a requisites for self-care to bring relief.

Self-Care Deficit

Self-care deficit refers to a relationship between the human properties therapeutic self-care demand and self-care agency in which constituent developed self-care capabilities within self-care agency are nonoperable or not adequate for knowing and meeting some or all components of the existent or projected therapeutic self-care demand.

Nursing agency: It refers to the complex property or attribute of persons educated and trained as nurses that is enabling when exercised for knowing and helping others, know their therapeutic self-care demands, for helping others meet or in meeting their therapeutic self-care demands, and in helping other regulate the exercise or development of their self-care agency or their dependent care agency. Therapeutic demand is a humanly constructed entity, with an objective basis in information that describes in individual structurally, functionally, and developmentally.

Nursing System

Nursing system refers to a continuing series of actions produced when nurses link one way or a number of ways in helping to their own actions or the actions of the persons under care that are directed to meet these persons' therapeutic self-care demands or to regulate their self-care agency. Self-care agency is the complex acquired ability to meet one's continuing requirement for care them regulated life processes, maintains or promotes integrity of human structures and functioning, human development and promotes well-being.

Three types of nursing system (described by Orem) are as follows:

1. **Wholly compensatory nursing systems:** These are needed when the nurse should be compensating for a patients total inability for (or prescription against) engaging and self-care activities that require ambulation and manipulation of movements.
2. **Partially compensatory nursing system:** It exists when both nurse and patient perform care measures or other actions involving manipulative tasks or ambulation.
3. **Supportive educative nursing system:** These are for situations when the patient is able to perform or can and should learn to perform required measures for externally or internally oriented self-care but cannot do so without assistance. The methods of assistance will include acting or doing for guidance, i.e. teaching, supporting, and providing a developmental environment.

In Orem's self-care deficit theory, nursing care becomes necessary when client is unable to fulfill biological, psychological, developmental and/or social needs. The goal of nursing is to care for and help client within total self-care. She viewed person/patient in an individual unable to continuously maintain self-care in sustaining life and health, in recovering from disease or injury or in coping with their effects.

According to Orem, health is an ability to meet self-care demands that contribute to the maintenance and promotion of structural integrity, functioning, and development. Illness occurs when a individual is incapable of maintaining self-care as a result of health related limitations. She perceived environment that any setting in which a patient has unmet self-care needs. And nursing is service of deliberately selected and performed actions to assist individuals to maintain self-care, including structural integrity, functioning, and development. The nurse determines why a client is unable to meet these needs, what must be done to enable the client to meet them and how much self-care the client is able to perform.

Philosophy of Nursing described by Orem

Action, provision and management of it on continuous basis in order to sustain life and health, recover from disease or injury and cope with their effects. Self-care is a requirement of every person—man, women and child. When self-care is not maintained, illness, disease or death will occur. Nurses sometimes manage and maintain required self-care continuously for persons who are totally incapable. In other instance, nurses help persons to maintain required self-care by performing some but not all care measures, by supervising others who assist patients and by instructing and guiding individuals as they gradually move toward self-care.

Orem suggests that a person needs nursing when the person has a health related self-care deficit. The areas of nursing practice are:

1. Entering into and maintaining nurse-client relationships with individuals families or groups.
2. Determining if and how clients can be helped through nursing.
3. Responding to clients' requirements and needs.
4. Giving direct help to clients and families.
5. Coordinating and integrating nursing with the clients' daily living, other healthcare activities and social or educational services required.

KING'S THEORY (1971)

Imogene M King earned her diploma in nursing from St John's hospital of Nursing in St Louis in 1945 and earned MSN at St Louis University and Doctor of Education degree from Columbia University, New York.

Concepts

The major concepts in her theory of goal attainment are interaction, perception, communication, transaction, role, stress, growth and development, and time and space. The definition of these concepts by King is as follows:

Interaction: It is defined as a process of perception and communication between person and environment, and between person to person, represented by verbal and nonverbal behaviors, which are goal directed. Each individual in an interaction (nurse and client) brings different knowledge, needs, goals, postexperiences and perceptions which influence the interactions.

Perception: It is defined as 'each persons' representation of reality. This includes import and transformation of energy, and processing, storing, and exporting informations. Perceptions are related to postexperiences, concept of self-socioeconomic group, biological inheritance and educational background.

Communication: It is a process whereby information is given from one person to another either directly or indirectly. It is the information component of the interactions. The exchange or verbal and non-verbal signs and symbols between nurse and client or between client and environment are communications.

Transaction: It is defined as purposeful interaction that leads to goal attainment. It includes observable behavior of human beings interacting with their environment, the valuation components of human interaction.

Role: It is defined as a set of behaviors expected to persons occupying a position in a social system; rules that define rights and obligations in a position. If expectations of role differ, then role conflict and role confusion exists.

Stress: It is a 'dynamic state' whereby a human being interacts with the environment. It involves an exchange of energy and information between the person and the environment for regulation and control of stressors and energy response of an individual to person, objects and events. An increase in the stress of the individual leads to narrow perception and decrease rationality and also affects nursing care.

Growth and development: These are defined as continuous changes in the individuals at the cellular, molecular and behavioral levels of activities that conducive in helping individuals to move toward maturity.

Time: It is defined as a sequence of events moving onward to the future—time is duration between one event and another as uniquely experienced by each human being.

Space: It is defined as existing in all directions and is the same everywhere. It is immediate environment in which nurse and client interact.

King's Assumptions

King's personal philosophy about human beings and life influenced her assumptions. Her theory of goal attainment based on those assumptions that focus on nursing is human beings interacting with their environment leading to a state of health for individuals, which is an ability to function in social roles. Her assumptions are nursing, person's health and environment as given below:

1. **Nursing** is an observable behavior found in healthcare system in society. The goal of nursing is to help individuals maintain their health, so that

they can function in their roles. Nursing is viewed as an interpersonal process of action, reaction, interaction and transaction. Perception of nurse and client also influences the interaction process.

2. **Person's health:** Persons refer to individuals that they are social beings, sentient beings, rational beings, perceiving beings, controlling being, purposeful beings, action-oriented beings and time-oriented beings.

   Health is viewed as a dynamic state in the life cycle; illness is interference in the life cycle. Health implied continuous adaptation to stress in the internal and external environment through optimum use of one's resources to achieve maximum potential for daily living. Health is the function of nurse, patient, physician, family and other interaction.

3. **Environment:** King states that an understanding of the ways that human beings interact with their environment to maintain health is essential for nurses. Adjustment to life and health care influenced by an individual's interaction with environment.

King's theory focuses on the interpersonal relationship between client and the nurse. The nurse-client relationship is vehicle for the nursing process, which is a dynamic interpersonal process in which the nurse and client are affected by each other's behavior, as well as by the health care system. The nurses goal is to use communication to assist the client in re-establishing maintaining positive adaptation to environment.

TRAVELBEE'S THEORY (1961)

Joyce Travelbee was a psychiatric nurse practitioner, educator and writer, born on 1926. She had basic nurse preparation and 1946 at Charity Hospital, School of Nursing and earned BSN from Lavisinia State University and MSN from Yale in 1954.

Major concepts defined by Travelbee in her theory are as follows:

1. Nursing is defined as an 'interpersonal process whereby the professional nurse practioner assists an individual, family or community to prevent or cope with the experience of illness and suffering and if necessary, to find meaning in these experiences'. Nursing is an interpersonal process because it is an experience that occurs between the nurse and an individual or group of individuals.
2. Person defined as human being, both the nurse and patient are human beings.
3. Health refers to the criteria of subjective and objective health. A person's 'subjective' health states in an individually defined state of well-being in accordance with self-appraisal of physical, emotional and spiritual status. Objective health is an absence of discernible disease, disability or defect as measured by physical examination, laboratory test, assessment by spiritual director, or psychological counselor.

Travelbee viewed interpersonal process as human-to-human relationship formed during illness and 'experience of suffering'. The goal of nursing is to assist individual or family to prevent or cope with illness, regain health, find meaning in illness or maintain maximum degree of health.

NEUMAN'S THEORY (1972)

Betty Neuman was born on 1924, completed her initial nursing education at Akron, Ohio in 1947, then earned master degree in mental health in 1966 and received doctorate degree in clinical psychology in 1985. She was a pioneer of nursing involvement in mental health.

The major concepts identified in her model are holistic client approach, open system, basic structure, environment, created environment, stresses, lines of defence and resistance, degree of reaction, prevention as intervention, and reconstruction. Further included the concepts of scholastic approach, content, process input and output, negontrophy, entropy, stability, wellness and illness.

To Neuman, the persons are dynamic composite of physiological, socio-cultural and developmental variables that function as an open system. As an open system, the person interacts with adjusts to and it adjusted by the environment, which is viewed as stressor. Stressors disrupt the system. She includes intrapersonal, interpersonal and extrapersonal stressor.

Neuman believes that nursing is concerned with the whole person. She views nursing as a 'unique profession in that it is concerned with all of the variables affecting an individual response to stress'. Because the nurses perception influences the care program. Neuman equates health to wellness and defines health and/or wellness as 'the condition in which all parts and subparts (variables) are in harmony with the client. So, health is a dynamic equilibrium on the normal line of defence. Illness occurs due to reaction to stressor with lines of resistance, internal and external stressors and restrictive factors are the environment. The reduction of the stressors through prevention acts at three levels of nursing.

The goal of nursing is to assist individual, families and groups in attaining and maintaining maximal level of total wellness. The nurse assesses managers and evaluates client systems. Nursing focuses on the variables affecting the client response to the stressor. Nursing action are earned out on three levels. When the stressor is identified but no reaction has occurred; interventions can decrease the degree of reaction or increase the line of defense. This is called primary prevention. When the reaction has already happened, secondary prevention is carried out with intervention aimed at treating symptoms and reducing reactions. After active treatment, tertiary prevention strengthens the lines of defense through education and uses the systems total resources to prevent further occurrence.

Neuman model is applicable to all phases of the nursing process. It can be applied across all clinical areas and is especially useful for individuals and families. It is a holistic approach because each system or subsystem cannot be isolated; rather, the influence of each system on the whole must be considered. The three levels of prevention are useful guidelines for planning nursing interventions.

ROY'S THEORY (1979)

Sister Callista Roy, a member of the Sisters of St Joseph of Carondeler, was born on 14th Oct, 1939 in Los Angeles, California. She was the receiver of BA in Nursing, MSc Nursing and MA in Sociology and PhD in Sociology.

The major concepts defined by Roy are as follows:

1. **Person:** According to Roy, a person is a biopsychosocial being in constant interaction with a changing environment. She defined the person, the recipient of nursing care, as a living complex, adaptive system with internal processes (the cognator and regulator) acting to maintain adaptation in the four adaptive modes, i.e. physiological needs, self-concept, role functions and interdependence. The person as a living system is 'a whole' made up of parts or subsystems that function as a unity for some purpose, patient is a person or family with unusual stressor or ineffective coping mechanism.
2. **Health:** It is a state and a process of being and becoming an integrated and whole person. Lack of integration represents lack of health.
3. **Environment:** According to Roy environment is all the conditions, circumstances, and influences surrounding and affecting the development and behavior of persons or groups. Factors in the environment that affect the person are categorized as focal, contextual and residual stimuli.
4. **Nursing:** It is defined broadly as 'a theoretical system of knowledge which prescribes a process of analysis and action related to the care of the ill or potentially ill person'.

Roy differentiates nursing as a science from nursing as a practice discipline. Nursing science is a developing system of knowledge about person that observes, classifies and relates the processes by which persons positively affect their health status. Nursing as a practice discipline is nursing scientific body of knowledge used for the purpose of providing an essential service to people, that is, promoting ability to affect health positively.

Roy's goal of nursing is to help man adapt to change in physiological needs, self-concept, role-function and interdependent relations during health and illness. Nursing fills a unique role as a facilitator of adaptation by assessing behavior in each of these four adaptive modes and intervening by managing the influencing stimulants.

As defined by Roy, response to a decrease in body integrity creates a need state, and the individual responds with an act or behavior. The physiologic mode involves oxygenation, and circulation, fluid and electrolyte balance, nutrition, rest and activity and regulations of temperature, hormones and sensory function. The self concept mode concerned with perceptions of one's physical self and personal self including personality, moral ethical beliefs and values. The interdependent mode involves social relationships, including both the need to be interdependent and the need for support by others. The role function involves the behaviors of a person in each role taken on life.

In this model, all nursing activities are aimed at promoting the individuals adaption to health and illness in all four adaptive modes. The nurse determines what demands are causing problems for a client and assess how well the client is adapting to them. Nursing care is then directed at helping the client adapt.

LEININGER'S THEORY (1978)

Madeleine M Leininger is the founder of transcultural nursing, and a leader in transcultural nursing and human cure theory.

Concept

The major concepts defined in her theory are as follows:

Care: It refers to phenomenon related to assistive, supportive or enabling behavior toward or for another individual (or group) with evident or anticipated needs to ameliorate or improve a human condition or life way.

Caring: It refers to action directed towards assisting, supporting or enabling another individual (or group) with evident or anticipated needs to ameliorate or improve a human condition or life way.

Culture: It refers to the learned, shared and transmitted values, beliefs, norms and life way practices of a particular group that guides thinking, decisions, actions and patterned ways.

Cultural care: It refers to the cognitively known values, beliefs and patterned expressions that assist, support, enable another individual or group to maintain well-being, improve a human condition or life way, face death and disabilities.

Nursing: It is a learned humanistic art and science that focuses upon personalized (individual group) care behaviors, functions and processes directed toward promoting and maintaining health behaviors or recovery from illness which have physical, psychocultural and social significance or meaning of those being assisted generally by a professional nurse or one with similar role competencies.

The goal of nursing is to provide care consistent with nursing emerging science and knowledge with caring as a central focus. According to the theory carrying is central and unifying domain for nursing knowledge and practice.

WATSON'S THEORY (1979)

Jean Harman Watson was born in Southern West Virginia. She earned a BSc in 1964, MS in psychiatric mental health nursing in 1966 and PhD in educational psychology and counseling in 1973. Watson's philosophy of caring attempts to define outcome of nursing activity in regard to the humanistic aspects of life. Her theory and philosophy of caring is based on the values of kindness, concern, love of self and others and respect for the spiritual dimensions of the person.

Human Caring in Nursing

Watson defined human caring in nursing as "an art and a science in which caring is a human- to-human process demonstrated through a therapeutic inter-personal interactions". The action of nursing is directed at understanding the inter-relationships with health, illness and human behavior. Nursing is concerned with promoting and restoring health and preventing illness.

Formation of a humanistic altruistic system of values: These values are learned early in life but can be greatly influenced by nurse education. This factor can be defined as satisfaction through giving and extension of the sense of self.

Instillation of faith and hope: This factor incorporating humanistic and altruistic values facilitates the promotion of holistic, nursing care and positive health within the client population. It also describes the nurses' role in developing effective nurse-client interrelation and in promoting wellness by helping the client adopt health seeking behavior.

Cultivation of sensitivity to onesself and to others: The recognition of feelings leads to self-actualization through self-acceptance for both the nurse and the client. As nurses acknowledge their sensitivity and feelings, they become more genuine, authentic and sensitive to others.

Development of helping trust and relationship: This relationship between the nurse and client is crucial for transpersonal caring. A trusting relationship promotes and accepts the expression of both positive and negative feelings. It involves congruence, empathy, non-possessive warmth, and effective communication.

Promotion and acceptance of the expression of positive and negative feelings: The sharing of feeling is a risk taking experience for both nurse and client. The nurse must be prepared for either positive or negative feelings. The nurse must recognize that intellectual and emotional understandings of a situation differ.

Systematic use of scientific problem solving method of decision making: Use of the nursing process brings a scientific problem solving approach to nursing care.

Promotion of interpersonal teaching learning: It is an important factor in which nurse facilitates the process of teaching-learning techniques that are designed to enable the client to provide self-care, determining personal needs, and to provide opportunities for their personal growth.

Provision for supportive, protective and/or corrective mental, physical, sociocultural and spiritual environment: The nurses must recognize the influences that internal and external environment have on the health and illness of individual. Accordingly, they should make arrangement to create such conducive environment for the patient in positive direction.

Assistance with gratification of human needs: The nurse recognizes the biophysical, psychophysical, psychosocial and interpersonal needs of self and client. Client must satisfy lower order needs before attempting to attain higher order ones, i.e. food elimination, ventilation (biophysical lower needs), activity/inactivity, sexuality (lower psychological needs), achievement, affiliation and self-actualization (higher ones).

Allowance for existential phenomenological force: Phenomenology describes data of the immediate situation that help people understand the phenomena in question. This analysis of human existence in a situation provides a thought provoking, experience leading to better understanding of ourselves and others.

As stated above each factor describes the earning prices of how client attain or maintains health or dies peacefully. Caring represents all of the factors the nurse uses to deliver health care to the client.

CONCLUSION

Nursing practice theories have the most limited scope and level of abstraction and are developed for use within a specific range of nursing situations. Nursing practice theories provide frameworks for nursing interventions, and predict outcomes and the impact of nursing practice. The claim that knowledge about clients, client problems, and nursing therapeutics is enough to make nursing practice scientific is refuted on the basis that practice theories in nursing must encompass not only theories addressing these aspects but also those dealing with practice issues pertaining to the nurse-agent in action. A comprehensive framework specifying two dimensions of focus for practice theories is proposed to examine different types of practice theories in nursing and it is further used to frame a science of nursing practice as a subset of nursing science at large. Knowledge development for a science of nursing practice is then examined within four possible paradigms founded on different ontological and epistemological views.

CHAPTER

15

Metaparadigms of Nursing

INTRODUCTION

A metaparadigm is a concept that is extremely general, one that serves to define an entire world of thought. 'Meta' means 'that which is behind,' in Greek, and refers to that which undergirds something else, serving as a conceptual basis. In her seminal (1984, cited in Slevin) work, 'Analysis and Evaluation of Conceptual Models of Nursing,' Jacqueline Fawcett developed the basic four metaparadigms of nursing. More recently, these have been revised by Basford and Slevin (2003) and serve to underpin the entire conceptual universe of the nursing profession.

DEFINITION

1. The **nursing metaparadigm** embodies the knowledge base, theory, philosophy, research, practice, educational experience and literature identified with the profession. These given concepts vary in accordance to the experiences and views of different nursing theorists.
2. The nursing paradigm is a model that describes the relationship between person, health and the environment. The model has developed over a long period of time from the beliefs and practices of healthcare professionals.
3. Nursing metaparadigm (Fig. 15.1) is a nursing statement or group of statements that identifies phenomena which encompass a series of philosophical assumptions and also guides the approach to those assumptions. It has four interrelated central concepts, which are person, environment, health, and nursing. Nursing metaparadigm serves to strengthen the entire conceptual field of the nursing profession.

CONCEPT OF MATAPARADIGM

A nursing program is identified as a single entity (program) when it can be demonstrated that all of the following criteria are met:

1. The program is within one governing organization that holds an appropriate institutional accreditation from an agency recognized by the Accreditation Commission for Education in Nursing (ACEN).

2. The program is within the jurisdiction of one State Board of Nursing and/or other identified regulatory body exclusive of clinical learning experiences.
3. There is one set of student learning outcomes for the program offered.
4. There is one nurse administrator who has responsibility and authority for the program which may include: hiring and evaluation of faculty; development or revision of the curriculum; assignment/approval of faculty responsibilities; establishment of program specific admission/progression criteria; and development and administration of the program budget.
5. The faculty can demonstrate that they function as a faculty of the whole within a set of established faculty policies through their organization and decision-making processes, and methods of input into the curriculum development, delivery and evaluation.
6. There is a systematic evaluation plan that addresses the student learning outcomes, program outcomes and the ACEN standards.
7. A single degree, certificate or diploma is offered to students successfully completing the program.
8. All students are governed by a single set of policies.

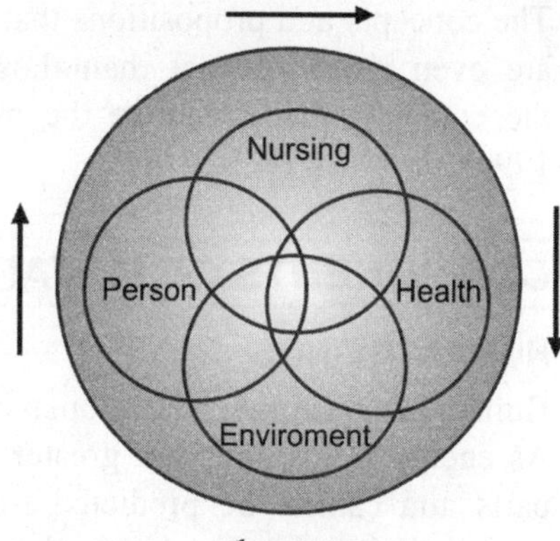

Figure 15.1: Metaparadigm of nursing

MEANING OF METAPARADIGM

Metaparadigm is the combination of two words, meta and paradigm. According to Mosby's (1994) definition, meta, can mean either 'after or next' or 'change or exchange.' Mosby's (1994) defines paradigm as 'a pattern that may serve as a model or example. Chin and Jacobs (1987) identify paradigm as, a generally accepted world view or philosophy, a framework or structure within which theories of the discipline are organized. According to Fawcett (1984), "a metaparadigm of a discipline is a group of statements identifying its phenomena in a global rather than specific way." Metaparadigm is 'the most global perspective of a discipline and acts as an encapsulating unit or framework, within which the more restrictive structures work'.

A metaparadigm is the most global perspective of a discipline and "acts as an encapsulating unit or framework within which the more restricted and structure develop" (Eckberg and Hill, 1979). Each discipline singles out phenomena of interest that it will deal with in a unique manner.

The concepts and propositions that identify and interrelate these phenomena are even more abstract than those in the conceptual models. These are the concepts that comprise the metaparadigm of the discipline (Fawcett, 1994).

COMPONENTS OF METAPARADIGM

HUMAN BEINGS

Human beings are viewed as open energy fields with unique life experiences. As energy fields, they are greater than and different from the sum of their parts and cannot be predicted from knowledge of their parts. Humans, as holistic beings, are unique, dynamic, sentient, multidimensional, capable of abstract reasoning, creativity, esthetic appreciation and self-responsible. Language, empathy, caring and other abstract patterns of communication are aspects of an individually high level of complexity and diversity and enable one to increase knowledge of self and environment. Humans are viewed as valued persons, to be respected, nurtured and understood with the right to make informed choices regarding their health.

For the purpose of study in nursing, biological, psychological, spiritual, intellectual and sociocultural dimensions of human beings and stages of human development are delineated as they affect behavior and health. These dimensions operate within and upon the human being in an open, interrelated, interdependent and interactive way. The nursing client is an open system, continually changing in mutual process with the changing environment. Recipients of nursing actions may be well or ill and include individuals, families and communities.

ENVIRONMENT

Environment is the landscape and geography of human social experience, the setting or context of experience as everyday life and includes variations in space, time and quality. This geography includes personal, social, national, global and beyond. Environment also includes societal beliefs, values, mores, customs and expectations. The environment is an energy field in mutual process with the human energy field and is conceptualized as the arena in which the nursing client encounters esthetic beauty, caring relationships, threats to wellness and the lived experiences of health. Dimensions that may affect health include physical, psychosocial, cultural, historical and developmental processes, as well as the political and economic aspects of the social world.

HEALTH

Health, a dynamic process, is the synthesis of wellness and illness and is defined by the perception of the client across the life span. This view focuses on the entire nature of the client in physical, social, aesthetic, and moral realms. Health is contextual and relational. Wellness, in this view, is the lived experience of congruence between one's possibilities and one's realities and is based on caring and feeling cared for. Illness is defined as they lived experience of loss or dysfunction that can be mediated by caring relationships. Inherent in this conceptualization is each client's approach to stress and coping. The degree or level of health is an expression of the mutual interactive process between human beings and their environment.

NURSING PRACTICE

Nursing is an academic discipline and a practice profession. It is the art and science of holistic health care guided by the values of human freedom, choice and responsibility. Nursing science is a body of knowledge arrived at through theory development, research and logical analysis. Nursing and other supporting theories are essential to guide and advance nursing practice. The art of nursing practice, actualized through therapeutic nursing interventions, is the creative use of this knowledge in human care. Nurses use critical thinking and clinical judgment to provide evidence-based care to individuals, families, aggregates, and communities to achieve an optimal level of client wellness in diverse nursing settings/contexts. Clinical judgment skills are therefore essential for professional nursing practice.

Human caring as the moral ideal of nursing is the central focus of professional practice. It involves concern and empathy, and a commitment to the client's lived experience of human health and the relationships among wellness, illness and disease. The nurse, as a person, is engaged as an active partner in the human care transactions with clients across the life span.

Human care and human care transactions seek to protect, enhance and preserve human worth and dignity. Human caring involves values, a will and a commitment to care, communication, knowledge, caring actions and consequences. Human care is an epistemic endeavor that defines both nurse and client and requires study, reflection and action. Caring is contextual, specific and individual and involves organized, specific practice that is related to caring for and about others. Caring is nursing's source of power.

NURSING AND METAPARADIGM

Nurses function autonomously and use power to shape the profession and empower clients through caring partnerships and other transactions. Within this framework, power is defined as the capacity to participate knowingly in the nature of change and is characterized by awareness, advocacy, choice, freedom to act intentionally, healing and involvement in creating changes.

Nurses use critical thinking to facilitate translation of knowledge and skill into professional nursing practice. The nursing process, a form of critical thinking, is a methodology for nursing practice, deliberate, systematic, and goal oriented. Deliberative behaviors for the process are observation, intuition, reflection, caring, empowering, communication, assessment, and choice of alternative actions. Nursing practice incorporates intellectual, interpersonal, communication and psychomotor skills in the care of individuals, families, aggregates and communities, regardless of setting, and emphasizes a collaborative relationship with other healthcare providers.

Multiple aspects of the complex role of the humanitarian nurse, such as learner, clinician and leader derive from the responsibility to provide diagnostic, technologic, supportive and therapeutic care; to protect the rights, safety and welfare of clients; to improve healthcare delivery, to influence health and social policy, and to contribute to the development of the profession. The goal of nursing is humanistic enhancement of health potential in human beings as well as caring for the well, ill and the dying. Excellence in nursing requires commitment, caring and critical thinking in terms of mastery, status and control over practice.

CONCLUSION

A metaparadigm is the broadest perspective of the discipline, a way to describe the concepts that concern the profession or domain. The metaparadigm for nursing describes those concepts that define the discipline of nursing. Since the early 1970's, four concepts (person, health, nursing, and environment) have been considered essential in describing the parameters of the profession. A metaparadigm is a concept that is extremely general, one that serves to define an entire world of thought. "Meta" means "that which is behind," in Greek, and refers to that which under-girds something else, serving as a conceptual basis. In her seminal (1984, cited in Slevin) work, "Analysis and Evaluation of Conceptual Models of Nursing," Jacqueline Fawcett developed the basic four metaparadigms of nursing. More recently, these have been revised by Basford and Slevin (2003) and serve to underpin the entire conceptual universe of the nursing profession. This paradigm refers to the sick individual not as a "patient," but as a "subject," a person in the full sense of the word. This includes families and social groups that have come to define the person as such. This person is unique and autonomous, and should be treated as such. A real person is not a mere object of professional care and surveillance.

SECTION IV
Nursing Process Application

GLOSSARY

1. **Advanced practice nurse:** A master's prepared nurse with specialization and licensure to practice as a nurse practitioner, nurse anesthetist, nurse midwife, clinical nurse specialist, clinical nurse leader or other advanced specialist role.
2. **Case manager:** A health professional, who advocates for the patient to receive the most appropriate treatment with acceptable quality in the most effective manner and appropriate setting at the best price.
3. **Nurse midwife:** A registered nurse, who has advanced education and certification to practice uncomplicated obstetrical care, including normal spontaneous vaginal delivery, without direct physician supervision.
4. **Nurse practitioner:** A registered nurse, who has advanced education and certification to carry out expanded healthcare evaluation and decision making regarding patient care; boundaries of independent practice are set by state laws.
5. **Nursing diagnosis:** A standardized statement about the health of a client for the purpose of providing nursing care; identified from a master list of nursing diagnosis terminology.
6. **Nursing process:** A system of assessing patients, diagnosing individual nursing care needs, planning care, implementing plans and evaluating care.
7. **Assessment:** It includes collection of objective and subjective data, organization of data and statement of the nursing diagnosis.
8. **Analysis:** It is the process by which the nurse organizes the data, identifies the client's health needs and problems and prioritizes those problems.
9. **Planning:** Based on analysis of data, is the development of individualized nursing care. It includes collaboration with the client for determining client/nursing goals, setting priorities and selection of therapeutic nursing interventions.
10. **Implementation:** It is the operationalization of selected nursing interventions. In addition to providing nursing care and/or management activities, in includes continued collaboration with the client to validate the plan of care and processing new information through continued data collection.

11. **Evaluation:** It consists of measuring the outcomes of therapeutic nursing interventions and the effectiveness of nursing care in relation to established criteria. The client's progress in relation to the achievement of established goals indicates whether optimal health has been attained or revisions in the plan need to occur.
12. **Nursing roles:** Competencies and skills performed by nurses in response to current and anticipated health needs of the client.
13. **Optimal health:** The highest potential degree of physical, psychosocial, and spiritual well-being that is within the client's capacity.
14. **Settings:** Geographical and/or situational environments where nurses practice. Settings may be traditional in which policies, procedures and protocols for providing health care may be established or nontraditional where policies, procedures and protocols are implied.
15. **Therapeutic communication skills:** The application of a dynamic process between two or more persons, in which there is an exchange of information, thoughts and feelings. The skills involved are accurate perception, interpretation and expression, in a style sensitive to the purpose and context of the interaction. This interaction may occur in various formats including verbal, nonverbal, tactile, artistic creations, test base or information technology.
16. **Therapeutic nursing interventions:** Holistic nursing actions that are implemented in an accurate, safe manner according to national standards and practice guidelines.
17. **Clinical diagnosis:** Diagnosis based on signs, symptoms and laboratory findings during life.
18. **Differential diagnosis:** The determination of which one of several diseases may be producing the symptoms.
19. **Medical diagnosis:** Diagnosis based on information from sources such as findings from a physical examination, interview with the patient or family or both, medical history of the patient and family and clinical findings as reported by laboratory tests and radiologic studies.
20. **Physical diagnosis:** Diagnosis based on information obtained by inspection, palpation, percussion and auscultation.

CHAPTER

16

Introduction to Nursing Process

INTRODUCTION

The nursing process is a problem-solving approach used by nurses to meet the needs of the patient. It is a deliberative method that relies on the use of cognitive, interpersonal and psychomotor skills.

The nursing process is the systematic, rational method of planning and providing nursing care. Its goal is to identify the client's health status, actual or potential healthcare problems, to establish plans to meet the individual needs and to deliver specific nursing interventions to meet those needs.

The nursing process is cyclical, i.e. the component of the nursing process follows a logical sequence, but more that one component may be involved at any given time. The nursing process provides a framework for accountability in nursing.

DEFINITION

1. The nursing process is cyclical, that is the component of the nursing process follows a logical sequence, but more than one component may be involved at any given time. The nursing process provides a framework for accountability in nursing.
2. The nursing process can be defined as an orderly, systematic way of identifying the clients(patient) problems, making plans to solve them, initiating the plans or assigning others to implement it and evaluating the extent to which the plan was effective in resolving the problems identified.
3. Nursing process is an evolving procedure consisting of five components by which a person's health status and needs are identified (assessment and diagnosis), plans are developed (planning), care is delivered (implementation) and outcomes are evaluated (evaluation) as the physical,

social and emotional problems of the person are resolved and/or new problems are identified.

STEPS IN NURSING PROCESS

The nursing process consists of five steps or components (Figs 16.1 and 16.2). These five steps of the nursing process are assessment, nursing diagnosis, planning, implementation and evaluation. The scientific nursing activities and responsibilities are associated with each steps of the nursing process.

ASSIGNMENT

It is collecting, verifying and organizing data about the client's health status. Data about physical, emotional, developmental, social, cultural, intellectual and spiritual aspects of the client's are obtained from a variety of sources and are the basis for actions; and decisions taken at a subsequent phases.

NURSING DIAGNOSIS

It is a process of making a clinical judgment about a client's potential or actual health problem. Nursing diagnosis is the statement of the judgment. In this phase, the nurse sorts, clusters the data and analyses, what are the actual and potential health problems, for which the client needs nursing assistance and what may be the contributing factors to this problem.

PLANNING

It involves a series of steps in which the nurse and client set priorities, formulate goals or expected outcomes and establish a written care plan for nursing interventions. The plan to resolve or minimize the identified problems of the client and to coordinate the care provided by all the health team members.

IMPLEMENTATION

It is putting the nursing care plan into action. During the implementation phase, the nurse continues to collect data and carries out the prescribed nursing activities or delegates the care to an appropriate person who validates the nursing care plan.

EVALUATION

It is assessing the client's response to nursing interventions and then comparing the response to predetermined standards. These standards are often referred to as 'outcome criteria'. The nurse determines the extent to which the goals

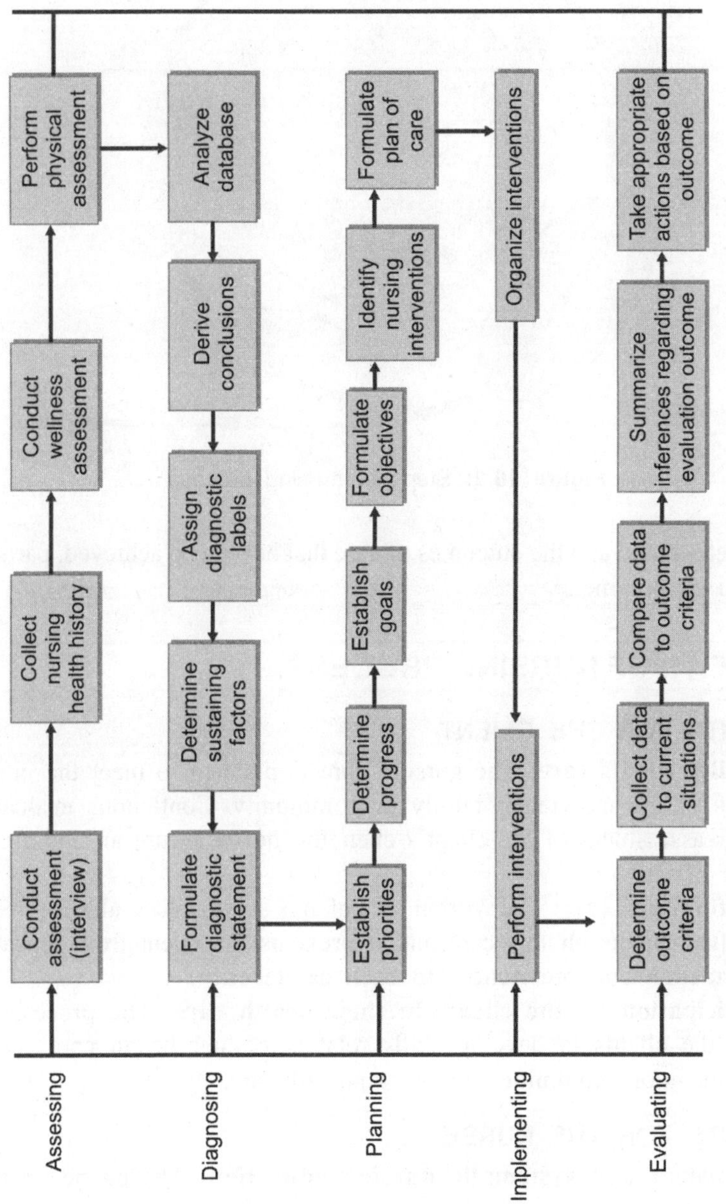

Figure 16.1: Steps and application of nursing process model

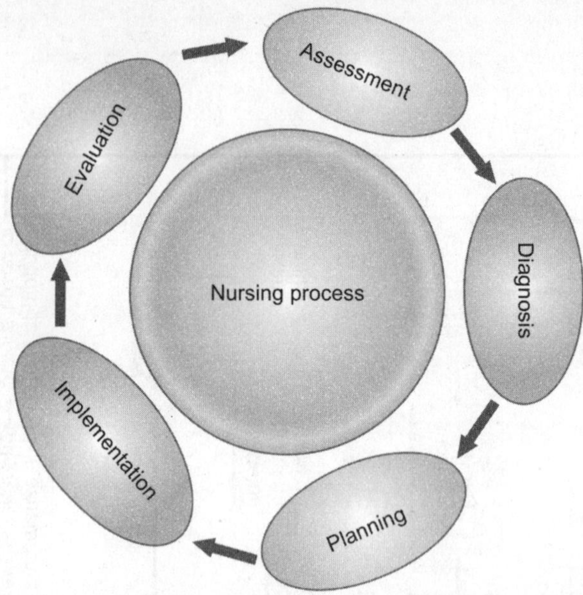

Figure 16.2: Steps of nursing process

are predetermined and the outcomes of care that have been achieved, partially achieved or not met.

BENEFITS OF NURSING PROCESS

BENEFITS FOR THE CLIENT

1. **Quality clients care:** The nursing care is planned to meet the unique needs of the individual, family or community. Continuous evaluation and reassessment of the client's changing needs ensure an appropriate level of care.
2. **Continuity of care:** The written care plan is accessible to all the persons involved in the client's care and it prevents the client from repeating information and preferences to each caretaker.
3. **Participation by the clients in their health care:** The process can help the clients to develop skills related to their health care and to become more committed to the goals of care.

BENEFITS FOR THE NURSE

1. **Consistent and systematic nursing education:** The agency, which accredits nursing education programs requires all graduates to be competent in using the nursing process.
2. **Job satisfaction:** Well written care plans has given the nurses to be

confident about that nursing interventions, which are based on correct identification of the clients problems, thus preventing the uncoordinated, trial and error nursing.
3. **For professional growth:** By elevating the effectiveness of the nursing interventions the nurse learns, which interventions are most effective and which one can be adapted to meet the needs of other clients.
4. **Meet professional standards:** Learning and implementing the nursing process while providing client care is a basic requirement for professional nursing competence.

FRAMEWORK FOR ACCOUNTABILITY

1. Accountability is the condition of being answerable and responsible to someone for specific behaviors that are part of the nurse's professional role.
2. The nursing process provides a framework for accountability and responsibility in nursing and maximizes accountability; and responsibility for standards of care.
3. Nurses are accountable to the client (public), to their professional statuary nursing body, to colleagues, to the employing agency and to themselves.
4. The nursing process provides a framework for accountability in all areas. A professional nurse is accountable for activities in all five phases of the nursing process.

ADVANTAGES OF NURSING PROCESS

When used effectively, the nursing process offers many advantages:
1. Nursing process is patient-centered, helping to ensure the patient's health problems and his/her response to them are the focus of care.
2. It enables nurse to individualize care for each patient.
3. It promotes the patient's participation in their care, encourages independence and concordance; and gives the patient a greater sense of control—important factors in a positive health outcome.
4. Nursing process improves communication by providing nurses with a summary of the patient's recognized problems or needs.
5. It promotes accountability for nursing activities, which in turn promotes quality assurance.
6. It promotes critical thinking, decision-making and problem-solving.
7. Nursing process is outcome-focused and encourages the evaluation of results.
8. It minimizes errors and omissions in care planning.

CONCLUSION

The nursing process is a scientific method used by nurses to ensure the quality of patient care. While the scientific method is a process for creating and performing experiments objectively, the nursing process is a method for creating and implementing patient care plans. Perception and intuition are an important part of this process, as opposed to being strictly scientific and only considering data. The nursing process is cyclical. This means that it never truly ends. Patients always have needs and are always at risk. As such, the process is always being used to help assess and meet those needs. The process that serves as an organizational framework for the practice of nursing. It encompasses all of the steps taken by the nurse in caring for a patient—assessment, nursing diagnosis, planning, implementation, and evaluation. The rationale for each step is founded in nursing theory. The process requires a systematic approach to the person's situation, beginning with assessment and including an evaluation and reconciliation of the perceptions by the person, the person's family, and the nurse. A plan for the nursing actions to be taken may then be made, and, with the participation of the person and the person's family, the plan may be set. The plan developed with the person and the person's family is then implemented. The outcome is evaluated with the person and the person's family. The steps follow each other at the start of the process but may need to be taken concurrently in some situations. The process does not reach completion with evaluation. The steps are begun again, allowing recurrent evaluation of the assessment, plan, goals, and actions.

CHAPTER

17

Nursing Assessment

INTRODUCTION

The first step of nursing process is assessment. Assessment is the collection of data about the client from a variety of sources. Assessment is the continuous process carried out during all phases of the nursing process. It may be used during the diagnosis phase to validate a diagnosis. A 'systematic, dynamic process by which the nurse, through interaction with the client, significant others, and health care providers, collects and analyzes data about the client. Assessment is broader than observing and data gathering. It includes the application of processes such as critical thinking and professional judgments used in prioritizing, identifying immediate and anticipated need, analyzing medical and nursing interventions aimed at appropriate outcomes, and providing for holistic continuum of care', American Nurses Association (ANA), Nursing Scope and Standards of Practice.

DEFINITION

1. The first step of nursing process is assessment. Assessment is the collection of data about the client from a variety of sources. Assessment is the continuous process carried out during all phases of the nursing process. It may be used during the diagnosis phase to validate a diagnosis.
2. Assessment is collecting, verifying and organizing data about the client's health status. Data about physical, emotional, developmental, social, cultural, intellectual and spiritual aspects of the client's are obtained from a variety of sources and are the basis for actions and decisions taken at a subsequent phases.

PREREQUISITES TO ASSESSMENT

1. **Beliefs:** The nurse's belief encompasses a caring philosophy about the client's responsibilities and health and illness, and the role of nursing in health care. These philosophies do not blossom overnight, but are molded during the course of nursing education by nurses, other students, instructors and clients.

2. **Knowledge:** The knowledge base for nurses is extensive and nurses are required to use information from sciences such as nursing, anatomy, physiology, microbiology, pharmacology, chemistry and nutrition. Using all of these sciences as guidelines, the nurse can analyze data collected about the client.
3. **Skill:** A variety of skills are required to perform a complete assessment of the client. They include psychomotor and interpersonal.

Psychomotor skills are the technical skills required in many phases and nursing process. During the assessment phase, the most common skills are those of physical assessment such as inspection, palpation and auscultation.

Interpersonal skills are important in all phases of nursing process, but are a critical component of the assessment phase. The term therapeutic relationship is often used to describe the communication techniques that allow the client and family to share views openly.

DATA COLLECTION

Data collected from a patient includes both objective and subjective data. Objective data are detectable by an observer. Examples of objective data are blood pressure recording, checking body temperature, detecting cyanosis in a patient. Subjective data are apparent only to the patient concerned. Examples of subjective data are feeling of pain, itching, etc.

SOURCES OF DATA

Sources of data are as follows:

1. **Client:** The chief source of data is usually the client unless the client is too ill, young or confused to communicate clearly. The client can provide subjective data that no one else can offer.
2. **Significant others:** Significant others are supporting person, who knows the client well and often provide data. They might convey information about the stress, the client was experiencing before the illness, family attitudes to illness and health; and the client's home environment.
3. **Health personnel:** Health personnel are often the sources of information about a client's health. Nurses, physicians, social workers and physiotherapist are included in health personnel. Physician who knows the client's home setting may provide valuable data about the family and the environmental stress.
4. **Medical records:** Medical records are often a source of a client's present and past health and illness patterns. This record can provide nurses with information about a client's coping behaviors, health practices, previous illness and allergies.

5. **Other records and reports:** Other records and reports can also provide information pertinent to health, laboratory and tests are frequently ordered as part of the physician's initial examination to aid in a medical diagnosis.
6. **Literature:** The review of nursing and related literature such as professional journals and reference texts can provide additional information for the database.

METHODS OF DATA COLLECTION

Methods of data collection of the patients includes:

1. **Observation:** The nurse observes mainly through sight, all of the senses are engaged during careful observations. Observation has two aspects:
   a. Noticing the stimuli
   b. Selecting organizing and interpreting the data, i.e. perceiving them. Observation is a conscious, deliberate skill that is developed only through effort and with an organized approach.
2. **Interviewing:** The nurse interviews the patient and his/her significant others, obtain data by asking relevant questions. Interview is a planned communication or conversation with a purpose. Interviewing can be viewed as a process in the nursing health history, which is the primary tool for data collection during the assessment phase of the nursing process.
3. **Examination:** Nurses perform physical assessment to obtain the objective data needed to complete the assessment phase of the nursing process. A complete database of both subjective and objective data allows the nurse to formulate nursing diagnosis, to develop client goals and intervene to promote health; and prevent disease.

GUIDELINE FOR DATA COLLECTION

1. **Initial history:** The data collected in this step usually include the historical data (pat illness), current data (the current complaint) and demographic data (date of birth, gender, address). It is helpful to address the client's chief complaint early in the interview process.
2. **Symptom analysis:** When a client expresses a problem, the nurse conducts a complete analysis of a symptom. This process begins with symptoms analysis, which is the collection of subjective data about the problem. Symptoms analysis requires the client to identify the location of the symptoms, describe the symptoms, severity of the pain, and timing of the symptoms (including onset, duration and frequency).

   Aggravating and relieving symptoms and any associated symptoms. It is crucial that the nurse be able to perform a complete symptoms analysis. The data obtained can guide the nurse in detecting, what the problem is and what degree of priority is should be given.

3. **Approaches to history taking:** There are various approaches that can be used to provide a systematic guide to assessment. Gordon has devised functional health patterns and the North American Nursing Diagnosis Association (NANDA) has devised human response patterns based on patterns of unitary persons.
4. **Physical examination:** Physical examination of the client is the second portion of assessment. Examination allows the nurse to gain objective data through the use of inspection, percussion, palpation and auscultation. These data further define the client's response to the disorder, provide a baseline of data for further comparison and elaborate on the subjective data provided in the client's history.

PHYSICAL EXAMINATION

Assessment of physical findings should confirm data obtained in nursing history. Baseline information is obtained on admission. The proper examination proceeds logically from head to be starting with general appearance, blood pressure, pulse, hands, head and neck, heart, lungs, abdomen, legs and feet.

DEFINITION

Physical examination is defined as a complete assessment of patient's physical and mental status.

PURPOSE

The purpose of physical examination of patient is:

1. To understand the physical and mental well being of the patient.
2. To detect disease in its early stage.
3. To determine the cause and the extent of disease.
4. To understand any changes in the condition of diseases, any improvement or regression.
5. To determine the nature of the treatment or nursing care needed for the patient.
6. To safeguard the patient and his/her family by noting the early signs, especially in case of a communicable disease.
7. To contribute to the medical research.
8. To find out whether the person is medically fit or not for a particular task.

METHODS OF PHYSICAL EXAMINATION

Inspection

Visual examination of the body is called inspection. It is the observation with the naked eyes to determine the structure and functions of the body. It means looking with eyes, it reveals any rash, scar, color, size, shape, contour or symmetry of body parts. The quality of inspection depends on the time spent by the nurse to be thorough and systematic. In a hurry, we may overlook significant findings and make an incorrect conclusion. The following principles should be kept in mind for making accurate inspections:

1. Good lighting and exposure are essential.
2. Inspect each area for size, shape, color, symmetry and proposition and find out any deviations from normal.
3. Use additional lights for examining body cavities, e.g. oral.
4. Use sense of olfaction along with visual to detect abnormalities, e.g. bad breath indicates unhygienic mouth conditions, acidotic smell is significant of diabetic acidosis (Fig. 17.1).

Palpation

It is the feeling of the body or a part with the hands to note the size and positions of the organs. In palpation the finger pads are used and not the finger tips. Palpation is an assessment technique in which the examiner feels with his/her fingers and one or both hands. Skill and gentleness are important. The degree of pressure applied during palpation varies, depending on tenderness of the area and the depth of palpation required. It reveals any swelling, coldness, hotness, stiffness, hardness, smoothness, roughness, pain, vibration, firmness and flaccidity.

The following points are to be kept in mind while doing palpation:

1. The client should be relaxed and comfortable. Observe non-verbal signs of discomfort during palpation.
2. Palpation to be done with warm hands, short fingernails and a gentle approach.
3. Palpation to be done slowly and gently.
4. For light palpation the hand is depressed about 1cm (1/2 inch) and for deeper palpation it should be approximately 2.5 cm (1 inch).
5. Use appropriate parts of the hands for doing various palpations.

Percussion

It is the examination by tapping with the fingers on the body to determine the condition of the internal organs by the sounds that are produced. It is done by placing a finger of the left hand firmly against a part to be

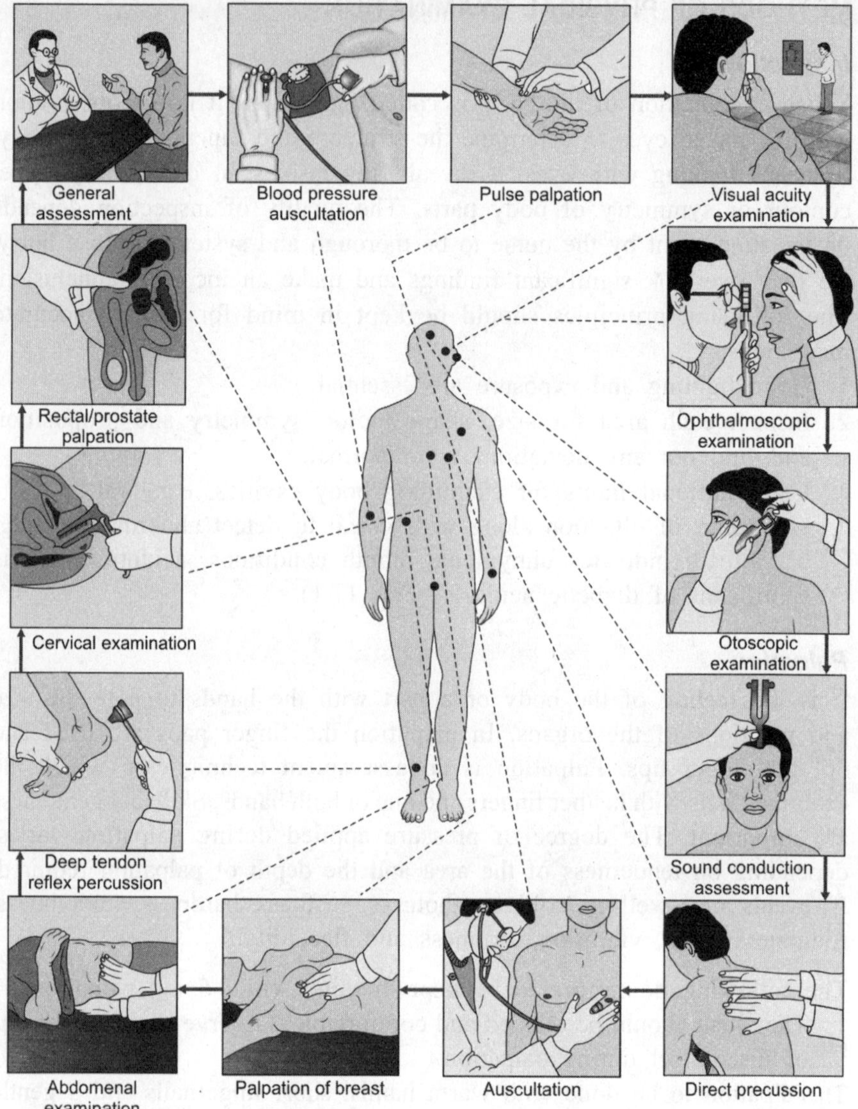

Figure 17.1: Head to toe examination of the patient

examined and tapping with the finger tips of the right hand. It means striking/tapping with fingers. It elicits sounds, which indicate whether the underlying tissues are solid or filled with air or fluid. The sounds may be:

1. **Resonance:** A low pitched and loud sound heard over the normal lung tissues.
2. **Hyperresonance:** Very loud, very low pitch sound longer than resonance and is of booming quality signifies emphysema.

3. **Tympany:** A drum-like sound heard over the air-filled tissues such as gastric air bubble.
4. **Dull:** A medium-pitched sound with a medium duration without resonance heard over solid tissues such as heart, liver.
5. **Flat:** A high-pitched sound with a short duration without resonance heard over complete solid tissues such as hand, thigh.

Methods of percussion: The percussion can be done by two methods. These are:

1. **Direct percussion:** Striking the body surface directly with one or two fingers, e.g. ascitic thrill.
2. **Indirect percussion:** Placing the middle finger of the non-dominant hand firmly against the body surface and striking the distal joint of now-dominant finger with the middle fingers of the dominant hand (Figure 17.1 showing indirect percussion).

Auscultation

Auscultation means listening with stethoscope/placing ear against the body. It reveals sounds produced within the body and the blood vessels such as heartbeats, bowel sounds, while auscultation frequency loudness, quality and duration of the sound to be noted.

Manipulation

Manipulation is the moving of a part of the body to note its flexibility. Limitation of movements is discovered by this method.

Testing of Reflexes

The response of the tissues to external stimuli is tested by means of percussion hammer, safety pin, wisp of cotton, hot and cold water, etc.

HEAD TO TOE EXAMINATION

The examination is carried out in an orderly manner focusing upon one area of the body at a time. The observation of the patient starts as the patient walks into the examination room, e.g. a limp may be noted as the patient walks in. The following observations are made.

GENERAL APPEARANCE

1. Nourishment: Well-nourished or under nourished.
2. Body build: Thin or obese.
3. Health: Healthy or unhealthy.
4. Activity: Active or dull (tired).

MENTAL STATUS

1. Consciousness: Conscious, unconscious, delirious, talking incoherently.
2. Look: Anxious or worried, depressed, etc.

POSTURE

1. Body curves: Lordosis, kyphosis, and scoliosis.
2. Movement: Any limp.

HEIGHT AND WEIGHT

Record the height and weight.

SKIN CONDITIONS

1. Color: Pallor, jaundice, cyanosis, flushing, etc.
2. Texture: Dryness, flaking, wrinkling or excessive moisture.
3. Temperature: Warm, cold and clammy.
4. Lesions: Macules, papules, vesicles, wounds, etc.

HEAD AND FACE

1. Shape of the skull and fontanel.
2. Skull circumference.
3. Scalp: Cleanliness, condition of the hair, drandruff, pediculi, infections like ringworm.
4. Face: Pale, flushed, puffiness, fatigue, pain, fear, anxiety, enlargement of parotid glands, etc.

EYE

1. Eyebrows: Normal or absent.
2. Eyelashes: Infection, sty.
3. Eyelids: Edema, lesions, ectropion, entropion.
4. Eyeballs: Sunken or protruded.
5. Conjunctiva: Pale, red, purulent.
6. Sclera: Jaundiced.
7. Cornea and iris: Irregularities and abrasions.
8. Pupils: Dilated, constricted reaction to light.
9. Lens: Opaque or transparent.
10. Fundus: Congestion, hemorrhagic spots.
11. Eye muscles: Strabismus (squint).
12. Vision: Normal, myopia, hypermetropia.

ARTICLES APPROPRIATE FOR SPECIFIC EXAMINATION

1. **Eye:** Torch, ophthalmoscope, snellens chart, wisp of cotton.
2. **Ear:** Head mirror, light bulb fixed on the wall or a table lamp and a torch, a tuning fork.

3. **Nose:** Nasal speculum, forceps, a head mirror and a light bulb.
4. **Throat:** Tongue depressor, a laryngeal mirror, a kidney tray, a paper bag, throat swabs in a container. Torch gauze pieces in a bowl.
5. **Chest and abdomen:** Stethoscope, tape measure.
6. **Vaginal:** Sterile vaginal speculum, gloves, a kidney tray, a bowl with swabs (sterile), and an antiseptic lotion.
7. **Rectal:** Proctoscope, gloves, finger cots, a kidney tray, water-soluble jelly.
8. **Neurological:** A percussion hammer, safety pins, a wisp of cotton, hot or cold water.

Ears

1. External ear: Discharges, cerumen obstructing the ear passage.
2. Tympanic membrane: Perforations, lesions, bulging.
3. Hearing: Hearing acuity.

Nose

1. External nares: Crusts or discharges.
2. Nostrils: Inflammation of the mucus membrane, septal deviations.

Mouth and Pharynx

1. Lips: Redness, swelling, crusts, cyanosis, angular stomatitis.
2. Odor of the mouth: Foul smelling.
3. Teeth: Discoloration and dental caries.
4. Mucous membrane and gums: Ulceration and bleeding, swelling, pus formation.
5. Tongue: Pale; dry, lesions, sords, furrows, tongue tie, etc.
6. Throat and pharynx: Enlarged tonsils, redness and pus.

Neck

1. Lymph nodes: Enlarged, palpable.
2. Thyroid gland: Enlarged.
3. Range of motion: Flexion, extension and rotation.

Chest

1. Thorax: Shape, symmetry of expansion, posture.
2. Breathe sounds: Sigh, swish, rustle, wheezing, rales, crepitations, pleural rub, etc.
3. Heart: Size and location, cardiac murmurs.
4. Breasts: Enlarged lymph nodes.

Abdomen

1. Observation: Skin rashes, scars, hernia, ascites distension, pregnancy, etc.
2. Auscultation: Bowel sounds, fetal heart sounds.

3. Palpation: Liver margin, palpable spleen, tenderness at the urea of appendix, inguinal hernias.
4. Percussion: Presence of gas, fluid or masses.

Extremities

Movement of joints, tremors, clumbing of fingers, ankle edema, varicose veins, reflexes, etc.

Back

Spina bifida curves.

Genital and Rectum

1. Inguinal lymph glands: Enlarged, palpable.
2. Patency of urinary meatus and rectum (in infants).
3. Descent of the testes.
4. Vaginal discharges.
5. Presence of sexually transmitted diseases (STD).
6. Hemorrhoids.
7. Enlargement of the prostate gland.
8. Pelvic masses.

Neurological Tests

1. Coordination tests.
2. Reflexes.
3. Equilibrium tests.
4. Tests for sensations.
5. Role of the nurse in the physical examination.

PREPARATION OF THE ENVIORNMENT

1. Maintenance of privacy.
2. A separate examination room is needed.
3. Keep the doors closed. The relatives are not allowed.
4. Drape the patient according to the parts that are exposed.
5. Lighting: As far as possible natural light should be available in the examination room, because if a patient is jaundiced, it may not be detected in the artificial light. There should be adequate lighting.
6. Comfortable bed or examination table: The patient should be placed comfortably throughout the examination. There should be provision for the maintenance of a suitable position, e.g. a lithotomy position may be maintained when examining the genitalia. To maintain this position, a special examination table with stirrup rods is needed.
7. The room should be warm and without draft.

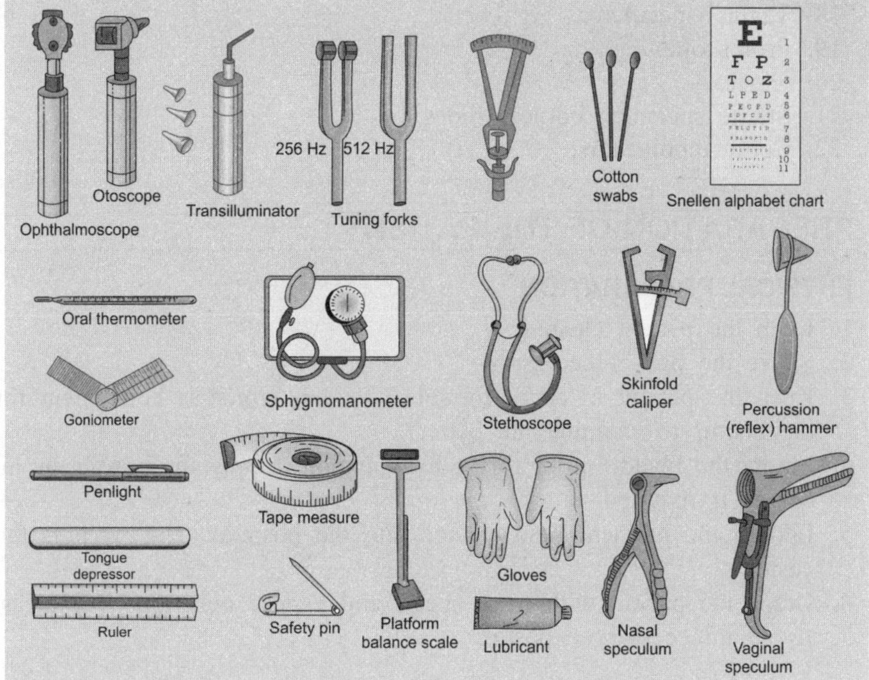

Figure 17.2: Equipments used in medical diagnosis

PREPARATION OF THE EQUIPMENT

All the articles needed for the physical examination are kept ready for the examination at hand (Fig. 17.2).

1. Sphygmomanometer.
2. Stethoscope.
3. Foetoscope.
4. TPR tray.
5. Tongue depressor.
6. Pharyngeal retractor.
7. Laryngoscope.
8. Tape measure.
9. Flash light.
10. Weighing machine.
11. Opthalmoscope.
12. Otoscope.
13. Tuning fork.
14. Nasal speculum.
15. Percussion hammer, safety pins.
16. Cotton wool, cold and hot water.
17. Test tubes.

18. Vaginal speculum.
19. Protoscope.
20. Gloves.
21. Sterile specimen bottles, slides.
22. Cotton applicators.

PREPARATION OF THE PATIENT

PHYSICAL PREPARATION

1. Keep the patient clean.
2. Shave the part if necessary.
3. Keep the patient in a comfortable position, which is convenient for the doctor to examine the patient.
4. Empty the bladder prior to the examination. Empty the bowels by an enema if required.
5. Loosen the garments and change into the hospital dress, if it is the custom.
6. Drape the patient with extra sheets and expose only the need areas.
7. Avoid unnecessary exposure.

MENTAL PREPARATION

1. The patient may be quite new to the hospital situation and he/she may be anxious about his/her illness.
2. Patient may have false ideas about the medical examination.
3. It is the duty of the nurse to allay patient anxieties and fears by proper explanations.
4. Explain the sequence of the procedure to gain patient's confidence and co-operation.
5. As far as possible, a nurse should remain with a female patient during the physical examination.

ASSISTING IN EXAMINATION

TO TAKE HEIGHT AND WEIGHT

1. To measure the length of the baby who cannot stand, place the baby on a hard surface, with the soles of the feet supported in an upright position.
2. The knees are extended and the measurement is taken from the soles of the feet to the vertex of the head.
3. The head should be in such a position that the eyes are facing the ceiling.
4. After a child can stand, the height can be measured, if the child with the heels back and head against a wall.

5. A small flat board held from the top of the head to the wall, will give an accurate measure of the height that is the distance from the floor to the board.
6. The weight of a person who can stand is generally measured by a standing scale.
7. The patient stands on the platform and the weight is noted on the dial.
8. Usually the weight is taken without shoes.
9. To take the weight of the baby, a baby weighing scale is used, in which there is a container, where the baby can be laid.
10. It is important to weigh a baby unclothed, weigh the clothes separately and subtract this weight.

TO MEASURE THE SKULL CIRCUMFERENCE

The skull is measured at its greatest diameter from above the eyes to the occipital protuberance.

EXAMINATION OF THE EYES

1. Examination is done in a lying or sitting position.
2. The examiner frequently uses a head mirror that reflects light to the patient's face.
3. First examination is one of inspection to determine the movements of the eyes, reaction to light, accommodation to near and far objects.
4. For detailed examination of the internal parts of the eye an ophthalmoscope is used.

EXAMINATION OF THE EARS

1. The patient may be placed either in a lying or sitting position with the ear to be examined turned towards the examiner.
2. Articles used for the examination are a head mirror, ear speculum of various sizes, cotton tipped applicators and autoscope.
3. Tuning fork is used to test the hearing.
4. A child needs to be carefully restrained.
5. Young children sit on their mother's lap with their legs restrained between the mother's knees and their arms held against their back.
6. The mother then holds the child's head against the chest.
7. Very small infants can be laid on the examination table.

EXAMINATION OF THE NOSE, THROAT AND MOUTH

1. The patient is usually seated with the head resting against the back of the chair.
2. For the examination of the throat, a tongue depressor and a good light are needed.

3. For examination of the nose, a nasal speculum and a head mirror are used. Sometimes the autoscope is also used.

EXAMINATION OF THE NECK

The neck needs to be palpated for lymph nodes. In order to assess the thyroid glands, the patient is asked to swallow saliva.

EXAMINATION OF THE CHEST

1. While examining the anterior chest, the patient is placed in a horizontal recumbent position.
2. The chest is examined in several ways.
3. It is percussed to determine the presence of fluid or congested areas.
4. The physician listens to the sound within the chest by means of a stethoscope.
5. To examine the posterior chest, the patient is placed in a sitting position.
6. The heart and lungs are examined by percussion and auscultation.
7. The breasts are examined by palpation for the presence of lumps or growths.
8. The axillae are palpated for enlarged lymph nodes.
9. During the examination, the patient's face is turned away from the doctor.

EXAMINATION OF THE ABDOMEN

1. Extremities are inspected, palpated and moved.
2. A fine tremor suggestive of hyperthyroidism can be observed, if the patient is asked to hold the arms out in front of him for a few minutes.

Care of After Examination

1. Assist him to dress and help him to remain in a comfortable position in the bed.
2. Aftercare: Wash the equipment with soap and water, rinse, dry and sterilize, as needed.
3. Replace the equipments in their usual places.
4. Label specimens properly and send them to the laboratory immediately.

Nurse's Responsibilities during Physical Examination

1. A separate examination room is needed. Keep the doors closed, screen the patient and provide privacy if he is not in a separate room. Relatives are not allowed.
2. Drape the patient according to the parts that are to be examined. Natural light should be available in the examination room.
3. There should be adequate lighting in the room. The patient should be comfortable throughout the examination.

4. There must be provision for the maintenance of a suitable position, e.g. Lithotomy position. The room should be warm.
5. The nurse must stay in the room at all times while the doctor examines a female patient.
6. During the examination of a male patient's genitals, the nurse must leave the room. Take the patient's temperature, pulse, respiration and blood pressure, if recent readings are not available.
7. Give health teaching to the patient as need arises.

CONCLUSION

The first step of the nursing process is assessment. During this phase, the nurse gathers information about a patient's psychological, physiological, sociological, and spiritual status. This data can be collected in a variety of ways. Generally, nurses will conduct a patient interview. Physical examinations, referencing a patient's health history, obtaining a patient's family history, and general observation can also be used to gather assessment data. Patient interaction is generally the heaviest during this evaluative phase.

CHAPTER

18 Nursing Diagnosis

INTRODUCTION

The second step of the nursing process is often referred to as analysis, as well as need (or problem) identification or nursing diagnosis. Although all these terms may be used interchangeably, the purpose of this step of the nursing process is to draw conclusions regarding a client's specific needs or human responses of concern, so that effective care can be planned and delivered.

Today, the use of the nursing process and nursing diagnoses is rapidly becoming an integral part of an effective system of nursing practice. It is a system that can be used within existing conceptual frameworks, because it is a generic approach adaptable to all academic and clinical settings. In addition, as mentioned in the first chapter, organizing schemata of nursing problems other than North American Nursing Diagnosis Association (NANDA) are used within the profession.

DEFINITION

1. The nursing diagnosis is a conclusion drawn from the data collected about a client that serves as a means of describing the health need amenable to treatment by nurses. A uniform or standardized way of identifying, focusing on and labeling specific phenomena allows the nurse to deal effectively with individual client responses.
2. Nursing diagnosis is defined as "a clinical judgment about individual, family or community experiences/responses to actual or potential health problems/life processes. A nursing diagnosis provides the basis for selection of nursing interventions to achieve outcomes for which the nurse has accountability."
3. The process of assessing potential or actual health problems, including those pertaining to an individual patient, a family or community that fall within the scope of nursing practice; a judgment or conclusion reached as a result of such assessment or derived from assessment data.
4. A nursing diagnosis is a standardized statement about to the health of a client (individual, family or community) for the purpose of providing nursing care. One organization for defining standard diagnoses is the North American Nursing Diagnosis Association now known as NANDA-International.

CONCEPT OF NURSING DIAGNOSIS

1. Nursing diagnosis is actual or potential problems that are amenable to resolution by nursing actions are identified as nursing diagnosis.
2. The five national conferences on the classification of nursing diagnosis held in 1970's and the early 1980's have provided an impetus for the identification and classification of nursing diagnosis according to symptomatology.
3. When developing the nursing diagnosis for a particular patient, the nurse must first identify the commonalities among the assessment data collected. These common features lead to the categorization of related data that reveal the existence of a problem and the need for nursing intervention. The patient's nursing problem is then defined as the nursing diagnosis.
4. It must be remembered that nursing diagnosis are not medical diagnosis, they are not medical treatments prescribed by the physician; they are not diagnostic studies; they are not the equipment utilized to implement medical therapy.
5. Nursing diagnoses that are succinctly stated in terms of the specific problems of the patient will guide the nurse in the development of the nursing care plan.

MEANING OF NURSING DIAGNOSIS

Nursing diagnosis is a statement of a health problem or of a potential problem in the client's health status that a nurse is licensed and competent to treat. Four steps are required in the formulation of a nursing diagnosis. A database is established by collecting information from all available sources, including interviews with the client and the client's family, a review of any existing records of the client's health, observation of the client's response to any alterations in health status, a physical assessment and a conference or consultation with others concerned in the client's care. The database is continually updated. The second step includes analysis of the client's responses to the problems, healthy or unhealthy and classification of those responses as psychologic, physiologic, spiritual or sociologic. The third step is the organization of the data, so that a tentative diagnostic statement can be made that summarizes the pattern of problems discovered. The last step is confirmation of the sufficiency and accuracy of the database by evaluation of the appropriateness of the diagnosis to nursing intervention and by the assurance that given the same information, most other qualified practitioners would arrive at the same nursing diagnosis. In use, each diagnostic category has three parts—the term that concisely describes the problem, the probable cause of the problem and the defining characteristics of the problem. A number of nursing diagnoses have been identified and are listed as accepted by the NANDA and they are updated and refined at periodic meetings of the group.

NURSING DIAGNOSIS CLASSIFICATION

The North American Nursing Diagnosis Association-International system of nursing diagnosis provides four categories.

1. **Actual diagnosis:** A clinical judgment about human experience/responses to health conditions/life processes that exist in an individual, family, or community'.
   An example of an actual nursing diagnosis is sleep deprivation.
2. **Risk diagnosis:** Describes human responses to health conditions/life processes that may develop in a vulnerable individual/family/community. It is supported by risk factors that contribute to increased vulnerability. An example of a risk diagnosis is Risk for shock.
3. **Health promotion diagnosis:** A clinical judgment about a person's, family's or community's motivation and desire to increase wellbeing and actualize human health potential as expressed in the readiness to enhance specific health behaviors, and can be used in any health state.
   An example of a health promotion diagnosis is readiness for enhanced nutrition.
4. **Syndrome diagnosis:** A clinical judgment describing a specific cluster of nursing diagnoses that occur together and are best addressed together and through similar interventions. An example of a syndrome diagnosis is relocation stress syndrome.

STRUCTURE OF DIAGNOSIS

There are five types of nursing diagnoses in the NANDA system.

1. An actual diagnosis is a statement about a health problem that the client has and could benefit from nursing care.
   An example of an actual nursing diagnosis is: Ineffective airway clearance related to decreased energy and manifested by an ineffective cough.
2. A risk diagnosis is a statement about a health problem that the client does not have yet, but is at a higher than normal risk of developing in the near future.
   An example of a risk diagnosis is risk for injury related to altered mobility and disorientation.
3. A possible diagnosis is a statement about a health problem that the client might have now, but the nurse does not yet have enough information to make an actual diagnosis.
   An example of a possible diagnosis is possible fluid volume deficit related to frequent vomiting for three days and manifested by increased pulse rate.
4. A syndrome diagnosis is used when a cluster of nursing diagnoses are often seen together.
   An example of a syndrome diagnosis is: Rape-trauma syndrome related to anxiety about potential health problems and as manifested by anger, genitourinary discomfort and sleep pattern disturbance.

5. A wellness diagnosis is used to describe an aspect of the client, which is at a high level of wellness.

   An example of a wellness diagnosis is potential for enhanced organized infant behavior, related to prematurity and as manifested by response to visual and auditory stimuli.

DIAGNOSTIC REASONING

1. **Classification:** The initial step of data analysis is classification of the data. Data need to be organized in order to be clearly analyzed and the most logical means to organize data is to classify them. The body systems approach functional health pattern approaches are two convenient methods of classification. When these methods are used for taking a history and performing a physical examination, the data are already classified.
2. **Validation:** The next step of data analysis is validation. In this step, the nurse verifies the diagnosis by speaking to the client. The nurse can validate finding with the family, especially if the client is unable to communicate. For example, the nurse could ask about scars or wounds and therefore, expand the database on the client. The nurse can also validate the diagnosis by comparing it to textbook material or by talking to other nurses.
3. **Inductive versus deductive reasoning:** The nurse may use inductive or deductive reasoning to interpret data. Inductive reasoning begins with a set of facts from which a conclusion is drawn. Inductive reasoning is the use of cues to draw a conclusion.

   Deductive reasoning begins with the facts that the client is on bed rest and taking narcotics; and concludes (deduces) that the client is at an increased risk.

NURSING AND MEDICAL DIAGNOSIS

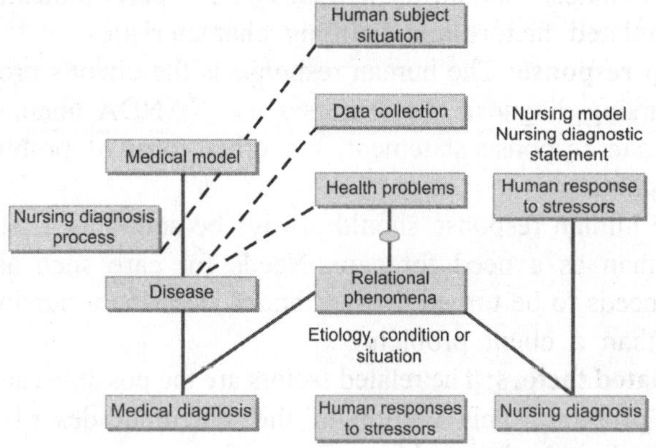

Figure 18.1: Nursing and medical diagnosis

ERRORS IN DIAGNOSIS

1. **Incomplete data:** Common cause of incomplete data occurs during the interview phase of assessment. Some clients withhold information intentionally because some they feel embarrassed or are unsure, how the nurse would react to the information.
2. **Inaccurate interpretation:** Data from the client can be misinterpreted in several ways. The problem can be diagnosed in several ways. The problem can be diagnosed before the data are completely collected. Sometimes the nurse can have a personal prejudice about the client.
3. **Lack of knowledge or experience:** Less clinical experience and knowledge may result in inaccurate data processing. Failure to recognize a problem is a common experience for most nurses. The inexperienced nurse may overlook important data or fail to realize the significance of the data.

IMPORTANCE OF NURSING DIAGNOSIS

1. The diagnosis is anything abnormal or that concerns the client or strengthens of the client. Diagnoses within the realm of nursing are the response of the client to a state of health or illness and include physical, psychological, spiritual and educational areas.
2. These nursing diagnosis and their treatment are within the legal scope of nursing practice. The actual conditions that nurses are educated to handle and licensed to treat are called nursing diagnosis.
3. The role of the nurses can vary greatly between settings; there has always been difficulty in describing the work in nursing. NANDA has provided national leadership in the development of standardized statements or nursing diagnosis, to describe human response to actual or potential health problems, which nurses treat.

WRITING OF NURSING DIAGNOSIS

A nursing diagnosis should be written in three parts indicating the human response, related factors and defining characteristics.

1. **Human response:** The human response is the client's problem attached as a nursing diagnosis. Most nurses use NANDA nursing diagnosis as the human response statement, but other form of problem statements are possible.

   The human response should always be stated as a response to care rather than as a need for care. Needs for care such as needs to be fed or needs to be turned every 2 hours, describe a nursing intervention rather than a client problem?
2. **The related factors:** The related factors are the possible causes or etiology of the problem. This section of the statement describes the factors associated with the problem. These factors may be environmental, psychological, physiological, sociocultural or spiritual.

Because these factors direct the nursing actions aimed at resolving, preventing or reducing the problem, the related factor should be directed at an aspect of the client response on which the nurse have an impact.

3. **The defining characteristics:** Are the data indicating the problem is present. When the client is at risk of developing a problem, the risk factors are identified rather than defining characteristics.

TEN RULES OF WRITING NURSING DIAGNOSIS

1. Write the diagnosis in terms of the client's response rather than nursing need.
2. Use 'related to', 'rather than' 'due to' or 'caused by' to connect the first two parts of the statement.
3. Write the diagnosis in legally advisable terms.
4. Write the diagnosis without value judgments.
5. Avoid reversing the parts of the statement.
6. Avoid using single cues as the first part of the statement.
7. The two parts of the statement should not mean the same thing.
8. Express the related factor in terms that can be changed.
9. Do not include the medical diagnosis in the nursing diagnosis.
10. State the diagnosis clearly and concisely.

COLLABORATIVE PROBLEMS

1. As nurses have continued to work with nursing diagnosis, shortcomings of the system have been identified.
2. Carpenito defines collaborative problems as the psychological complications that have resulted or may result from the pathophysiologic and treatment related conditions and from other situations.
3. Nurses monitor to detect the onset and status of complications and collaborate with physicians in treatment.

CONCLUSION

The diagnosing phase involves a nurse making an educated judgment about a potential or actual health problem with a patient. Multiple diagnoses are sometimes made for a single patient. These assessments not only include an actual description of the problem (e.g. sleep deprivation) but also whether or not a patient is at risk of developing further problems. These diagnoses are also used to determine a patient's readiness for health improvement and whether or not they may have developed a syndrome. The diagnoses phase is a critical step as it is used to determine the course of treatment.

CHAPTER

19

Nursing Planning

INTRODUCTION

The next step in the nursing process is planning activities to promote healthy client responses or prevent, correct or reduce unhealthy client responses.

Planning and setting expected outcomes begins by determining the priority of human response. It is (in five-step nursing process) a category of nursing behavior in which a strategy is designed to achieve the goals of care for an individual patient, as established in assessing and analyzing. Planning includes developing and modifying a care plan for the patient, cooperating with other personnel, and recording relevant information. To develop the plan, the nurse anticipates the patient's needs according to established priorities; involves the patient and the patient's family; and significant others in designing the plan; uses all information necessary for managing the patient's care, including recorded information from other health professionals and the age, sex, culture, ethnicity and religion. Plans for the patient's comfort, activity, and function; and chooses nursing measures that are necessary to deliver care as planned. With the cooperation of other health personnel, the nurse coordinates care for the benefit of the patient and identifies resources in the healthcare facility or community for social or health assistance as needed by the client or the patient's family. All information relevant to the management of the patient's care plan is recorded. Planning follows analyzing and precedes implementing in the five-step nursing process (Fig. 19.1).

DEFINITION

It involves a series of steps in which the nurse and client set priorities, formulate goals or expected outcomes and establish a written care plan for nursing interventions. The plan to resolve or minimize the identified problems of the client and to co-ordinate the care provided by all the health team members.

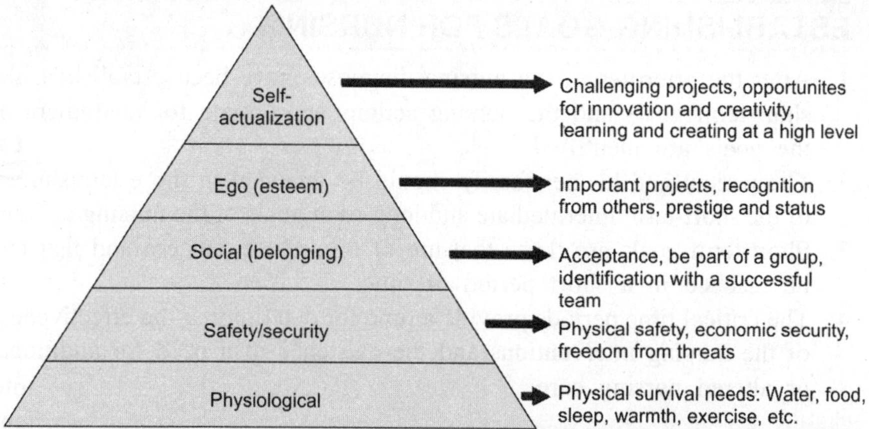

Malsow's hierarchy of needs is shown above. The pyramid illustrates the five levels of human needs. The most basic are physiological and safety/security, shown at the base of the pyramid. As one moves to higher levels of the pyramid, the needs become more complex.

Figure 19.1: Maslow's hierarchy of needs

PHASES OF PLANNING

Phases of nursing planning are as follows:

1. Assessment of priorities to nursing diagnosis.
2. Specification of short-term, intermediate and long-term goals of nursing action.
3. Identification of specific nursing interventions appropriate for attaining the goals.
4. Documentation of the nursing diagnosis, goals, nursing interventions and expected outcomes in the nursing care plan.

STEPS IN PRIORITIES

Impardent priorities regarding nursing diagnosis is described in following steps:

1. The assignment of priorities to the nursing diagnosis should be a joint effort by the nurse and the patient or patient's family members.
2. Consideration must be given to the urgency of the problems. The most critical receiving the highest priorities.
3. Maslow's hierarchy of needs provides a useful framework for the determination of priority problems. The use of this hierarchy requires that high priorities be given to physical needs.

ESTABLISHING GOALS FOR NURSING

1. After the priorities of the nursing diagnoses have been established, the short-term goals and the nursing actions appropriate for attainment of the goals are identified.
2. The patient and his/her family should be included in the establishment of the short-term intermediate and long-term goals of the nursing actions.
3. Short-term goals are those that are of immediate concern and that can be reached in a short period of time.
4. The critical time periods provide a time for determining the effectiveness of the nursing interventions and the existence of a need for additional or altered nursing care.

TEAM NURSING

1. Ideally the accomplishment of all aspects of the planning phase of the nursing process is a group effort.
2. The nurse collaborates with other members of the nursing team, with the patient and his/her family and with appropriate resource persons from the health care agency and community agencies.
3. It is also important to remember that the patient is part of a family. The family members have need that arises from the patient's illness.
4. Another aspect of care planning takes into the account the fact that the patient comes from the community. Community agencies have an interest in the patient and are involved in planning.

FORMULATING NURSING CARE PLAN

The nursing care plan serves to communicate the following information to all members of the nursing team:

1. Nursing diagnosis and their priorities.
2. The goals of the nursing interventions.
3. The nursing interventions, which are expressed in the form of nursing orders.
4. The outcomes criteria, which identify the expected behavioral outcomes for the patient.
5. The critical time period within which each outcome must be met.

CONCLUSION

Once a patient and nurse agree on the diagnoses, a plan of action can be developed. If multiple diagnoses need to be addressed, the head nurse will prioritize each assessment and devote attention to severe symptoms and high risk factors. Each problem is assigned a clear, measurable goal for the expected beneficial outcome. For this phase, nurses generally refer to the evidence-based Nursing Outcome Classification, which is a set of standardized terms and measurements for tracking patient wellness. The Nursing Interventions Classification may also be used as a resource for planning.

CHAPTER

20

Nursing Implementation/ Intervention

INTRODUCTION

Implementation as a phase of the nursing process involves putting the plan of care into effect. The nurse coordinates her activities with those of others responsible for contributing to patient care and delegates responsibility to other professional and technical caregivers as appropriate. During implementation the care plan is tested for effectiveness. Nursing interventions may not have had the desired effect or a change in the patient's condition, may present more critical problems that have a higher priority, thus requiring revision of the plan and different interventions. Nursing interventions are the actual implementation of the care plan. Nursing interventions are designed to promote, maintain or restore the client's health.

DEFINITION

1. Nursing intervention is an action for which nurses are responsible that is intended to benefit a patient or client.
2. Nursing interventions are actions undertaken by a nurse to further the course of treatment for a patient. In several nations, professional nursing organizations have created complex classification systems for such interventions, creating a standardized system that can be used by all nurses to provide a high level of care. The goal is to improve the health and comfort of the patient.

MEANING OF INTERVENTION

Nurses carry out nursing interventions during the implementation phase of the nursing process. Some examples of nursing interventions would be, administer pain medication as needed, turn and reposition every two hours or perform range of motion exercises. An order may be required of certain nursing interventions before they can be carried out. A standing order would be an example of this. Standing orders are made by doctors in case certain situations arise, such as giving a medication when the patient shows signs of agitation or insomnia. Some interventions are actually carried out by other licensed healthcare professionals, for example a physical or respiratory therapist. The nurse records all interventions performed as well as the patient's response and outcome. This information is also relayed at the end of the shift to the nurse who will be caring for the patient next during the oncoming shift.

Nursing intervention is an act by a nurse that implements the nursing care plan or any specific objective of that plan, such as turning a comatose patient to avoid the development of decubitus ulcers or teaching insulin injection technique to a patient with diabetes before discharge from the hospital. The patient may require intervention in the form of support, limitation, medication or treatment for the current condition or to prevent the development of further stress. As stress increases, the need to adapt and the need for nursing intervention increase.

CHARACTERISTICS OF NURSING INTERVENTION

Nursing interventions have following seven characteristics:

1. Be congruent with the overall plan of care.
2. Be based on scientific principles.
3. Be individualized to the client.
4. Be designed to provide a safe and therapeutic environment.
5. Consider the need for teaching and learning.
6. Use resources appropriately.
7. Be clearly communicated.

STAGE OF NURSING INTERVENTION

Nursing intervention has four stages. The first is the assessment, in which the nurse determines what the problem is, as for instance in the case of someone with a nail in his/her foot. After the assessment, the nurse formulates an appropriate intervention plan, which in the case of this fictional patient would involve removal of the nail, irrigation of the wound, the administration of prophylactic antibiotics and a tetanus shot. After planning, the nurse implements the treatment he/she has formulated and then evaluates the patient to determine the outcome of the interventions, and to decide if additional interventions need to be undertaken.

PROVING SELF-CARE

The nurse should identify what skills are required for providing the intervention. It is important to remember that when a skill is delegated to another healthcare team member, the registered nurse remains legally responsible for the client's outcome.

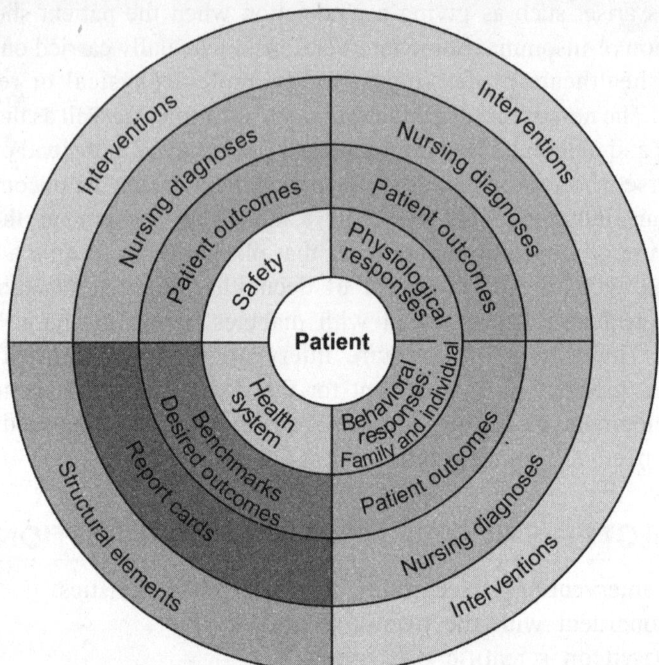

Figure 20.1: Steps of nursing process

Nurses can work alone or as part of patient care teams and interventions work in the same way in both cases. When a patient is admitted to the hospital, for example, nurse may have medical orders from a doctor, such as a standing order for medication, but the nurses also formulate a plan, which may include things like regularly checking patient vitals, monitoring fluid output and educating the patient and his or her family about the situation

Another aspect of providing self-care is continuous monitoring for complication. There are many complications that can allow surgery, medication administration and disease states. While the care is being given, the nurse continues to assess the client and evaluate his/her response to the care.

The nurse also needs to consider his/her which of the interventions could be modified, if the client shows no progress toward the desired outcome.

RATIONALE

At times, the scientific rationale for an intervention is required on a student care plan or listed within a standardized plan of care. It is important that the care given has its basis in scientific study, not in habit or old wives tales. The use of rationale assists in identifying the professional nurse from other healthcare providers.

NURSING ROLES

According to Benner's Helper role, care providing falls into seven categories—teaching and coaching, diagnostic and patient monitoring; management of rapidly changing conditions, administering and monitoring therapeutic regimens, monitoring and ensuring quality of healthcare practices, and organizational and work role competencies. Nursing interventions can include things like counseling, referrals, patient advocacy, the administration of medication, and the performance of minor medical procedures. As in all medical care, the primary concern is keeping the patient stable enough to receive treatment, while the secondary concern is evaluating all patient needs and deciding on a course of action. When a patient comes in with an obstructed airway and a broken leg, for instance, the airway must be secured before the broken leg can be treated. Nurses are also unafraid to call in support from other medical professionals when they need it.

In nursing schools, students are usually taken through a number of theoretical cases in which they are presented with a hypothetical assessment, and asked to come up with a nursing plan, which includes specific interventions. Nursing students also discuss routine interventions that are used on a regular basis and learn about how to assess patients, how to work with other medical staff to achieve a treatment plan, and how to interact with patients and their families to ensure that everyone stays informed, comfortable and happy.

CONCLUSION

The implementing phase is where the nurse follows through on the decided plan of action. This plan is specific to each patient and focuses on achievable outcomes. Actions involved in a nursing care plan include monitoring the patient for signs of change or improvement, directly caring for the patient or performing necessary medical tasks, educating and instructing the patient about further health management, and referring or contacting the patient for follow-up. Implementation can take place over the course of hours, days, weeks, or even months.

Nursing intervention: Any act by a nurse that implements the nursing care plan or any specific objective of that plan, such as turning a comatose patient to avoid the development of decubitus ulcers or teaching insulin injection technique to a patient with diabetes before discharge from the hospital. The patient may require intervention in the form of support, limitation, medication, or treatment for the current condition or to prevent the development of further stress. As stress increases, the need to adapt and the need for nursing intervention increase. Implementing consist of doing and documenting the activities that are the specific nursing actions needed to carry out the interventions. Common determinants for implementation relate to knowledge, cognitions, attitudes, routines, social influence, organization, and resources.

CHAPTER

21 Nursing Evaluation

INTRODUCTION

The last step in the process is evaluation. Evaluation examines the degree of goal attainment and basically asks, "Did the client achieve the goal he/she was supposed to?" and if not why not? Evaluation begins with collecting data about the client's health status, closely re-examining the outcome criteria. The degree of outcome attainment is determined and a revised plan of care is established, if needed.

MEANING OF EVALUATION

During the evaluation phase of the nursing process, the nurse assesses whether the patient's goals have been achieved and to what degree. Some goals are met partially or not at all and in these cases the nurse must determine what nursing actions should be implemented to bring about full achievement of goals. Goals that are met fully must be assessed to determine whether the implementation of nursing actions is necessary to continue or not. The evaluation is also documented. Evaluation is continuously done and depends upon all other phases of the process.

EVALUATION WILL ANSWER THE FOLLOWING QUESTIONS

1. Were the nursing diagnoses accurate?
2. Did the patient meet the outcome criteria?
3. Did the patient meet the criteria within the critical time periods?
4. Have the patient's nursing problems been resolved?
5. Have the patient's nursing needs been met?
6. Should the nursing interventions be retained, altered or discontinued?
7. Have new problems evolved, for which nursing interventions have not been planned or implemented?
8. What factors influenced the achievement or lack of achievement of the goals?
9. Do priorities need to be reassigned?
10. Should changes be made in the goals and outcome criteria?

FORMAL EVALUATION MODELS

Formal evaluation can be viewed as informal. There is also a formal method of evaluation through a system called quality assurance.

1. Quality assurance is the planned and systematic evaluation of care given to group of clients. The organization most actively involved in formal quality assurance is the joint commission for accreditation of health care organizations.
2. Quality assurance programs in nursing are viewed as evaluation system composed of three dimensions—structure, process and outcome.
3. The structural dimension: Focuses on the organization within which nursing care is provided.
4. The process dimension: Focuses on patient welfare and end results of the care provided to the patient.

EXPLANATION FOR EVALUATION PROCESS (FIG. 21.1)

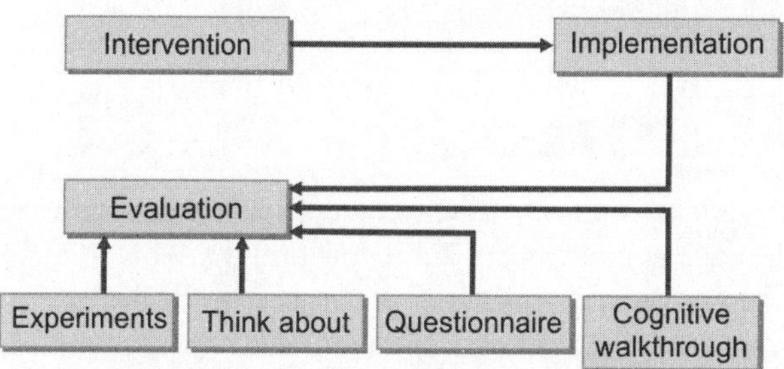

Figure 21:1: Evaluation process

OUTCOME CRITERIA

Goals for accountability and quality assurance in nursing are being realized. The American Nurses Association (ANA) has developed basic standards that provide a general model for nursing practice by which the quality of nursing practice may be evaluated. Record keeping has been revised to provide a problem-oriented approach to documentation of data. The use of outcome criteria as validations of the nursing process has become an accepted trend. The nursing audit has become an accepted method for comparing results of the actual nursing performance with the established criteria.

CONCLUSION

Evaluation, the final step of the nursing process, is crucial to determine whether, after application of the nursing process, the client's condition or well-being improves. The nurse applies all that is known about a client and the client's condition, as well as experience with previous clients, to evaluate whether nursing care was effective. The nurse conducts evaluation measures to determine if expected outcomes are met, not the nursing interventions. The expected outcomes are the standards against which the nurse judges if goals have been met and thus if care is successful. Providing health care in atimely, competent, and cost-effective manner is complex and challenging. The evaluation process will determine the effectiveness of care, make necessary modifications, and to continuously ensure favorable client outcomes. Nurse must have intellectual and technical skill to monitor the effectiveness of nursing interventions. Nurse must have knowledge and skill of collecting subjective data and objective data.

SECTION V
Quality Patient Care

GLOSSARY

1. **Accounting system:** The series of tasks and records of an entity by which transactions are processed as a means of maintaining financial records.
2. **Analytical procedures:** Consist of the analysis of significant ratios and trends including the resulting investigation of fluctuations and relationships that are inconsistent with other relevant information or deviate from predictable amounts.
3. **Audit evidence:** The information obtained by the auditor in arriving at the conclusions on which the audit opinion is based.
4. **Audit risk:** The risk that auditors may give an inappropriate audit opinion on financial statements.
5. **Audit staff:** The personnel involved in an audit other than the audit engagement partner.
6. **Auditing:** A systematic process of objectively obtaining and evaluating evidence in respect of certain assertions about economic actions and events to ascertain the degree of correspondence between those assertions and established criteria and reporting the results to interested parties over a particular period of time.
7. **Auditor:** The person with final responsibility for the audit. This term is also used to refer to an audit firm.
8. **Goodwill:** The difference between the value of a business as a whole and the aggregate of the fair values of its separable net assets.
9. **Governance:** Describes the role of persons entrusted with the supervision, control and direction of an entity by ensuring that the entity achieves its objectives, financial reporting and of reporting to interested parties.
10. **Incoming auditor:** The auditor, who is to take over from the current auditor and did not audit the prior period's financial statements.
11. **Independent audit:** Providing reasonable assurance that published audited financial reports are free from material misstatement and are in accordance with legislation and relevant accounting standards.
12. **Internal audit:** An appraisal or monitoring activity established by management and the directors for the review of the accounting and internal control systems as a service to the entity.

13. **Principal auditor:** The auditor with responsibility for reporting on the financial statements of an entity when those financial statements include financial information of one or more components audited by other auditors.

CHAPTER

22

Quality Assurance

INTRODUCTION

The Joint Commission on the Accreditation of Healthcare Organizations (JCAHO) advocates that each hospital is required to conduct a comprehensive integrated Quality Assurance Program to ensure continuing control of quality care for patients. The need for nursing quality assurance active is spelt out in the nursing standards of JCAHO manual. It states that "the Nursing Service Department" has a planned and systematic process for the monitoring and evaluation of the quality and appropriateness of patient care and for resolving identified problems. Nursing manager's understanding of the concept of quality assurance will enhance their role in implementing and evaluating standards of care.

DEFINITION

1. Quality assurance (QA) is the process of establishing a target degree of excellence for nursing intervention and taking action to ensure that each patient receives the agreed upon-level of care.
2. Quality assurance is a judgment concerning the process of care based on the extent to which that tare contributes to valued outcomes.

   — *Donabedian 1982*
3. Quality assurance is the measurement of provision against expectations with declared intention and ability to correct any demonstrated weakness.

   —*Shaw*
4. Quality assurance is a management system designed to give maximum guarantee and ensure confidence that the service provided is up to the given accepted level of quality, the standards prescribed for that service, which is being achieved with a minimum of total expenditure.

   —*British Standards Institute*

CONCEPT OF QUALITY ASSURANCE

Duality assurance is a dynamic process through which nurses in both academic and clinical practice assume accountability for quality of care they provide

(George, Veigas and Isaac, 1984). It is a guarantee to the society that members of the nursing profession are regulating services provided by nurses. Kozier et al. (2004) define quality assurance as the defining of nursing practice through well written nursing standards and the use of those standards as a basis for evaluation on improvement of client care.

OBJECTIVES OF QUALITY ASSURANCE

Quality assurance whether in health or education had two main objectives:

1. To provide technical assistance in designing and implementing effective strategies for monitoring quality and correcting systemic deficiencies.
2. To refine existing methods for ensuring optimal quality health care through an applied research program (Decker, 1985 and Schroeder, 1984).

APPROACHES TO QUALITY ASSURANCE

In quality assurance, there are three approaches from which nursing care can be evaluated to assure quality nursing practice:

1. Structure.
2. Process.
3. Outcome.

Since each of these interaction elements contributes to the quality of nursing care delivered, an improvement in any of the three tends to produce favorable change in the other two.

STRUCTURAL ELEMENT

Structural element includes the physical setting, instrumentality and conditions through which nursing care is administered, such as philosophy, objectives, policies, procedures, records, organizational structures, financial resources, equipment and expectations, and attitudes of patients and employees.

PROCESS ELEMENT

Process element includes steps of the nursing process itself—assessment, diagnosing, planning, implementation and evaluation and; all subsystems within the nursing process, such as taking a health history, performing a physical examination, making a nursing diagnosis, determining nursing care goals, writing a nursing care plan, performing each care, cure and coordination of tasks prescribed by the care plan, measuring patient care outcome and recording and reporting patient's response to treatment. It is the criteria for measuring nursing care to determine if nursing standards of practice are being met, so they are task oriented.

OUTCOME ELEMENT

It includes changes in patient health systems that result from nursing interventions. For example, modification in signs and symptoms, knowledge, attitudes satisfaction, skill level and compliance with treatment regimen, and established patient outcome criteria.

STEPS IN QUALITY ASSURANCE

Quality assurance is the systematic process of evaluating the quality of care given in a particular unit or institution. It involves the following steps:

SETTING STANDARDS

A standards is a desired quantity, quality or level of performance with reference to a criterion against which performance is to be measured. The nursing profession through the American Nurses Association (ANA), itself has designated generic standards of nursing practice. In addition, each patient care unit must designated standards specific to the patient population served. These standards are the foundation upon which all other measures of QA are based.

For example, every patient will instruments are developed and selected to collect evidence that indicates standards are being met. There are three basic forms of nursing audits: structure, process and outcome. Standards define nursing care customers as well as nursing activities of structural resources needed. They are used for planning nursing care as well as for evaluating it.

ASSIGN RESPONSIBILITY

Assign responsibility to individual or committee.

DELINEATE SCOPE OF CARE

Develop an inventory including the type of patients served, the conditions and diagnoses treated, the treatment or activities performed, the type of practitioners providing care, the site where care is provided. This will provide bases for subsequent steps in the evaluation process.

IDENTIFY IMPORTANT ASPECTS OF CARE

Unit personnel should ask themselves "which of the things we do are most important?" the answer should lead to identifying important aspects of care (criteria). Priority should be given to those aspects of care, which occur frequently affect large number of patients involves risk or serious consequences or will deprive patient from substantial benefit if the care is not provided correctly or problematic behavior.

DETERMINING CRITERIA

Criteria must be determined that will indicate if the standards are being met and to what degree they are met. Criteria must be general and specific to the individual unit. A criterion is the value-free name of a variable that is known to be reliable indicator of quality. For example, a criterion to demonstrate that the standard regarding care plan for every patient is being met would be: "A nursing care plan is developed and written by a registered nurse within 12 hours of admission." This criterion provides a measurable indicator to evaluate performance.

DATA COLLECTION

Sufficient observations and random samples are necessary for producing reliable and valid information. A useful rule is that 10% of the institutional patient population per month should be sampled.

Data collection methods include:

- Patients' observations and interviews
- Nurses observations and interviews
- Review of charts.

EVALUATING PERFORMANCE

The methods include:
1. Reviewing documented records.
2. Observing activities as they take place.
3. Examining patients.
4. Interviewing patients, families and staff.

Records are most commonly used as source for evaluation, but they are not as reliable as direct observations. It is quite possible to write in the patient's chart activities that were not done or to not record these things that were done. Also, the chart indicates the care provided, but it does not demonstrate the quality of that care. Examples for evaluating performance.

For the stated criteria example: This step will be recorded to examine to determine if care plans were written on each patient within 12 hours of admission and, if so that standards had been met.

To measure quality of the care plan: Every care plan will include patient education appropriate to the patient's medical diagnosis, nursing diagnosis, interventions planned and discharge planning.

Problem identification: Analysis and reporting of the data gathered from the evaluation process will lead to problem identification and isolation, and the evidence is gathered through round, observation and records. The nurse manager's responsibility is to look for patterns or trends of deviation from normal, further data collection and analysis could be done for the identified problems.

Problem solution: Once problem has been defined and isolated, plans are made to solve them on a priority bases. Those that are critical, which involves safety and welfare of the patient take first priority. Other factors use in determining priority will include severity, frequency, benefit, cost and liability.

The first step is that the nursing unit must determine how much deviation from the standard is acceptable before changes are made. In the example of developing a written nursing care plan for every patient as a standard, the unit should decide if 45 out of 50 patients admitted have a care plan recorded within 12 hours of admission and the other 5 have recorded care plans within the next 6 hours, is this deviation acceptable? If not, then how should this be corrected?

- Is the unit short-staffed?
- Have there been an unusually large numbers of admissions recently?
- Are a number of new graduates being oriented on the unit?

After collecting all pertinent information about the possible causes, the Nurse Manager after consultation with staff and/or supervisor should make plans for correcting deficiencies in performance.

- What needs change? Structural element?
- Process element?
- Outcome element?

Monitoring and feedback: Follow-up on how effective changes have been in improving performance is very necessary step in the QA process.

If in the example prescribed, the nurse manager found that the next 50 patients had care plans recorded within 12 hours, then the performance had improved relative to that standard. If it had not improved, then another approach would need to be taken, or possibly, the criterion should be evaluated for appropriateness for that unit.

QUALITY ASSURANCE METHODS

The purpose of a nursing QA Program is to measure and improve the quality of patient care delivered in the organization. Therefore, a variety of QA methods have been used. These include:

Nursing audit: It is a method for evaluating quality of nursing care through the appraisal of the nursing process or customers of care as it is reflected in the patient care records. There are two types of audits:

1. Concurrent and
2. Retrospective audit.

Peer review: It is a process by which nurses evaluate one another's job performance against accepted standards.

Patient care profiles analysis: The analysis of longitudinal or cross-sectional complications of data about patients with a particular diagnosis or problem.

Quality circles: A quality circle is a small group of 5 to 15 employees who perform similar work and meet for one hour each week to solve problems related to their work.

Patient satisfaction (client feedback): Patient satisfaction is used as one of several indicators of quality.

QUALITY ASSURANCE CYCLE

In practice, QA is a cyclical, iterative process that must be applied flexibly to meet the needs of a specific program. The process may begin with a comprehensive effort to define standards and norms as described in steps 1–3 or it may start with small-scale quality improvement activities (steps 5–10). Alternatively, the process may begin with monitoring (step 4). Some teams may even choose to simultaneously begin in two places. For instance, comprehensive monitoring and focused problem solving may start as a coordinated, parallel effort. The ten steps in the QA process are discussed in the following section.

1. **Planning for quality assurance:** This first step prepares an organization to carry out QA activities. Planning begins with a review of the organizations scope of care to determine which services should be addressed.
2. **Setting standards and specifications:** To provide consistently high-quality services, an organization must translate its programmatic goals

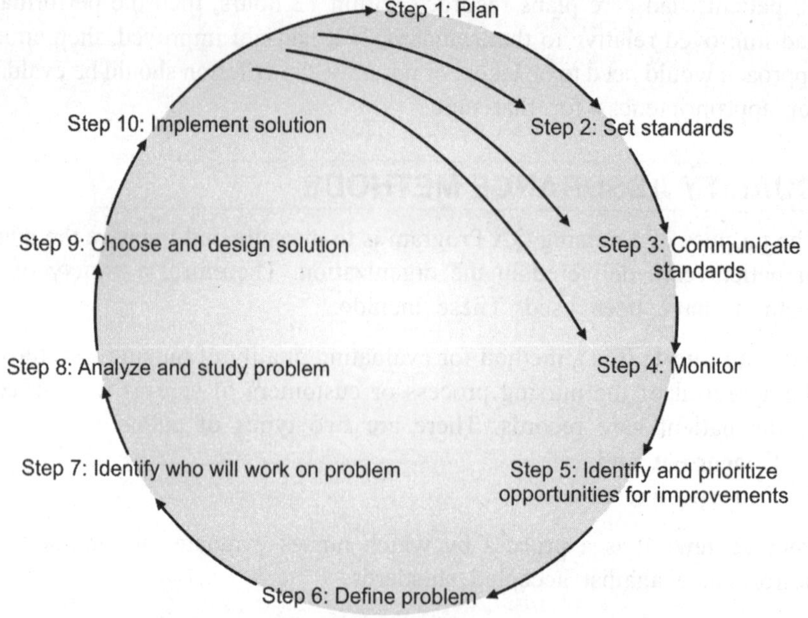

Figure 22.1: Steps in quality assurance

and objectives into operational procedures. In its widest sense, a standard is a statement of the quality that is expected. Under the broad rubric of standards there are practice guidelines or clinical protocols, administrative procedures or standard operating procedures, product specifications and performance standards. For some programs, setting standards and specifications involves a simple review of current guidelines and standard operating procedures to ensure that they are up-to-date.

3. **Communicating guidelines and standards:** Once practice guidelines, standard operating procedures and performance standards have been defined, it is essential that staff members communicate and promote their use. This will ensure that each health worker, supervisor, manager, and support person understands what is expected from him/her. This is particularly important if ongoing training and supervision have been weak or if guidelines and procedures have recently changed. Assessing quality before communicating expectations can lead to erroneously blaming individuals for poor performance when fault actually lies with systemic deficiencies. Additionally, QA efforts that begin with a surprise examination are likely to cause suspicion rather than support.
4. **Monitoring quality:** Monitoring is the routine collection and review of data that helps to assess whether program norms are being followed or whether outcomes are improved. By monitoring key indicators, managers and supervisors can determine whether the services delivered follow the prescribed practices and achieve the desired results.
5. **Identifying problems and selecting opportunities for improvement**: Program managers can identify quality improvement opportunities by monitoring and evaluating activities. Other means include soliciting suggestions from health workers, performing system process analyses, reviewing patient feedback or complaints and generating ideas through brainstorming or other group techniques. Once a health facility team has identified several problems, it should set quality improvement priorities by choosing one or two problem areas on which to focus. Selection criteria will vary from program to program.
6. **Defining the problem:** Having selected a problem, the team must define it operationally as a gap between actual performance and performance as prescribed by guidelines and standards. The problem statement should identify the problem and how it manifests itself. It should clearly state where the problem begins and ends and how to recognize when the problem is solved. Developing a problem statement is a crucial step in the QA process and its apparent simplicity is deceptive.
7. **Choosing a team:** Once a health facility staff has employed a participatory approach to selecting and defining a problem, it should

assign a small team to address the specific problem. The team will analyze the problem, develop a quality improvement plan and implement and evaluate the quality improvement effort. The team should comprise those who are involved with, contribute inputs or resources to and/or benefit from the activity or activities in which the problem occurs. This ensures the involvement of those most knowledgeable about the process.

8. **Analyzing and studying the problem to identify the root cause:** Achieving a meaningful and sustainable quality improvement effort depends on understanding the problem and its root causes. Given the complexity of health service delivery, clearly identifying root causes requires systematic, in-depth analysis. Analytical tools such as system modeling, flow charting and cause and effect diagrams can be used to analyze a process or problem.

   Analytical tools alone will not always provide enough information. A problem-solving team may need to conduct an in-depth examination. Such studies can be based on clinical record reviews, health center register data, staff or patient interviews, service delivery observations.
9. **Developing solutions and actions for quality improvement**: The problem-solving team should now be ready to develop and evaluate potential solutions. Unless the procedure in question is the sole responsibility of an individual, developing solutions should be a team effort. It may be necessary to involve personnel responsible for processes related to the root cause.
10. **Implementing and evaluating quality improvement efforts:** Implementing quality improvement requires careful planning. The team must determine the necessary resources and time frame; and decide who will be responsible for implementation. It must also decide whether implementation should begin with a pilot test in a limited area or should be launched on a larger scale. The team should select indicators to evaluate whether the solution was implemented correctly and whether it resolved the problem it was designed to address. In-depth monitoring should begin when the quality improvement plan is implemented. It should continue until either the solution is proven effective and sustainable or the solution is proven ineffective and is abandoned or modified. When a solution is effective, the teams should continue limited monitoring.

ROLE OF NURSE IN QUALITY ASSURANCE

Nurses are responsible for managing the caseload of client with needs of varying degrees of urgency. Using the resources available, they must provide priority services that will promote the highest possible level of person and group functioning and health. Some quality improvement activities for nurses include daily prioritizing care needs, seeking supervision or skills development for a difficult case, systematizing charting, so that needed documentation is effectively completed, proposing better ways to organize care of chronically ill client or establishing new agency procedures. All these actions demonstrate that nurses are valuating their work and looking for ways to improve care. Staff meetings, quality circle meeting, peer review and case conferences are common settings for nurses to bring the lessons of their practices to the larger group for examination and potential adoption.

It is the role of nursing administrator to develop a formalizing tractor to develop a formalized quality program that includes a three pronged focus based on a classic approach to quality management.

1. Review organizational structure, personnel and environment.
2. Focus on standards of nursing care and methods of delivering nursing care.
3. Focus on the outcomes of care.

Thus, any activities the nurse engages in to realize these goals contribute to the quality management program.

CONCLUSION

Nursing has clearly been concerned with defining and measuring quality long before the current national and State-level emphasis on quality improvement. Florence Nightingale analyzed mortality data among British troops in 1855 and accomplished significant reduction in mortality through organizational and hygienic practices. She is also credited with creating the world's first performance measures of hospitals in 1859. In the 1970s, Wandelt reminded us of the fundamental definitions of quality as characteristics and degrees of excellence, with standards referring to a general agreement of how things should be (to be considered of high quality). Patient safety is the cornerstone of high-quality health care. Much of the work defining patient safety and practices that prevent harm have focused on negative outcomes of care, such as mortality and morbidity. Nurses are critical to the surveillance and coordination that reduce such adverse outcomes. Much work remains to be done in evaluating the impact of nursing care on positive quality indicators, such as appropriate self-care and other measures of improved health status.

CHAPTER

23 Nursing Standards

INTRODUCTION

A standard is a means of determining what something should be. In nursing education, the standard refers to the established criteria for the provision of nursing education. In case of nursing practice, standards are the established criteria for the practice of nursing. Standards are having permanent value. A nursing standard can be a target.

Standard is an established rule as basis of comparison in measuring or finding capacity, quality context and value of objects in the same category. Standard is a broad statement of quality. It is a definite level of excellence as adequately required, aimed at or possible. Standard is a predetermined baseline condition as level of excellence that comprises a model to be followed and practiced. It is used as a measurement tool.

DEFINITION

'A standard is a model of established practice, which has general recognition and acceptance among registered professional nurses and is commonly accepted as correct standards of practice are agreed on levels of competence as determined by the American Nurses Association (ANA) and specially nursing organization'. —*American Medical Association (AMA), 1996.*

'Standards are defined as authoritative statements that describe a common level of care as performance by which the quality of practice can be determined or measured. Standard help define professional practice'. —*Hubes, 1996.*

PURPOSES OF STANDARDS

In order to provide a high quality of nursing education is necessary that nurse educators develop standard education and appropriate evaluation tools.

1. Standards give direction and provide guidelines.
2. Standards provide a baseline for evaluating quality care nursing education and thereby quality care.
3. It helps to plan for the faculty recruitment, development of infrastructure and others.

4. It aids in curriculum planning, implementation and evaluation.
5. It assists in planning for student welfare activities, staff welfare activities.
6. Standards help improve quality of nursing care, increase effectiveness of care and improve efficient.
7. A standard may help to improve documentation of nursing care.
8. Standards may help to determine the degree to which standards of nursing care maintained.
9. Standards help supervisors to guide nursing staff improve performance.
10. Standards may help to improve basis for decision making.
11. Standards may help justify demands.
12. Standards may help clarify nurse's area of accountability.
13. Standards may help nursing to define clearly different levels of care.

IMPORTANCE OF STANDARDS

1. It is an authoritative statement by which the quality nursing practice, service and education can be judged.
2. In nursing practice, standards are established for the practice of nursing.
3. It is a guideline, a recommended path to safe control and aid to professional performance.
4. It provides a baseline for evaluating quality of nurse care, increases effectiveness of care and improve efficiency.
5. Standards, help supervisors to guide nursing staff improve performances.
6. Standards may help to clarify nurses' area of accountability.
7. Standards may help nursing to clearly define different levels of care.
8. Standard is a device for quality assurance as quality control.

SOURCES OF NURSING STANDARDS

1. Professional organization or association, e.g. Trained Nurses Association of India (TNAI).
2. Licensing bodies, e.g. statutory bodies, Indian Nursing Council (INC), State Nursing Council (SNC), etc.
3. Universities and boards, e.g. The Tamil Nadu Dr MGR Medical University.
4. Institutions/healthcare agencies, e. g. university hospitals, health centers.
5. Department of institutions, e.g. department of nursing.
6. Patient care units, e.g. specific patients' unit.
7. Government units at national, state and local level.
8. Individual standards, e.g. personal standards.

CHARACTERISTICS OF STANDARDS

1. Statement must be broad.

Table 23.1: Joint Commision of American Hospital (JCAH) Nursing Services Standards

Standard	Emphasis
Standard I	The nursing department/service shall be directed by a qualified nurse administer and shall be appropriately integrated with the medical staff; and with other hospital staffs that provide and contribute to patient care. The administrator of the nursing department/ service shall be a qualified, registered nurse with appropriate education, experience, and licensure and demonstrated ability in nursing practice and administration.
Standard II	The nursing department/service shall be organized to meet the nursing care needs of patients ad to maintain established standards of nursing practice. The nursing department/service shall have a written organizational plan that delineates lines of authority, accountability and communication. The manner in which the nursing department/service is organized shall be consistent with the variety of patient services offered and the scope of nursing care activities. Reviewing and approviding policies and procedures. Establishing standards of nursing care accounting for professional and administrative nursing staff activities. Implementing the approved policies of the nursing department/service. Appointing committees as needed. Encouraging nursing staff personnel to participate in staff education programs.
Standard III	Nursing department/service assignments in the provision of nursing care shall be commensurate with the qualifications of nursing personnel and shall be designed to meet the nursing care needs of patient. A sufficient number of qualified registered nurses shall be on duty at all times to give patients the nursing care that requires the judgemet and specialized skills of a registered nurse.
Standard IV	Individualized, goal-directed nursing care shall be provided to patients through the use of the nursign process. The nursing process (assessment, planning, intervention, evaluation) shall be documented for each hospitlized patient from admission through discharge.
Standard V	Nursing department/service personnel shall be prepared through appropriate education and training programs for their responsibilities in the provision of nursing care. Education/training programs for nursing department/service personnel shall be ongoing and designed to augment their knowledge of pertinent new developments in patient care and to maintain current competence.The scope and complexity of program shall be based on the documented educational needs of nursing staff personnel and the resources availabel to meet those needs.
Standard VI	Written policies and procedures that reflect optimal standards of nursing shall guide the provision of nursing care. Written standards of nursing practice and reflected policies; and procedures shall define and describe the scope and conduct of patient care provided by the nursing staff. These standards, policies and procedures shall be reviewed at least annually, revised as necessary, dated to indicate the time of the last review, signed by the responsible reviewing authority and implicated.
Standard VII	As part of the hospitals quality assurance program, the quantity of an appropriateness of the patient care provided by the nursing department/ service are monitored and evaluated and identified programs are resolved. The nursing department/service has a planned and systematic process for monitoring and evaluation of the quality and appropriateness of patient care; and for resolving identified problems.

2. Must be realistic, acceptable and attainable.
3. Standards of nursing care must be developed by members of the nursing profession, preferably nurses practicing at the direct care level with consultation of experts in the domain.
4. It should be phrased in positive terms.
5. Must be understandable and stated in unambiguous terms.
6. Must be reviewed and revised periodically.
7. May be directed toward an ideal, i.e. optional standards or only specify the minimal care that must be attained, i.e. minimum standard.
8. And one must remember that standards that are workable are objective, acceptable, achievable and flexible.

PURPOSES OF STANDARD EDUCATION

The purposes of publishing, circulating and enforcing nursing standards in education are to:
1. Improve the quality of nursing education.
2. Decrease the cost of nursing education.
3. Ultimately to improve the patient care.

CLASSIFICATION OF STANDARDS

BASED ON ORIENTATION

Nursing care standards in hospital can be divided into ends and means standards.
1. **End standards:** The end standards are patient oriented; they describe the change as desired in a patient's physical status or behavior.
2. **Mean standards:** The mean standards are nursing oriented, they describe the activities and behavior designed to achieve end standards.

   End standards require information about the patients. A mean standard calls for information about the nurses' performance.

BASED ON FRAME OF REFERENCE

Nursing care standards can be classified according to frame of references, relating to nursing structure, process and outcome.
1. **Structure standard:** A structural standard involves the set-up of the institution. The philosophy, goals and objectives, structure of the organization, facilities and equipment and qualifications of employees are some of the components of the structure of the organization. For example, recommended relationship between the nursing department and other departments in a healthy agency are structural standards, because they refer to the organizational structure in which nursing is implemented. It includes people, money, equipment, staffing policies, etc. The use

of standards based on structure implies that if the structure is adequate, reliable and desirable, standard will be met and quality care will be given.

2. **Process standard:** Process standards describe the behaviors of the nurse at the desired level of performance. A process standard involves the activities concerned with delivering patient care. These standards measure nursing action involving patient care. The standards are stated in action verbs that are in observable and measurable terms. For example, the patient demonstrates. The focus is on what was planned, what was done and what was communicated as recorded. In process standard, there is an element of professional judgment, i.e. determining the quality as the degree of skill. It includes nursing care technique, procedures, regimens and processes.
3. **Outcome standards:** Descriptive statements of desired patient care results are outcome standard, because patients results are outcome of nursing intervention. An outcome standard measures changes in the patient health status. This change may be due to nursing care, medical care or as a result of variety of services offered to the patient. Outcome standards reflect the effectiveness and results rather than the process of giving care.

Thus, structural standards are agency or group oriented process, standards are nurse oriented and whereas outcome standards are patient results oriented. Normative standards describe practices considered 'good' or 'ideal' by some authoritative group. Empirical standards describe practices actually observed in a large number of patient care settings.

CONCLUSION

"Nursing Standards of Care" pertain to professional nursing activities that are demonstrated by the nurse through the nursing process. These involve assessment, diagnosis, outcome identification, planning implementation, and evaluation. The nursing process is the foundation of clinical decision making and encompasses all significant action taken by nurses in providing care to all consumers. While "Nursing Standards of Professional Performance" describe the roles of all professional nurses, there are many other responsibilities that are hallmarks of professional nursing. These nurses should be self-directed and purposeful in seeking necessary knowledge and skills to enhance career goals. Other activities—such as membership in professional organizations, certification in specialty or advanced practice, continuing education and further academic education, are desirable methods of enhancing the nurse's professionalism. Accountability for one's practice as a professional rests with the individual nurse. Professional standards ensure that the highest level of quality nursing care is promoted. Excellent nursing practice is a reflection of sound ethical standards. Client care requires more than just the application of scientific knowledge. A nurse must be able to think critically, solve problems, and find the best solution for client's needs to assist clients in maintaining, regaining, or improving their health. Critical thinking requires the use of scientifically based and practice-based criteria for making clinical judgments. These criteria may be scientifically based on research findings or practice based on standards developed by clinical experts and quality improvement initiatives.

CHAPTER

24

Nursing Audit

INTRODUCTION

Audit is the instrument for quantify assurance. It developed in 19th century; the nursing audit is similar to an audit performed by accounting departments. It is a process that offers the nursing personnel in a health agency, the opportunity to create and enforce standards of nursing care; and to examine their own practice in systematic manner.

MEANING OF AUDITING

Auditing is broadly defined as a systematic process of objectively obtaining and evaluating evidence in respect of certain assertions about economic actions and events, to ascertain the degree of correspondence between those assertions and established criteria; and reporting the results to interested parties. Auditing usually covers a particular period of time. Auditing may be narrowly defined as a written report on the examination of financial statements for a particular period of time.

DEFINITION

1. Nursing audit is the systematic, critical analysis of the quality of clinical/ community care. It is an official examination of nursing records for the purpose of evaluation verification and betterment of nursing care.
2. Nursing audit is a systematic formal and written appraisal by nurses of the quality of the content and process of nursing service from care record for discharged patients.
3. Nursing audit is the systematic critical analysis of the quality of clinical care. It is an official examination of nursing records for the purpose of evaluation.
4. Nursing audit is a process of collecting information from nursing reports and other documented evidence about patient care and assessing the quality of care by the use of quality assurance programmer.

OBJECTIVE OF NURSING AUDIT

1. To justify the cost incurred on human and material resources.
2. To study the quality of patient care against defined criteria.
3. To take remedial actions toward cost-effectiveness.
4. To assess the competence of nursing staff.
5. To prevent repetition of mistakes and to bring to notice the deficiencies in hospital care and in correcting the causative factors.

To bring to notice the overall objective of nursing audit is quality assurance of delivered care in relation to change in the health status of the patient and cost-effectiveness.

TYPES OF AUDIT

1. **Nursing management audit:** This type is more structure oriented focusing on administrative aspects of the nurse's responsibilities and nurses that the health facilities are suitably equipped to provide care.
2. **Retrospective audit:** This is the evaluation of nursing care by examining the records and charts of discharged patients.
3. **Concurrent audit:** It is the evaluation of the nursing care by the observation and retrospective method during the delivery of care. The best method of audit depends on the objective of audit.

CHARACTERISTICS OF AUDIT

1. Audit looks at the entire process of care including administration and not just at clinical management.
2. Compares the care, which actually is given. Standard procedures are agreed to decide, which care should be given.
3. Concentrates on finding solutions for the problems identified.

PRINCIPLES OF AUDITING

Fundamental principles are those according to which the books of business accounts are audited. These principles can be changed according the desire of the auditor. We discuss the main principles of auditing under these headings:

1. **Planning:** It is the basic principle of auditing. The auditor should plan before starting the work. In planning, auditor decides accounting about the system and internal control procedure.
2. **Honesty:** Honesty and sincerity is the second important principle of auditing. The loyalty of auditor to work and profession must be beyond the doubts.
3. **Impartiality:** In case of audit, the attitude of the auditor must be impartial. Keeping in view this principle his/her personal views may not be included in the audit report.

4. **Secrecy:** Secrecy must be maintained by the auditor during the process of audit. He cannot disclose any information to the third party.
5. **Evidence:** During the audit, the auditor can collect the evidence through the working papers. Auditor can frame his/her opinion on the audit evidence. The nature and source of evidence must be kept in view by the auditor.
6. **Consistency:** It is an important principle of auditing. In case of selecting the rates of depreciation and valuation of stock, the accountant must follow the rates of the coming years. In this regard there should be consistency and changes are not acceptable.
7. **Legal frame work:** The business activities may run within the rules and legal formalities. To protect the rights of the interested parties rules must be applied.
8. **Working paper preparation:** The auditor collect documents providing evidence that audit was carried out according the principles. The auditor prepares the working paper and kept in this custody as a proof.
9. **Internal control:** The auditor will examine the accounting system and inter auditor control. To frame opinion, he/she keeps in view the evidence obtained from the books.
10. **Report:** According the principle of auditing, a report will be prepared by the auditor at the end. It may be conditional or unconditional. The auditor can draw conclusion and disclose the facts and figures about the business for general information.

TECHNIQUES OF AUDITING

Techniques of auditing means the procedure and method, which is adopted by the auditor in checking the accounts. Following are the important techniques of audit:

1. **Examination of record:** This technique is commonly used by the auditors. The inspection of books and documents is made to verify the validity of data.
2. **Inquiry:** The auditor can also use the technique of inquiry. He can get the information from resource persons inside or outside the enterprise.
3. **Sampling:** Auditor can select few items from whole accounting information. This technique enables the auditor to obtain and evaluate the evidence of some characteristics of the whole class. It is helpful in forming the conclusion.
4. **Confirmation:** To ensure the accuracy of the data, auditor can collect the information from the debtor. Confirmation is response to an inquiry to prove certain data recorded in the books.
5. **Compliance:** To check the arithmetical accuracy of accounting record, the balancing accounts can be compared with the vouchers to test the reliability of data.

6. **Compliance test:** These tests are designed to check the effectiveness and compliance of internal control. In obtaining the audit evidence, auditor is concerned with the existence of effective internal control.
7. **Use of computer techniques:** There are large number of audit techniques like audit software, test packs and mapping, which can be used by the auditor to test the accuracy of the data.
8. **Substantive test:** These are designed to obtain evidence that data produced by accounting system is accurate or not. It has two kinds:
   a. Test of detail transaction.
   b. Test of significant ratios and trends.
9. **Dependence on experts and auditors:** The auditor has to rely on the internal and other auditors to complete work. Auditor has also to rely on other experts like lawyers, engineers and doctors for their expert opinion about the business.
10. **Analytical review:** It consists of studying significant ratios, trends and investigating different changes. This review procedure is based on the expectations of relationship among the past and present data.

ETHICAL PRINCIPLES

In carrying out the audit of financial statements, auditors should comply with the ethical guidance issued by their relevant professional bodies. Ethics is more of a norm or a certain code of conduct expected of a group of individuals or a professional body. It dictates some degree of inward values expected of such groups of individuals or body. The ethical principles which govern the auditors' professional responsibilities include:
1. Integrity.
2. Objectivity.
3. Independence.
4. Professional competence and due care, professional behavior.
5. Confidentiality.

BENEFITS OF AUDIT

1. **Patient:** The fundamental principle behind nursing care audit to everyone involved in care.
2. **Nursing staff:** For nurses, nursing care audit offers the opportunity to concentrate on areas of care where their skills and efforts can have positive outcomes, greater senses of achievement, autonomy, responsibility and provides a means for self-improvement.
3. **Community:** The new purchases provide environment in the hospital and requires practitioners to quantify the work. They do nursing care

audit and allows nurses to measure the more intangible aspects of their work, in particular the quality care and so demonstrate the contribution.

NURSING AUDITOR

1. **Internal auditor:** The nursing experts from within the hospital are deputed for internal audit and the auditing is done within the agency or hospital.
2. **External auditor:** Nursing and the medical administrations from the ministry other agencies of professional association like Trained Nurses Association of India (TNAI), undertake the nursing audit in the desired agency or hospital.

NURSING AUDIT SYSTEM

Nursing audit refers to the assessment of the quality of clinical nursing. For nursing auditing, questions are asked such as, Is nursing properly practiced? Are assessment of structure of care, facilities, equipments and manpower resources available conducive to the delivery of quality care? While assessment of outcome care, auditors also asks, what effects, the nursing care have on alteration of the health status of the recipient of care.

ADVANTAGES OF NURSING AUDIT

1. Can be used as a method of measurement in all areas of nursing.
2. Several functions are easily understood.
3. Scoring system is fairly simple.
4. Results are easily understood.
5. Assesses the work of all those involved in recording care.
6. May be a useful tool as part of a quality assurance program in areas where accurate records of care are kept.

DISADVANTAGES OF NURSING AUDIT

1. Appraises the outcomes of the nursing process, so, it is not so useful in areas where the nursing process has not been implemented.
2. Many of the components overlap making analysis difficult.
3. Is time consuming.
4. Requires a team of trained auditors.
5. Deals with a large amount of information.
6. Only evaluates record keeping.
7. Only serves to improve documentation, not nursing care.

AUDIT COMMITTEE

Before carrying out an audit, an audit committee should be formed, comprising of a minimum of five members, who are interested in quality assurance, are clinically competent and able to work together in a group. It is recommended that each member should review not more than 10 patients each month.

RELIABILITY OF AUDIT EVIDENCE

The reliability of audit evidence is influenced by its source, which may either be internal or external and by its nature, which may be visual, documentary or oral. The auditor must be aware of the following matters in assessing the reliability of audit evidence:

1. Audit evidence from external sources (for example, confirmation received from a third party) is more reliable than that obtained from the entity's records.
2. Audit evidence obtained from the entity's records is more reliable when the related accounting and internal control systems operate effectively.
3. Audit evidence obtained directly by auditors is more reliable than that obtained by or from the entity.
4. Audit evidence in the form of documents and written representations are more reliable than oral representations.
5. Original documents are more reliable than photocopies, telexes or facsimiles.

PROCEDURE FOR OBTAINING AUDIT EVIDENCE

Auditors normally obtain audit evidence by inspection, observation, enquiry, confirmation, computation and analytical procedures. The choice of one or a combination of the procedures, which the auditor may adopt is dependent, in part, upon the period of time during which the audit evidence sought is available and the form in which the accounting records are maintained.

INSPECTION

Inspection involves the following:

1. Examination of records, documents or tangible assets.
2. Provision of audit evidence of varying degrees of reliability depending on their nature and source; and the effectiveness of internal controls over their processing.

Three major categories of documentary audit evidence are listed below in descending degree of reliability as audit evidence:

1. Evidence created and provided to auditors by third parties.
2. Evidence created by third parties and held by the entity.
3. Evidence created and held by the entity.

Inspection provides reliable audit evidence about the existence of the tangible assets inspected, but not necessarily as to the ownership or value of such assets.

OBSERVATION

The auditor by observation looks at a procedure being performed by others. For example, the auditor observes the counting of stock by the entity's staff or the performance of internal control procedures as part of the conduct of an audit.

ENQUIRY AND CONFIRMATION

Enquiry involves seeking information within and outside the entity. Enquiry may be formal or informal. Responses to enquiries obtained from third parties may confirm or disprove information previously made available to the auditor.

Confirmation involves obtaining response to an enquiry to corroborate information previously made available to the auditors in the course of the audit.

Examples of Direct Confirmation

1. Confirmation of debts by communication with debtors.
2. Confirmation of legal cases by communication with the entity's solicitors.
3. Confirmation of bank balances by communication with the entity's bankers, etc.

COMPUTATION

The auditor uses computation to check the arithmetical accuracy of source documents and accounting records. Computation also involves performing independent calculations.

ANALYTICAL PROCEDURES

Analytical procedures consist of the analysis of relationship between:

1. Items of financial data.
2. Items of financial and non-financial data, derived from the same period.
3. Comparable financial information deriving from different periods or different entities.

Analytical procedures are used to identifying consistencies and predicted patterns or significant fluctuations and unexpected relationships and the results of investigations performed.

DOCUMENTATION

Documentation is the duty of the auditor to document matters, which are important in providing evidence to support the audit opinion and evidence that the audit was carried out in accordance with auditing standards, accounting standards and relevant regulations.

CONCLUSION

Nursing audit is the process of collecting information from nursing reports and other documented evidence about patient care and assessing the quality of care by the use of quality assurance programs. A profession concerns for the quality of its service constitutes the heart of its responsibility to the public. An audit helps to ensure that the quality of nursing care desired and feasible is achieved. This concept is often referred to as quality assurance. Before carrying out an audit, an audit committee should be formed, comprising of a minimum of five members who are interested in quality assurance, are clinically competent and able to work together in a group. It is recommended that each member should review not more than 10 patients each month and that the auditor should have the ability to carry out an audit in about 15 minutes. If there are less than 50 discharges per month, then all the records may be audited, if there are large number of records to be audited, then an auditor may select 10 per cent of discharges.

CHAPTER

25

Total Quality Management

INTRODUCTION

Total quality management (TQM) is the optimization and integration of all the functions and processes of a business in order to provide for excited customers through a process of continuous improvement. The 1990's are the decade of globalization. In order, for companies to be competitive in this environment they have seen the imperative need for quality. However, through the decades leading to the 1990's there have been many "Experts" who have explicitly underlined the need for TQM systems in companies, but due to many factors these ideas have either gone unheeded or been buzzword for a short time. It is possible that TQM, is once again a buzzword and a marketing tool, but nevertheless it is a tool that is being extensively used in the 1990s to help companies gain and maintain a competitive edge over their rivals.

DEFINITION

1. Total quality management (TQM) refers to management methods used to enhance quality and productivity in business organizations. TQM is a comprehensive management approach that works horizontally across an organization, involving all departments and employees; and extending backward and forward to include both suppliers and clients/customers.
2. Total quality management is a management philosophy that seeks to integrate all organizational functions (marketing, finance, design, engineering and production, customer service, etc.) to focus on meeting customer needs; and organizational objectives.

OBJECTIVES OF TOTAL QUALITY MANAGEMENT

1. Process improvement.
2. Defect prevention.
3. Priority of effort.

4. Developing cause-effect relationships.
5. Measuring system capacity.
6. Developing improvement checklist and check forms.
7. Helping teams make better decisions.
8. Developing operational definitions.
9. Separating trivial from significant needs.
10. Observing behavior changes over a period of time.

TOTAL QUALITY MANAGEMENT TOOLS

1. **Quality improvement teams:** These are small groups of employees who work on solving specific problems related to quality and productivity, often with stated targets for improvement. Quality improvement teams are proving to be highly successful at tracking down the causes of poor quality as well as taking remedial action.
2. **Benchmarking:** This is the process of identifying the best practices and approaches by comparing productivity in specific areas within ones' own company to other organizations both within and outside the industry.
3. **Statistical process control:** This is a statistical technique that uses periodic random samples taken during actual production to determine whether acceptable quality levels are being met or whether production should be stopped in order to take remedial action. Because most processes produce some variation, statistical process control (SPC) uses statistical tests to determine when variations fall outside a narrow range around the acceptable quality level. The emphasis when using SPC is on defect prevention rather than trying to inspect the quality into the product.

TOTAL QUALITY MANAGEMENT PRINCIPLES

1. **Add values to the process:** Every action by every employee should add value to the process or product in every way all the time. Enhance your work by your actions.
2. **Deliver quality on time, all the time:** Develop a pattern of delivering perfect products and services on time. Rate your sources by their ability to do this.
3. **Base business relationships on mutual trust and confidence:** Providers and suppliers build trust and confidence through quality and deliverability. Customers build it by quick payment and clear lines of communication. Reliability, forthrightness and honesty are the basis of forming business relations.
4. **Train individuals and teams to solve problems:** Teach problem -solving tools/techniques and teaming as the means to solve quality, safety, productivity and deliverability problems.

5. **Empower employees to be responsible:** For quality, safety, productivity and deliverability. Empowering means giving workers responsibility for their actions affecting their work. Share governance.
6. **Deed ownership of process to employees:** Who have proven their capability. Reward and reinforce empowerment with incentives, job security and equity sharing. Make employees owners of the process, not attendants.
7. **Implement the new technology**: Use modern information resources, internet, databases, telecommunications, applications software and project scheduling as tools to improve productivity. Use SPC to eliminate errors and defects; and continually improve the system.
8. **Collect, measure and evaluate data:** Before making decisions. "It never hurts to turn the light on" (J DeSimone). Make decisions based on evidence, "If you can't measure it, you can't evaluate it."
9. **Apply the 80/20 principle:** Use this problem-solving tool to put problems into 'trivial many' and 'vital few' categories. Record the causes and frequencies of problems on a tally sheet. Develop this into a Pareto chart, which plots the frequencies (most to least important) of the problems. About 20% of the causes create at least 80% of the problems. It is important to resolve vital problems first.
10. **Develop win-win scenarios:** Create solutions that will benefit all parties. Cooperation that develops synergism is the best solution.
11. **Develop a master plan:** Good design precedes good craftsmanship. A well-designed plan tracks and benchmarks an action through to its completion. "Quality begins at the design level." (Marty Madigan).
12. **Plan for all contingencies:** Prepare all solutions by developing alternatives. If necessary, flowchart plans dealing with all possible alternatives. Apply 'if-then-else' type of logic to problems.
13. **Make zero defects and accidents:** Use the tools of TQM, SPC and problem-solving to achieve these goals by detecting and eliminating the causes.
14. **Qualify your sources and supplies:** Use quality and deliverability as the basis for selecting the source of your materials and services.
15. **Deliverability:** The right product at the right place at the right time. In world-class just-in-time (JIT) delivery systems, source parts are used without delay and inspection in the process.
16. **Meet the needs of customers:** Customers are anyone affected by your work: coworkers, team members, management and especially the end-users. They are the rationale for your work. The justification for your work is to deliver products or services that meet or exceed their requirements.
17. **Improve continuously and always:** Institute continuous improvement and life-long education, principles based on the 14 points by W Edwards

Deming. Optimize your curve. They constitute an ever expanding continuum. Add to this list.

ELEMENTS OF TOTAL QUALITY MANAGEMENT

Total quality management (TQM) is a management approach that originated in the 1950s and has steadily become more popular since the early 1980s. Total quality is a description of the culture, attitude and organization of a company that strives to provide customers with products and services that satisfy their needs. The culture requires quality in all aspects of the company's operations, with processes being done right the first time and defects, and waste eradicated from operations.

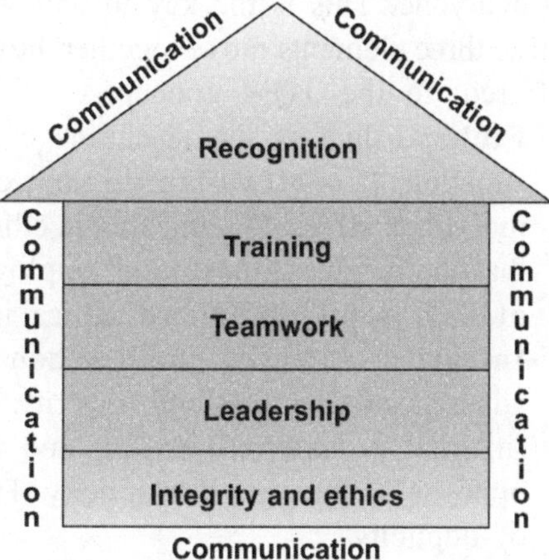

Figure 25.1: Key elements of total quality management

To be successful implementing TQM, an organization must concentrate on the eight key elements (Fig. 25.1):

1. Ethics.
2. Integrity.
3. Trust.
4. Training.
5. Teamwork.
6. Leadership.
7. Recognition.
8. Communication.

This paper is meant to describe the eight elements comprising TQM.

KEY ELEMENTS

Total quality management has been coined to describe a philosophy that makes quality driving force behind leadership, design, planning and improvement initiatives. For this, TQM requires the help of those eight key elements. These elements can be divided into four groups according to their function. The groups are:

a. **Foundation:** It includes ethics, integrity and trust.
b. **Building bricks:** It includes training, teamwork and leadership.

c. **Binding mortar:** It includes communication.
d. **Roof:** It includes recognition.

FOUNDATION

Total quality management is built on a foundation of ethics, integrity and trust. It fosters openness, fairness and sincerity and allows involvement by everyone. This is the key to unlocking the ultimate potential of TQM. These three elements move together, however, each element offers something different to the TQM concept.

1. **Ethics:** Ethics is the discipline concerned with good and bad in any situation. It is a two-faceted subject represented by organizational and individual ethics. Organizational ethics establish a business code of ethics that outlines guidelines that all employees are to adhere to in the performance of their work. Individual ethics include personal rights or wrongs.
2. **Integrity:** Integrity implies honesty, morals, values, fairness and adherence to the facts and sincerity. The characteristic is, what customers (internal or external) expect and deserve to receive. People see the opposite of integrity as duplicity. TQM will not work in an atmosphere of duplicity.
3. **Trust:** Trust is a by-product of integrity and ethical conduct. Without trust, the framework of TQM cannot be built. Trust fosters full participation of all members. It allows empowerment that encourages pride ownership and it encourages commitment. It allows decision making at appropriate levels in the organization, fosters individual risk taking for continuous improvement and helps to ensure that measurements focus on improvement of process and are not used to contend people. Trust is essential to ensure customer satisfaction. So, trust builds the cooperative environment essential for TQM.

BRICKS

Basing on the strong foundation of trust, ethics and integrity, bricks are placed to reach the roof of recognition. It includes:

1. **Training:** Training is very important for employees to be highly productive. Supervisors are solely responsible for implementing TQM within their departments and teaching their employees the philosophies of TQM. Training that employees require are interpersonal skills, the ability to function within teams, problem solving, decision making, job management performance analysis; and improvement, business economics; and technical skills. During the creation and formation of TQM, employees are trained so that they can become effective employees for the company.
2. **Teamwork:** To become successful in business, teamwork is also a key element of TQM. With the use of teams, the business will receive quicker and better solutions to problems. Teams also provide more

permanent improvements in processes and operations. In teams people feel more comfortable bringing up problems that may occur and can get help from other workers to find a solution and put into place. There are mainly three types of teams that TQM organizations adopt.

a. **Quality improvement teams or excellence teams (QITs):** These are temporary teams with the purpose of dealing with specific problems that often recur. These teams are set up for period of 3–12 months.
b. **Problem solving teams (PSTs):** These are temporary teams to solve certain problems and also to identify; and overcome causes of problems. They generally last from 1 week to 3 months.
c. **Natural work teams (NWTs):** These teams consist of small groups of skilled workers who share tasks and responsibilities. These teams use concepts such as employee involvement teams, self-managing teams and quality circles. These teams generally work for 1–2 hours a week.

3. **Leadership:** It is possibly the most important element in TQM. It appears everywhere in organization. Leadership in TQM requires the manager to provide an inspiring vision, make strategic directions that are understood by all and to instill values that guide subordinates. For TQM to be successful in the business, the supervisor must be committed in leading his employees. A supervisor must understand TQM, believe in it and then demonstrate their belief and commitment through their daily practices of TQM. The supervisor makes sure that strategies, philosophies, values and goals are transmitted down throughout the organization to provide focus, clarity and direction. A keypoint is that TQM has to be introduced and led by top management. Commitment and personal involvement is required from top management in creating and deploying clear quality values; and goals consistent with the objectives of the company; and in creating and deploying well defined systems, methods and performance measures for achieving those goals.

BINDING MORTAR

1. **Communication:** It binds everything together. Starting from foundation to roof of the TQM house, everything is bound by strong mortar of communication. It acts as a vital link between all elements of TQM. Communication means a common understanding of ideas between the sender and the receiver. The success of TQM demands communication with and among all the organization members, suppliers and customers. Supervisors must keep open airways where employees can send and receive information about the TQM process. Communication coupled with the sharing of correct information is vital. For communication to be credible the message must be clear and receiver must interpret in the way the sender intended.

Ways of Communication

There are different ways of communication such as:

a. **Downward communication:** This is the dominant form of communication in an organization. Presentations and discussions basically do it. By this the supervisors are able to make the employees clear about TQM.
b. **Upward communication:** By this the lower level of employees are able to provide suggestions to upper management of the affects of TQM. As employees provide insight and constructive criticism, supervisors must listen effectively to correct the situation that comes about through the use of TQM.

   This forms a level of trust between supervisors and employees. This is also similar to empowering communication, where supervisors keep open ears and listen to others.
c. **Sideways communication:** This type of communication is important because it breaks down barriers between departments. It also allows dealing with customers and suppliers in a more professional manner.

ROOF

Recognition

Recognition is the last and final element in the entire system. It should be provided for both suggestions and achievements for teams as well as individuals. Employees strive to receive recognition for themselves and their teams. Detecting and recognizing contributors is the most important job of a supervisor. As people are recognized, there can be huge changes in self-esteem, productivity, quality and the amount of effort exhorted to the task at hand. Recognition comes in its best form when it is immediately following an action that an employee has performed. Recognition comes in different ways, places and time.

Ways: It can be by way of personal letter from top management. Also by award banquets, plaques, trophies, etc.

Places: Good performers can be recognized in front of departments, on performance boards and also in front of top management.

Time: Recognition can given at any time like in staff meeting, annual award banquets, etc.

TOTAL QUALITY MANAGEMENT PROCESS

Total quality management views an organization as a collection of processes. It maintains that organizations must strive to continuously improve these processes by incorporating the knowledge and experiences of workers. The simple objective of TQM is "Do the right things, right the first time, every time". TQM is infinitely variable and adaptable.

PLANNING PHASE

Planning is the most crucial phase of total quality management. In this phase employees have to come up with their problems and queries, which need to be addressed. They need to come up with the various challenges they face in their day-to-day operations and also analyze the problem's root cause. Employees are required to do necessary research and collect relevant data, which would help them find solutions to all the problems.

DOING PHASE

In the doing phase, employees develop a solution for the problems defined in planning phase. Strategies are devised and implemented to overcome the challenges faced by employees. The effectiveness of solutions and strategies is also measured in this stage.

CHECKING PHASE

Checking phase is the stage where people actually do a comparison analysis of before and after data to confirm the effectiveness of the processes and measure the results.

ACTING PHASE

In this phase employees document their results and prepare themselves to address other problems.

Total quality management is now becoming recognized as a generic management tool, just as applicable in-service and public sector organizations. There are number of evolutionary strands, with different sectors creating their own versions from the common ancestor. TQM is the foundation for activities, which includes:

1. Commitment by senior management and all employees.
2. Meeting customer requirements.
3. Reducing development cycle times.
4. Just in time/demand flow manufacturing.
5. Improvement teams.
6. Reducing product and service costs.
7. Systems to facilitate improvement.
8. Line Management ownership.
9. Employee involvement and empowerment.
10. Recognition and celebration.
11. Challenging quantified goals and benchmarking.
12. Focus on processes/improvement plans.
13. Specific incorporation in strategic planning.

CONCLUSION

Total quality management is a management approach centered on quality, based on the participation of an organization's people and aiming at long term success (ISO 8402:1994). This is achieved through customer satisfaction and benefits all members of the organization and society. In other words, TQM is a philosophy for managing an organization in a way which enables it to meet stakeholder needs and expectations efficiently and effectively, without compromising ethical values. Total quality management is a continuous process of reducing or eliminating errors in manufacturing, streamlining supply chain management, improving the customer experience and ensuring that employees are up-to-speed with their training. Total quality management aims to hold all parties involved in the production process as accountable for the overall quality of the final product or service.

CHAPTER

26 Role of Professional Bodies

INTRODUCTION

Many professional bodies perform professional certification to indicate a person possesses qualifications in the subject area and sometimes membership in a professional body is synonymous with certification, but not always. Sometimes membership in a professional body is required for one to be legally able to practice the profession. Many professional bodies also act as learned societies for the academic disciplines underlying their professions.

MEANING OF PROFESSIONAL ASSOCIATION

Generally, the association means the combination of the people of same category for their common interest. They will meet as and when the need arises and when their common interest is affected; and when their common interest is to be developed. Through the association, the employees and workers solve many problems. Professional body or professional organization, also known as a professional association or professional society, is an organization, usually nonprofit that exists to further a particular profession, to protect both the public interest and the interests of professionals.

Associations are organizations of persons with common interests. Merton defined a professional association as, "an organization of practitioners, who judge one another as professionally competent and have united together to perform social functions, which they cannot perform in their separate capacity as individuals." Associations exist in all profession and in all parts of the world. Associations serve their individual members through a variety of services.

Professional associations provide a vehicle for nurses to meet present and future challenges; and work toward positive profession wide changes that keep pace with societal changes. As for as the educational institution is concerned, the employee associations are formed among the teachers and office staff to promote their own welfare.

VITAL ROLE OF REGULATORY BODIES

1. To ensure the public's light to quality healthcare service.
2. To support and assist professional members.
3. Set and enforce standards of nursing practice.
4. Monitor and enforce standards for nursing education.
5. Set the requirements for monitor and enforce standards of nursing practice.
6. Set the requirements for registration of nursing professionals.

CHARACTERISTICS OF PROFESSIONAL BODIES

1. Professional bodies are relatively permanent.
2. It is voluntary in nature.
3. It is an instrument of defence against exploitation.
4. It is an association of educated persons.
5. It is for the common purpose.

PRINCIPLES OF PROFESSIONAL BODIES

1. Unity is strength.
2. Collective bargaining.
3. Promotion of common interest.
4. Career advancement.
5. Opportunity for the self-career development.
6. Economic security.
7. Security of service.

BENEFITS OF PROFESSIONAL BODIES

1. Developing leadership skills.
2. Recognition through certification. Certification is a formal, but voluntary process of demonstrating expertise in particular areas of nursing.
3. Legislative lobbying power. Association lobbies the government to influence the laws affecting nursing.
4. Other benefits—publications, continuing nursing education, discounts in train, eyeglasses, goods and services.
4. To negotiate collective bargaining to get the dues in terms of finance and nonfinance.
5. To get along with their fellow workers in a better way and to gain respect in the eyes of their peers.
6. To safeguard the common interest of the professionals.
7. To promote public relations.

IMPORTANCE OF PROFESSIONAL BODIES

THE PUBLIC

Serve public by establishing codes of ethics and standards of practice, socializing new members to these codes and standards, and enforcing codes and standards in practice.

THE PROFESSION

Serve by being the mechanism through which the collective interests of its members are pressed collectively and focused politically. Collective action means the activities are undertaken on behalf of a group of people, who have common interests. Professional association help nurses use collective action to push for political responses to benefit consumers of health care and members of the profession.

INDIVIDUAL MEMBERS

Serve by providing continuing education and ensuring mechanisms for a professional work place. They work by forming relationships with the public and other professions and by ensuring that the professions work is properly understood; and supported by the public, government officials and other healthcare professionals.

TYPES OF ASSOCIATION

1. **Broad purpose professional association:** Trained Nurses Association of India is one of the nurses association in India. The purpose of establishment of TNAI is wide and it is discussed later in this chapter.
2. **Specialty practice association:** Nurses, who work in a particular specialty area can establish an organization, e.g. Association of Nurse Midwives, American Association of Critical Care Nursing, Emergency Nurses Association and Association of Rehabilitative Nurses.
3. **Special interest association.** This association includes National Black Nurses Association, Jamaican Nurses Association, National Hispanic Nurse Association and Transcultural Nursing Society. These were established to serve the interest of the particular group.

TRAINED NURSES ASSOCIATION OF INDIA (TNAI)

Nurses' charter: In 1937, the adopted the nurses' charter, which formed the basis for TNAI's representations to government and other employing authorities on vital matters like upgrading, development and standardization of nursing education (basic and post basic), improvement of living and service conditions for nurses throughout India and registration of qualified nurses. Sustained efforts of the TNAI also brought about the constitution of the Indian Nursing Council and also State Nursing Councils, which established a uniform system of nursing education in the country and nurses qualified from recognized institutions could practice in any part of the country. The Indian Nursing Council Act was passed by an ordinance on December 31, 1947. The council was established in 1949.

STANDARDIZATION OF NURSING EDUCATION

In the early days, TNAI assisted in the formulation of basic nursing curricula and in later years, the association was instrumental in promoting the establishment of degree courses and post-certificate programers in teaching and administration. As early as 1933, an Education Committee was appointed. The Committee of Nurses appointed through the TNAI to advise the Bhore Committee (The Health Survey and Planning Committee, 1941–1944) took up again the question of establishing degree courses, which were accepted by the government. The colleges of nursing were established in Delhi and Vellore (Tamil Nadu) in 1946. The recent educational activities of the association are conducting educational conferences and workshops. Various conferences and workshops were organized on various nursing topics from time to time by TNAI.

SERVICE CONDITION FOR NURSES

The association is officially recognized by the government of India as a service organization. The voice of the association is accepted as the voice of nurses in India and the resolutions adopted by it and presented to the various authorities are well received and generally accepted for implementation, sooner or later.

INDIAN NURSING COUNCIL ACTIVITIES

The Indian Nursing Council (INC), which was authorized by the Indian Nursing Council Act of 1947, was established In 1949 for the purpose providing uniform standards in nursing education and reciprocity in nursing registration throughout the country. The only national legislation directly related to nursing practice, also provides a basis from which rules for nursing practice can be developed. Among other responsibilities, this Act gives authority to the INC for prescribing curricula for nursing education and recognizing qualifications of institutions with teaching programs for nursing.

This means that the INC has authority to control nursing education and what the nurse is prepared to do. It is important because legal responsibility does finally depend upon what you should be able to do and how you should do it as well as what you are not prepared to do. The INC uses this authority in nursing education, but it delegates authority for control of nursing practice to the State Nurses Registration Councils.

FUNCTIONS OF INDIAN NURSING COUNCIL

1. It provides uniform standards of nursing education and reciprocity in nursing registration.
2. It has authority to prescribe curriculum for nursing education in all states.
3. It has authority to recognize program for nursing education or to refuse recognition of a program if it did not meet the standards required by the council.
4. To provide the registration of foreign nurses and for the maintenance of the Indian Nurses Register.
5. The INC authorizes State Nurses Registration Council and Examination Board to issue qualifying certificates.

The INC has been given heavy responsibilities for nursing practice and nursing education, but it has not been able to exert enough power to support high standards in nursing.

ROLE OF STATE GOVERNMENT

The state government controls nursing practice throughout the State Nurses Registration Acts. The State Nurses Registration Councils have authority to prescribe rules of conduct, to take disciplinary action and to maintain registers of nurses. Except for the uniform standards given by the INC, the State Nurse Practice Act is the important law affecting Nursing Practice Act that protects the public by broadly defining the legal scope of nursing practice.

FUNCTIONS

1. It registers nurse/midwives.
2. It serves as legal protections to the nurse.
3. It protects the public from incompetent nursing practice or poor nursing care.
4. It accredits and inspects schools of nursing and college of nursing.
5. It prescribes the rules of conduct, table disciplinary action.

INTERNATIONAL COUNCIL OF NURSES

The International Council of Nurses (ICN), founded in 1899 by Bedford Fenwick, is a federation of nonpolitical and self-governing national nurses association. The head quarters are in Geneva, Switzerland. The main purpose of the ICN is to provide a mean through which the national associations can share their interest in the promotion of health and care of the sick.

FUNCTIONS

1. To promote the development of strong national nurses associations.
2. To assist national nurses association to improve the standards of nursing and the competencies of nurses.
3. To assist national nurses associations to improve the status of nurses within their countries.
4. To serve as the authoritative voice for nurse and nursing internationally.

The ICN is the global voice of nursing. The governing body of the ICN is the council of national representative which is made up of the ICN Honorary officers and the presidents of the national members associations. The ICN code of ethics for nurses has four principle elements.

STATE REGISTRATION COUNCIL

Since the INC works in cooperation and coordination with the State Nursing Councils, it is necessary that one must say a few words about the State Nursing Councils. The training of nurses, midwives, health visitors and ANMs is to a large extent controlled by Nurses' Registration Councils in the respective states. State Nursing Council serves as a legal protection to the nurse and protects the public from incompetent nursing practices or poor nursing care.

Functions

1. Inspect and accredit schools of nursing in their state.
2. Conduct examinations.
3. Prescribe rules of conduct, take disciplinary actions, etc.
4. Maintain register of nurses, midwives, auxiliary nurse midwives (ANMs) and health visitors in the State.

The State Registration councils are autonomous to a great extent except that they do not have powers to prescribe syllabi for the various training courses, recognize examining bodies and to negotiate reciprocity. These powers are vested with the INC and State Councils ensure that the prescribed syllabi are followed and standards are maintained.

CONCLUSION

Professional bodies are organizations whose members are individual professionals. In some professions it is compulsory to be a member of the professional body, in others it is not. This usually depends on whether or not the profession requires the professional to have a 'licence to practice', or to be on a professional register, in order to do their job. This is related to how the profession is regulated, i.e. who is responsible for making sure that professionals are doing their jobs properly. The goal of advocacy efforts by professional associations is to educate association members, all professional nurses, and the public about the importance of broad-base membership, creative ideas, esprit de corps, and energetic participation in helping the profession improve and move to higher levels. In prior eras, visionary nurses realized the need for associations in order to meet the changes occurring in the social, cultural, and economic sectors of their world. Elected association leaders today remain responsive to their members and incorporate members' input by devising new mechanisms to advance healthcare through the nursing profession, thus allowing members to contribute to the accountability and voice of the profession to society.

SECTION VI
Community Health Care

GLOSSARY

1. **Assimilation:** Individuals or group from one culture identifying more strongly with the dominant culture in values, activities and daily living.
2. **Clinical practice guidelines:** Systematically developed statements to assist practitioner and patient decisions about appropriate healthcare for specific clinical circumstances.
3. **Community based nursing:** Nursing care within the context of the clients family and community with a prevention focus that enhances the clients ability for self care, a collaborative effort to maintain continuity of care.
4. **Community development block:** Community development is a process, which is designed to promote better living of the whole community, with the active participation by the community itself along with governmental efforts.
5. **Community development:** Community development is a process to create conditions of economic and social progress of the whole community with its active participation and the fullest possible reliance upon the community's institutive.
6. **Community health nurse:** Community health nurse is person plays important role in helping people learn to care themselves and to work with other community residents to develop the capacity or infrastructure needed to ensure essential healthcare for everyone.
7. **Community health nursing:** Community health nursing is a synthesis of nursing and public health practice applied of promoting and preserving the health of people. The practice is general and compressive. It is not limited to a particular age group or diagnosis and continuing, not episodic.
8. **Community health:** A focus on sustaining all members of the community at their highest possible level of functioning for their individual happiness and their collective benefit. It is a science and art of preventing disease, prolonging life and promoting health; and efficiency through organized effort.
9. **Community hospital:** A short-stay general or specialty (e.g. women's, children's, eye, orthopedic) hospital, excluding those owned by the federal government.

10. **Community resources:** A collection of healthcare providers or supportive care providers who share common interests or a sense of unity.
11. **Community:** Community is a group of inhabitants living together in a somewhat localized area under the same general regulations and having common interests, functions, needs and organizations.
12. **Comprehensive health care:** Comprehensive health care is the combined (integrated) curative, preventive, promotive and restorative care made available to the people without distinctions of caste, creed or economic status from birth to death (from womb to tomb).
13. **Concept:** Concepts are the elements or components of a phenomenon necessary to understand the phenomenon and derived from impressions the human mind receives about phenomena through sensing the human environment.
14. **Family developmental task:** The usual and expected family psychological, cognitive or psychomotor skills at certain persons in life, failure to master a developmental task can lead to unhappiness and difficulty with later tasks.
15. **Family functions:** Active or behavior of families that maintains the unity of the family and meets the family's needs.
16. **Family health:** Family health is concerned for the most part with the care of well, families, with non-hospitalized sick persons and their families, with groups of people and with health problems that affect the community as a whole.
17. **Family structure:** The characteristics of individuals (age, gender, number) who make up the family unit.
18. **Family system theory:** A theory that says the family is a collection of people who are integrated, interacting and dependent and that the actions of the other members.
19. **Family:** Family is a group of two or more persons joined by ties of marriage, blood or adoption who constitute a single household, who interact with each other in their respective familial status, positions and roles, to create and maintain a common subculture.
20. **Five-year plan:** Five-year plan is a mechanism to bring about uniformity in policy formation in programs of national importance. It recognizes the health as an important contributory factor in the utilization of manpower and in the upliftment of the economic condition of the country.
21. **Health administration:** Health administration is a branch of public administration, which deals with matters relating to the promotion of health, preventive services, medical care, rehabilitation and the delivery of health services, the development of health manpower, and medical education and training.

22. **Health administration:** Health administration is the science and art of organizing and coordinating government agencies whose purpose is to improve the physical, mental and social well-being of the people.
23. **Health center:** It is defined as an institution for the promotion of health and welfare of the people in a given area, which seeks to achieve health work through coordination with welfare and relive organization.
24. **Health for all:** Health for all has been defined as attainment of a level of health that will enable every individual to lead a socially and economically productive life.
25. **Health programs:** National Health Programs are directly run by the ministers who can have a bearing in reduction of mortality and morbidity; and also have a salutary effect on efforts to improve the quality of life of a common man. It also reinforce the delivery of primary, secondary and tertiary healthcare throughout the country.
26. **Health:** A state of physical, mental and social well-being and the absence of disease or other disorders. It involves constant change and adaptation to stress.
27. **Healthcare delivery system:** Healthcare delivery system is a systematic and organized way of delivering or operating to provide healthcare facilities and services to the people. It may be broadly divided into private, voluntary and government agencies.
28. **Healthcare team:** Healthcare team refers to all of the personal in all of the departments of a healthcare facility, who provides healthcare services. They are doctors, nurses, technicians and paramedical staffs.
29. **Home visit:** Assessment, diagnosis, planning and evaluation of nursing care in the client's home.
30. **Models:** Models are graphic or symbolic representations of phenomena that objectify and present certain perspectives or points of view about nature or function or both.
31. **National health policies:** The National Health Policy (NHP) is the statement enunciated by the government of India about the manner in which the task related to health and allied subjects have to be performed in view of the actual needs and priorities.
32. **Nursing:** Nursing is an art, science and profession by which we render, serve to human being to help him/her to regain or to keep a normal state of body and mind; and when it cannot accomplish this, it help him/her for the relief from physical pain, mental anxiety or spiritual discomfort.
33. **Philosophy:** A philosophy is statement of belief and values about human being and their world.
34. **Policy:** Policy is the statement about the manner in which a given task is to be performed. It is a blueprint for future action. it enables the individuals responsible for doing it, perform it efficiently.

35. **Primary health care:** It is a essential health care based on practical, scientifically sound and socially accepted methods; and technology, made universally acceptable to individuals, and families in the community involving their full participation, and at a cost that the community and country can afford to maintain at every stage of their development.
36. **Primary health center:** Primary health center is an institution for providing comprehensive health care, e.g. preventive, promotive and curative services to the people living in a defined geographical area. It seeks to achieve its purpose by grouping under one roof or co-ordinate all the health work of that area.
37. **Primary nursing:** In primary nursing, a professional nurse has total responsibility for a particular patient or group of patients. The model's purpose is to provide continuity and coordination of care.
38. **Profession:** A profession is an occupation with moral principles that are devoted to the human and social welfare. The service is based on specialized knowledge and skill developed in a scientific and learned manner
39. **Quality care:** The degree of which health services for individuals and populations increase the likelihood of desired health outcomes and are consistent with current professional knowledge.
40. **Standards:** Standards are authoritative statements by which the nursing profession describes the responsibilities for which practitioners are accountable.
41. **Theory:** Theory refers to a set of logically interrelated concepts, statement, proposition and definitions, which have been derived from philosophical beliefs of scientific data and from which questions or hypothesis can be deduced, tested and verified.

CHAPTER

27

Primary Health Care

INTRODUCTION

The system of health care practiced in India presently includes treatment of illness, promotion of health and prevention of illness. Community participation is recognized as a major component. The stress is on the provision of these services to the people representing a shift from medical care to health care and from urban population to rural population.

DEFINITION

Primary health care is essential health care made universally accessible to individuals and families in the community, by means acceptable to them, through their full participation ands at a cost that the community, and country can afford. It forms an integral part both of the country's health system of which it is the nucleus and the overall social and economic development of the community.—*Alma Ata, 1978*.

HIGHLIGHTS OF DEFINITION

This definition highlights several attributes of primary health care. It stresses on:

1. Its essentiality by observing that primary health is essential health care.
2. Its 'accessibility' by observing "made universally accessible to individuals and families in the community.
3. Its 'acceptability' by observing by means acceptable to them.
4. Its 'patricianly' by observing 'acts a cost that the community and country can afford'.
5. Its 'affordability' by observing 'it forms an integral part both of the country's health system of which it is the nucleus and the overall social and economic development of the community'.
6. Its integrality by observing 'it forms an integral part both of the country's health system of which it is the nucleus and the overall social, and economic development of the community.'

ATTRIBUTES OF PRIMARY HEALTH CARE

1. **Accessibility:** Primary health care permeates uniformly to reach equitably to all segments of population.
2. **Acceptability:** Primary health care achieves acceptability through cultural assimilation of its policies and programs.
3. **Adaptability:** Primary health care system is highly flexible and adaptable. It believes in 'adaptation' rather than 'acceptance'
4. **Affordability:** Primary health care is affordable to consumer as well as providers.
5. **Availability:** Primary health care is always ready to respond to any demand at any time.
6. **Appropriateness:** Primary health care system evolves from the socioeconomic conditions, social values and health situation of a community, it is quite appropriate from all angles.
7. **Closeness:** Primary health center is close at hand to people at their door steps.
8. **Continuity:** Primary health service is a continuous service, which extends from 'womb' to 'tomb' and addresses the changing needs of an individual in all situations of health and disease.
9. **Comprehensiveness:** Primary health care is comprehensive and the curative needs of the community.
10. **Coordinativeness:** Primary health care is dependent on intersectoral coordination and community participation.

ELEMENTS OF PRIMARY HEALTH CARE

As per Alma-Ata declaration, primary health care includes:

1. Education concerning prevailing health problems and methods of identifying, preventing and controlling them.
2. Promotion of food supply and proper nutrition.
3. An adequate supply of water and basic sanitation.
4. Maternal and child health care including family planning.
5. Immunization against the major infectious disease.
6. Prevention and control of locally endemic diseases.
7. Appropriate treatment of common diseases and injuries.
8. Promotion of mental health.
9. Provision of essential drugs.

PRINCIPLES OF PRIMARY HEALTH CARE

1. **Equitable distribution:** Primary health care services must be shared equally by all people irrespective of their ability to pay (rich, poor, urban or rural).

2. **Community participation:** Primary health care must be a continuing effort to secure meaningful involvement of the community in the planning, implementation and maintenance of health services.
3. **Coverage and accessibility:** Primary health care implies providing health care services to all which are required by them. The care has to be appropriate and adequate in content; and in amount to satisfy the essential health needs of the people; and has to be provided by methods acceptable to them.
4. **Intersectoral coordination:** Primary health care requires joint efforts of other health related sectors such as agriculture, animal husbandry, food, industry, housing, social welfare, public works, communication and other sectors.
5. **Appropriate health technology:** The technology that is scientific, adaptable to local need and socially acceptable instead of costly methods, equipment and technology.
6. **Human resource:** Health resource is very essential to make full use of all the available resources including the human potential of the entire community.
7. **Referral system:** Referral system would be desirable to develop referring from one level to another with laid down procedures and policies.
8. **Logistics of supply:** The logistic of supply include planning and budgeting for the supplies required procurement or manufacture, storage distribution and control.
9. **Physical facilities:** The physical facilities for primary health care need to be simple and clean. It should have a specious waiting area with toilet facility.
10. **Control and evaluation:** A process of evaluation has to be built into assess the relevance, progress, efficiency, effectiveness and impact of the services.

LEVELS OF HEALTH CARE

In India, the complex of primary health centers and their subcenters through the agency of multipurpose health workers, village health guides/trained dais provide primary health care. Since India has opted for "Health for all by 2000 AD", the primary health care system has been recognized and strengthened to make the primary health care delivery system more effective (WHO Chronicle, 1977). The health care service is organized at three levels, i.e. primary, secondary and tertiary. These levels represent different types of care involving varying degrees of complexity.

PRIMARY CARE LEVEL

It is the first level of contact of individuals, families and community with the national health system, where primary health care (essential health care) is provided. As a level of care, it is close to the people, where most of their health problems can be dealt with and resolved. At this level, the health care will be most effective within the context of the needs and limitations of the area.

SECONDARY CARE LEVEL

The next higher level of care is the secondary (intermediate) health care level. At this level, problems that are more complex are dealt with. In India, this kind of care is generally provided in district hospitals and community health centers, which also serve as the first referral level facility (WHO Chronicle, 1969).

TERTIARY CARE LEVEL

The tertiary level is a more specialized level than secondary care level and requires specific facilities and attention of highly specialized health workers. This care is provided by the regional or central level institutions, e.g. Medical College Hospitals, All India Institutes, Regional Hospitals and Specialized Hospitals.

A fundamental and necessary function of the health care system is to provide a sound referral system. It must be a two-way exchange of information and returning patients to those who referred them for follow-up care (UNICEF-WHO Joint Committee on Health Policy, 1987). This will ensure continuity of care and inspire confidence of the consumer in the system.

HEALTH CARE AT VILLAGE LEVEL

The Government of India evolved a National Health Policy based on primary health approach in 1983. Steps for implementing the National Health Policy were undertaken during the sixth (1980–1985) and seventh (1986–1990) Five-Year Plans. One of schemes adopted to implement the policy was the training of local dais (traditional birth attendants) in the country to improve their knowledge in the elementary concepts of maternal and child health; and sterilization (asepsis) besides obstetric skills. The dais was trained for 30 working days at the primary health centre (PHC), subcenters or maternal child health (MCH) centers. During the training, the daises were to conduct two home deliveries under the guidance and supervision of the female health worker (FHW) or assistant nurse midwife (ANM). The emphasis during training was on asepsis, so that home deliveries are conducted under safe hygienic conditions thereby reducing the maternal and infant mortality.

After successful completion of training, each dai was provided with a delivery kit and a certificate. These dais were also expected to play a vital role in propagating small family norm, since they were more acceptable to the community. The national target was to train one local dai in each village.

HEALTH CARE AT SUBCENTER LEVEL

The subcenters are the peripheral outposts of the health care delivery system in rural areas. These were established on the basis of one subcenter for every 5,000 population in general and one for every 3,000 population in the hilly, tribal and backward areas. Each subcenter is manned by a male and a female multipurpose health worker. The functions of subcenters are limited to MCH, family planning and immunization and implementation of some aspects of national health programs such as Malaria Eradication Program.

PRIMARY HEALTH CENTER LEVEL

The primary health centers and its subcenters provide the infrastructure to provide health services to the rural population. The National Health Plan of 1983 proposed reorganization of PHC on the basis of one PHC for every 30,000–50,000 population in the plains and one PHC for every 20,000 population in hilly, backward and tribal areas for effective coverage.

In every community development block, there are one or more PHCs each of which covers 30,000 rural population with a 15 member of staffs.

COMMUNITY HEALTH CENTERS

Community health centers were established by upgrading the primary health centers (established earlier), each community health center covering a population of 80,000–1,25,000 (one in each community development block), with 30 beds and specialists in surgery, medicine, obstetrics and gynecology; and pediatrics with X-ray and laboratory facilities. A community health officer has been included in the 25 member staff in order to strengthen the preventive and promotive aspects of health care.

ROLE OF NURSE IN PRIMARY HEALTH CARE

1. Community health nurse work with population, community, family, individual. The focus is multiple or promoting health maintaining a degree of balance toward health.
2. Community health nurse focus on assessment of the impact of the socio-economical and cultural factors affecting health measures, the most

constantly be dealt with and take priority in order to make family assume health measures.

3. The community health nurse works with entire spectrum of health and illness conditions from optimal health to minor or severe conditions from acute to chronic illness.
4. The community health nurse works in all kinds of setting such as home, school, clinic, industry, etc.
5. The community health nurse works in school, where primary goal is health education and disease prevention.
6. The community health nurse works in industry is to improve the production and employees safety.
7. The community health nurse is responsible for assisting patients and families to coordinate health care, which necessitates contact with personnel from health, welfare and other significant community agencies.
8. Community health nurse has responsibilities in education—an training of individuals, auxiliaries and others.
9. The community health nurse involves in provision of direct services to patients both preventive and curative at the out patient, In-patient clinics and community.

CONCLUSION

Health care and its delivery system are changing rapidly in order to meet the needs and problems of the ever-changing society. Health problems have been and still are the basis for planning and for providing health services. Mortality and morbidity rates associated with preventable conditions are high due to lack of adequate environmental sanitation such as safe water supply, safe disposal of human excreta and refuse, control of flies, mosquitoes and other diseases vectors and adequate housing.

CHAPTER

28

Community-oriented Nursing

DEFINITION

1. Community health nursing defined as 'community health refers to the health status of the members of the community, to the problem affecting their health and to the totality of health care provided to the community.'
2. Community health refers to the health status of the members of the community, to the problems affecting their health and to the totality of health care provided for the community. —*Blum*
3. Community health or public health is defined as 'the art and science of maintaining, protecting and improving health of people through organized effects'. —*American Association of Public Health*
4. Public health is total development of individual and society. Public health is dedicated to the common attainment of the highest level of physical, mental and social well-being and longevity consistent with available knowledge and resources at given time and place.
5. Community health nursing is defined as, nursing services organized by a community or agency to carry out nursing aspects of community health program in the homes, schools, industries or in the health centers.

NATURE OF COMMUNITY HEALTH NURSING

The community is responsible for providing all facilities and total care to all. Such changes have led to the placement of the term public health with community health. Hence 'community health' encompasses all those process of prevention of disease, promotion and protection of health of all people.

Community health nursing implies making systematic assessment and diagnosis of health status of people and their problems, planning; and implementing comprehensive health care services for the entire community with their active cooperation and participation. In community health nursing, the major emphasis is laid on primary level prevention through community approaches.

The community health nursing implies sound preparation of community health personnel, so that they are knowledgeable and skillful. They need to acquire knowledge about community's structure, community dynamics, community approaches, population statistics and community health indicators, epidemiological aspects of health problems, health planning, administration; and delivery system.

The community health demands are places on the nurse and the nursing profession as a result of changes in society, especially changes in modern technology. Social consciousness and the quality, type and financing of health care. Emphasis has shifted from acute hospitalized based care to preventive community health care. All changes that affect the health care delivery system affect nursing.

PHILOSOPHY OF COMMUNITY HEALTH NURSING

Nursing contributes to the health services in a vital and significant way in the health care delivery system. It recognizes national health goals and is committed to participate in the implementation of national health policies and programs. It aims at identifying health needs of the people, planning and providing quality care in collaboration with other health professional and community groups.

1. The essential dignity and worth of the individual.
2. The right of an individual for basic necessities.
3. The right of the individual to help in times of need and crisis.
4. The great capacity for growth within all social beings.
5. The possession by individuals of potentialities and resources for managing their own lives.
6. The need for individuals to struggle and strive to improve their life and environment.
7. The importance of freedom to express one's individuality.

Individual's right of being healthy: Health is believed to be one of the rights of all human beings, nationally and internationally. Indians Constitution provides directives to ruling political party to design health care delivery system to promote and preserve this right by providing effective health services to all without any discrimination.

Working together toward common goal: Health is no longer considered in an isolated manner, but it is an integral part of socioeconomic, sociocultural; and political components. Willingness to share the responsibility of helping each other is the basis of modern concept of community health.

Social systems: Social systems have an impact on a community and consequently, the halts of that community. Social system includes a community's economy, education, religion, welfare, politics, recreation, legal system, health care, safety and transportization etc. should be shared with all people (proper distribution). These should not be any type of discriminations; rather weaker sections should be helped to have these means and facilities.

OBJECTIVES OF COMMUNITY HEALTH NURSING

Nursing seeks to help people understand the importance of all segments of their life and the environment to their well-being. Nursing uses scientific knowledge to perform activities to prevent illness and to help those with health problems to regain vigor and joy of life. Social change taking place in the community must be considered in planning health care. Nurses are key persons in providing health care in our changing society. Health education has for a long time been considered a major nursing responsibility. That responsibility is increasing with our social trends. Because nurses live in the community and have their own families, they are accessible to the people of the community. They are often called for help in emergencies or to give advice.

PRINCIPLES OF COMMUNITY HEALTH NURSING

Sound community health nursing and behavioral science preparation enables nursing students today to utilize scientific principles and concepts in carrying out a systematic nursing care at community setup. Scientific principles, which are drawn from all fields of learning, may be defined as comprehensive and fundamental laws, doctrines, truths or sets of facts that form the basis for established rules of action. The following are some main principles, which may used to guide for the community health nurse:

1. Effective health workers, irrespective of position or place or place of work, function as a team.
2. The community nurse should be a qualified person by a recognized school or college.
3. Health services should be based on the felt need of an individual, family and community.
4. Health services should make available to all people, irrespective of their stage, sex and status.
5. Community health nurses are accountable/responsible authorized health authority for her/his services.
6. Health services should be realistic in terms of available personnel and facilities.
7. Professional relationship and etiquette are essential in community health services.
8. Community health nurse must be a nonpolitical and nonsectarian in her/his relationship with people.
9. Evaluation and follow-up services is an important aspect in community health programs.

10. Facilities for further training and continuing education should be provided by the health authority.
11. Community health nurse should organize a periodical In-service education programs.
12. Community health nurse should organize and lead a team effectively and efficiently to provide best service to the community.
13. The family and community are the units of work. There should be adequate and accurate baseline data of the community is essential.
14. Supervision and guidance are needed to help the worker to produce a high quality of work.
15. Records and reports are essential in community health services.
16. The community health nurse should prepare update records and reports and sent to their higher level promptly.
17. The public health worker must never accept gifts or bribes.
18. Professional interest should be developed and maintained.
19. Job condition should be conductive to optimum satisfaction.

GOALS OF COMMUNITY HEALTH NURSING

1. To increase the capacity of families, groups and communities to cope with health and illness problems.
2. To support and supplement the efforts of other professional restoration and preservation of health.
3. To control or counteract as much as possible physical and social environmental conditions that threaten health or decrease the enjoyment of life.
4. To contribute to the reinforcement and improvement of nursing practice and public health practice, and service.

SCOPE OF COMMUNITY HEALTH NURSING

Community health nursing is concerned with the people who are sick as well as the healthy, young and old, male and female. At the same time, community health nurse is responsible for family centered care rather than an individual-oriented care. The community health nurse job is not only limited to the sick, but has equal responsibility to prevent the disease and to preserve; and promote the health of the people.

1. **Home care:** Nursing practice is applied in meeting the health needs of communities, families and individuals in their normal environment such as at home.
2. **Nursing homes:** The community health team who provides nursing care, treatment to the sick and health counseling given in nursing homes.
3. **Maternal and Child Health (MCH) and family planning:** The public health nurse plays a major role in the MCH and family planning services. It comprises antenatal, postnatal and child care services.

4. **School health nursing:** The school health nurse provides services to promote and protect the health of the school children. Nurse provides services like early detection of diseases, immunization, first- aid, dental health, school sanitation, maintenance of health records, health education, follow-up and referral services.
5. **Health care services:** The purpose of health care services to improve the health status of the population. It aims at mortality and morbidity reduction, increase in expectation of life, decreased in population growth rate, improvements in nutritional status, provision of basic sanitation, health manpower requirements and resource development; and certain other parameters such as food production, literacy rate, levels of poverty, etc.
6. **Industrial nursing services:** The nursing service at industrial area includes periodic health check-up, care of the sick, first aid, health counseling, industrial sanitation and safety, organization of services to women and children, rehabilitation of the ill and disabled workers and administration.
7. **Domiciliary nursing service:** Community health nurse focused at domiciliary nursing services includes maternity services health supervision, and disease prevention services; and service for illness and accidents.
8. **Geriatric nursing services:** Community health nurse should take care of old people in the community. The need of the geriatric nursing care is different and they need more care than the younger age groups.
9. **Mental health nursing service:** Mental health nursing services of a community health nurse includes early diagnosis and treatment, rehabilitation, psychotherapy, use of modern psychotropic drugs and after care services.
10. **Rehabilitation centers:** The community health nurse provides care in rehabilitation units. Nursing is an important component in the rehabilitation of the disabled.

COMMUNITY HEALTH NURSE

Community health nurse is a personnel, serving at the community level provide basic promotive, preventive curative and rehabilitative services directly to the community. The specific nursing activities, which are performed by the nurse will vary according to community needs and the structure of the primary health care system.

QUALITIES OF COMMUNITY HEALTH NURSE

1. A qualified community health nurse is one who has undergone basic general nursing, midwifery training and post basic education in community health nursing.

2. A community health nurse must have interest in people and in understanding human behavior.
3. Sincerity and ability to empathize are basic qualities required of a nurse.
4. A well poised nurse has a friendly disposition, honest, charitable, resourceful and cooperative and takes responsibilities with initiative.
5. Minimum essential skills of a nurse are observation, communication, interviewing, and bedsides supportive and technical skills.
6. Nurses must have abilities to make interpretations, make judgments and take decisions.

FUNCTIONS OF COMMUNITY HEALTH NURSE

Community health nurse functions vary according to the designation for which the nurse is employed and according to her education, and experience. Some community health nurses function on the staff level, while others serve in the capacity of administrator, supervisor or instructor in health organizations.

1. Community health nurse provides comprehensive health care to individuals, families and groups by teaching, counseling, and providing guidance.
2. Community health nurse develop goals to meet the need. She develops an action program, evaluates progress and plans again as needed.
3. Assistance to the family in improving environmental conditions that affect health, she helps plan a safe environment in the home, school and industry.
4. Providing supportive services to doctor such as early symptom detection and giving technical help.
5. Demonstration and teaching of skilled nursing care of the sick in the home.
6. Supervision of work of midwives, dais and other nursing personnel.
7. Helping in the adjustment of social and emotional conditions that affect health.
8. Coordination of work with other members of the health team working in the community.
9. Revising and revitalizing plan and programs.
10. Epidemiologic investigation in the field of communicable diseases such as tuberculosis, sexually transmitted diseases, leprosy, etc.
11. Organizing planned group classes in health with emphasis on applied nutrition, sanitation, child care and parent craft and family welfare services.
12. Development and utilization of facilities such as other branches of health and welfare services for making referrals and for promotion of sound and adequate health programs.
13. Nurse is responsible for planning, implementation and evaluation of a practical plan of nursing administration within the primary center and its associated subcenter.

14. The community health nurse involves in nursing research and collection of vital statistics.

COMMUNITY HEALTH CENTER (CHC)

Each block has one community health center (CHC) covering a population of 80,000–120, 000 population. Each CHC has services in surgery, medicine, obstetrics, gynecology, pediatric, dental and ear, nose, tongue (ENT). The services are rendered by a team of specialist, nurses and other personnel. Each community health center has three to four primary health centers. Community health works as a referral center for PHC's of the area. It is managed by 4 specialist doctors. At present there are 3215 community health centers (2005). At the community health center there are four specialist doctors—physician, surgeon, gynecologist and pediatrician. Each CHC has 30 beds, an X-rays room, a delivery room, operation theater and laboratory. The staffing of community health center is listed in Table 29.1.

Table 29.1: Staffing of community health center

Doctors	4
Nurses	7
Dresser	1
Pharmacist	1
Laboratory assistant	1
Radiographer	1
Ward boy	2
Cleaning worker	3
Dhobi	1
Gardener	1
Chowkidar	1
Ayah	1
D group servant	1
Total	25

If there is a vehicle, a driver can be appointed.

Maintenance of Community Health Center: The establishment and maintenance of community health centers are done under the Minimum Need Program (MNP) and Basic Minimum Service (BMS) of the State Governments. To strengthen the infrastructure of the rural health system, financial assistance is also available from Prime Minister's Rural Development Fellow Scheme Fund.

FUNCTIONS OF COMMUNITY HEALTH CENTER

1. Provides all preventive and curative health services.
2. Providing specialty services.
3. Caring and supervision of concerned PHCs.
4. Providing consultancy/referral services to PHCs.
5. Referring patients to teaching hospitals and district hospitals.
6. Providing reproductive and child health programs.
7. Implementation of all National Health Programs with active participation.

PRIMARY HEALTH CENTER

Primary health center is essential health care made universally accessible to individuals and families in the community by means acceptable to them, through their full participation; and at a cost that the community and country can afford. Primary health centers were started in 1952 as part of Community Development Program in order to provide comprehensive health care to people in rural areas. The community development blocks covering approximately 100 villages and about 80,000 populations. The primary health care consists of a main building and three subcenters.

Primary health center setup: Primary health center is the first contact print between people and doctor. Primary health center is established to cover 30,000 population in plains and 20,000 population in hilly/tribal areas. Establishment and maintenance of these centers are done under the Minimum Need Program of the state governments. The work of PHC is looked after by medical officer. There are four to six beds for patients and come diagnostic facilities for patients are also available at PHC.

CONCLUSION

Community health nursing is concerned with the people who are sick as well the healthy, young and old, male and female. At the same time, from the above points it is clear that community health nurse is responsible for family concerned care rather than an individual oriented care. Therefore one can say community health nursing practice primarily rests outside the therapeutic institutions. However, community health nursing links the hospital and community. Community health and community health nursing draw knowledge and practices from other disciplines such as medicine, surgery, pediatrics, obstetrics, gynecology, dentistry, health education and vital statistics.

CHAPTER

29

Family Health Care

INTRODUCTION

Family health is defined as "art and science of preventing disease, prolonging life and promoting health and efficiency of family through organized family efforts for the safe family environment; prevention and control of communicable diseases; reproductive and child health education of members in personal hygiene; seeking medical and nursing services for early diagnosis and treatment; development of social system and coping abilities to ensure normal development and optimum health status of family members".

DEFINITION

Nursing care directed to improving the potential health of a family or any of its members by assessing individual and family health needs and strengths, by identifying the health care of the family as a whole and those influencing the individual members by using family resources, by teaching and counseling and by evaluating progress towards stated goals.

DETERMINANTS/FACTORS OF FAMILY HEALTH

1. **Human biology:** It is composed of family size, structure, composition and characteristics, genetic inheritance, and self concept.
2. **Environment:** It is composed of physical, biological and social environment of the family.
3. **Lifestyle:** It is composed of daily living activities, behavioral and cultural practices including customs and traditions practiced by the family.
4. **Health and allied resources:** It includes health services, health related facilities, socioeconomic conditions, political system and health related services, etc.

GOALS OF FAMILY HEALTH CARE

1. Reduction of maternal, infant and child mortality and morbidity rates.
2. Family planning to space out children and ensure planned parenthood.

3. Improve nutritional status of all family members.
4. Health education of the family in all preventive, promotive, curative and rehabilitative aspects of health care.

OBJECTIVES OF FAMILY HEALTH CARE

1. Identify and appraises health problems of the family.
2. Ensure family's understanding and acceptance of the problem.
3. Provide prompted and proper services according to the health needs of the family.
4. Helps to develop the competence in the members to take care of their family as and when required.
5. Contributes desired materials to personal and social development of the family members.
6. Helps to promote the utilizing of available resources to maintain all aspects of health of the rehabilitative measure.

PRINCIPLES OF FAMILY HEALTH CARE

1. Establish good professional relationship with the family.
2. Provide proper health education and guidance to family to take care of themselves.
3. Collect all relevant information about family and community to identify problems; and set priorities.
4. Provide support to the family based on their needs.
5. Encourage and motivate family members to participate healthcare services to improve their health status.
6. Healthcare services should be provided to the family irrespective of sex, age, income, religion, etc.
7. Duplication of health services should be provided to the family irrespective of sex, age, income, religion, etc.
8. Proper health message to be communicated to family in every contact.

HOME VISIT

The community health nurse work with families in different settings including clinics, schools, support groups, office and the family home. Home visits give a more accurate assessment of the family structure and behavior in the natural environment.

Home visits also provide opportunities to observe the home environment and to identify barriers and support for reaching family health promotion goods. Health services in the home requires technical skills, knowledge of preventive and therapeutic measures, teaching ability, judgment and a full understanding of human relations.

Home visit refers to meeting the health needs of people at their doorsteps. Health services given at home for patient, family and the community in general for nursing service and health counseling.

CONCEPTS OF HOME VISITING

1. Home visiting provides opportunity to make direct observation on home environment, family structure, familial roles and relationships, lifestyle, cultural practices, group dynamics, etc. and make family health assessment.
2. In home visiting the members are relaxed, have more time and privacy and feel free to raise questions, seek clarifications; and sort out their problems.
3. It provides opportunities to make direct observation of care given by family members in planning and implementing family healthcare services.
4. It provides opportunities to contact and interact with most of the family members; and establish report with the family as a whole.
5. It also make possible to have active participation of family members in planning and implementing family health care.
6. It makes feasible to plan and provide comprehensive family health care with major emphasis on promotive and preventive care.

PURPOSES OF HOME VISITING

1. Home visiting is a routine part of a planned visiting program by a community health personnel.
2. It helps to investigate the source of infectious diseases.
3. To do follow-up on some problems identified in the health center, school, industry or hospital.
4. To assess the nutritional and immunization status, environmental hazards.
5. To give health education to the individual, family and community.
6. To supervise and guide other health workers.

PRINCIPLES OF HOME VISITING

1. **Need based:** Home visiting should be planned and conducted based on the identified needs of the people.
2. **Priority based:** The home visit should give to the existing problem in the family. It may be maternal and child health services or antenatal checkup.
3. **Regularity:** Plan for regular home visiting program based on family needs. It should be conducted at regular intervals.
4. **Flexibility:** The community health nurse should adopt a flexible approach based on prevailing circumstances at home.

5. **Scientific based:** Be sure of the scientific soundness of the subjects used for discussion. Use of technical skills includes hand washing an inspection.
6. **Analysis based:** Collect facts about the home, the patient and the environment and make on objective analysis of the facts as an initial step in visiting the home.
7. **Developing relationship:** Work with the person and family plan jointly. Home visiting helps to establish good working relationship in the family.
8. **Sensitivity:** The community health nurse should be sensitive to the persons feeling and needs at the time of the visit. Listen to the family and understand the other person's point of view.
9. **Educative:** Evaluate your own work remember the quality of care is more important than the number of hoe visits. It is essential to evaluate home visits from time to time.

STEPS IN HOME VISITING

1. **Initial phase:** The community health nurse should collect information from clinical and other records before planning for a visit. During home visit, nurse has to assess or observe and make a note in initial visit. The community health nurse should introduce and establish a friendly relationship by using simple language. Assess physical and environmental status, family's cultural background, occupation and income of family member, age, educational factors and psychological factors influences.
2. **Action phase:** The interpersonal relationship starts when nurses enter into the house. The nurse should use their effective communication skills to implement the nursing process. During home visit, nurse practice a variety of roles when interviewing in patient care. The community health nurse has to take a role as collaborator, consultant, coordinator, preventor of disease, promoter of health, health educator; and an epidemiologist; and takes steps to implement nursing process.

   During action phase the community health nurse provides nursing care. For example, taking temperature, physical examination and dressing, etc. Demonstrating and teaching, e.g. teaching insulin self-administration. Nurse makes diagnosis and tentative nursing care plan based on establishing priorities.
3. **Termination phase:** Nurse patient goals are reached, health is restored and the patient can function without actions. The nurse records the important events in the family and reports the problems of the family. Evaluation of home visit is a continuous process, through at the end of every visit community health nurse evaluate themselves.

ADVANTAGES OF HOME VISIT

1. The nurse can directly observe home and family atmosphere.

2. The nurse can directly observe the care given to patient by the family members.
3. It is possible to discover new health problems.
4. The family members will be more relaxed in their own surroundings.
5. The family gains confidence and feels to clear their doubts.
6. This helps to apply the gained knowledge and skills in the homes assisting and solving individual and families health problems.

CONCLUSION

The cardinal principle of community health nursing which must permeate all consideration of visit content is that family health work is the basis upon which all factors rest. The family is the unit of service in all generalized community health nursing services. The health of one member affects the welfare of every other member in the family. Every family is different and so the nurse must understand family ways, traditions and customs of people. The families are affected by every aspect of community life. Family health nurses help individuals and families cope with illness, chronic disability or times of stress. They spend a large part of their time working in patients' homes and with patients' families. Such nurses give advice on lifestyle and behavioral risk factors, and assist families with health matters. Through prompt detection, they can ensure early treatment of families' health problems. With their knowledge of public health and social issues and other social agencies, they can identify the effects of socioeconomic factors on families' health and refer them to the appropriate agency. They can facilitate early discharge from hospital by providing nursing care at home, and they can act as the lynchpin between the family and the family health physician, substituting for the physician when identified needs are more relevant to nursing expertise.

CHAPTER

30

Holistic Nursing

INTRODUCTION

The holistic nurse is an instrument of healing and a facilitator in the healing process. Holistic nurses honor each individual's subjective experience about health, health beliefs, and values. Holistic nurses may integrate complementary/alternative modalities (CAM) into clinical practice to treat people's physiological, psychological, and spiritual needs. Doing so does not negate the validity of conventional medical therapies, but serves to complement, broaden and enrich the scope of nursing practice; and to help individuals access their greatest healing potential. Florence Nightingale, who believed in care that focused on unity, wellness, and the interrelationship of human beings and their environment, is considered to be one of the first holistic nurses.

DEFINITION

Holistic nursing is defined as "all nursing practice that has healing the whole person as its goal"—*American Holistic Nurses' Association, 1998*

Description of holistic nursing: Holistic nursing is a specialty practice that draws on nursing knowledge, theories, expertise and intuition to guide nurses in becoming therapeutic partners with people in their care. This practice recognizes the totality of the human being—the interconnectedness of body, mind, emotion, spirit, social/cultural, relationship, context, and environment.

HOLISTIC TREATMENT MODALITIES

WHOLE MEDICAL SYSTEM

1. **Homeopathy:** A system of medicine which stimulates healing through the administration of substances prescribed according to three basic principles:
   i. Like cures like,
   ii. The more a remedy is diluted, the greater the potency.

iii. Illness is specific to the individual. Homeopathy is based on the belief that symptoms are signs of the body's effort to get rid of disease; treatment is based on the whole person, rather than on the symptoms.

2. **Osteopathic medicine:** A form of medicine that focuses on the relationship between the structure of the body and its function; and recognizes that both structure and function are subject to a range of disorders. In treatment of the individual, osteopaths use various forms of physical manipulation to facilitate the body's self-healing mechanism as well as more conventional medical therapies. Osteopaths are fully licensed to diagnose, treat and prescribe.

MANIPULATIVE AND BODY-BASED PRACTICES

1. **Acupressure:** Use of finger and hand pressure over specific points on the body to relieve pain and discomfort; and to influence the function of internal organs and body systems. Various approaches are used to release tension and restore the natural flow of energy in the body.
2. **Acupuncture:** Use of fine-gauged needles inserted into specific points on the body to stimulate or disperse the flow of energy. This ancient-oriental technique is used to alleviate pain or increase immunity by balancing energy flow. Massage, herbal medicine, and nutritional counseling are often used in conjunction with acupuncture.
3. **Alexander technique:** A series of lessons in rebalancing the body through awareness, movement and touch. As the student explores new ways of reorganizing neuromuscular function, the body is reacquainted with relaxed, healthy posture and direct, efficient movement.
4. **Amma therapy:** Amma is a form of oriental massage that focuses on the balance and movement of energy within the body.
5. **Aromatherapy:** Use of essential oils extracted from plants and herbs to treat physical imbalances as well as to achieve psychological and spiritual well-being. The oils are inhaled, applied externally or ingested.
6. **Body work:** Any therapy that involves touch and/or pressure on the body. Often the term is used as an umbrella to describe the use of two or more therapies by a single practitioner, either in separate sessions or during a single session, according to the needs of the client.
7. **Breema bodywork:** Breema incorporates simple, playful bodywork sequences along with stretch and movement exercises that help create greater flexibility, relaxed body, clear mind and calm, supportive feelings.
8. **Chiropractic medicine:** A healthcare system emphasizing structural alignment of the spine. Adjustments involve the manipulation of the spine and joints to re-establish: and maintain normal nervous system

functioning. Some chiropractors employ additional therapies such as massage, nutrition, and specialized kinesiology.

9. **Cranial osteopathy:** Gentle and almost imperceptible manipulation of the skull to re-establish its natural configuration and movement. Such correction can have a positive influence on disorders manifested throughout the body.
10. **Craniosacral therapy:** Diagnosis and treatment of imbalances in the craniosacral system. Subtle adjustments are made to the system through light touch and gentle manipulations.
11. **Dance therapy:** Therapy in which dance and music combine to allow the body, mind, soul, and spirit to be refreshed, uplifted, and experience the freedom that natural bodily movement allows.
12. **Feldenkrais method:** A method of instruction, through movement and gentle manipulation, to enhance self-image and restore mobility. Students are taught to notice how they are using their bodies, and how to improve their posture and move more freely.
13. **Jin Shin Jyutsu:** A bodywork technique, which balances body energy as it travels along specific pathways. Specific combinations of healing points are held with the fingertips to restore balance and harmony.
14. **Lymphatic therapy:** A vigorous form of massage that helps the body release toxins stored in the lymphatic system—excellent for the immune system and rebuilding the body.
15. **Massage:** The use of strokes and pressure on the body to dispel tension, increase circulation and relieve muscular pain. Massage can provide comfort and increased body awareness and can be an excellent method of releasing emotional as well as bodily tension.
16. **Movement therapy:** A guided series of movements and bodywork to open energy pathways and facilitate healing.
17. **M Technique:** A registered method of gentle, structured touch suitable for the very fragile or actively dying or when the giver is not trained in massage. It was created by a nurse for nurses.
18. **Neuromuscular therapy:** A massage therapy in which moderate pressure over muscles and nerves, as well as on trigger points, is used to decrease pain and tension.
19. **Physical therapy:** The treatment of physical conditions of body malfunction, damage or injury, using procedures designed to reduce swelling, relieve pain, strengthen muscles, restore range of motion and return functioning to the patient.
20. **Qigong:** An internal Chinese meditative practice that uses breathing techniques, gentle movement and meditation to cleanse, strengthen, and circulate the life energy.

21. **Shiatsu:** An energy-based system of bodywork using a firm sequence of rhythmic pressure held on specific points, designed to awaken acupressure meridians.
22. **Trigger point therapy:** A method of compression of sensitive points in the muscle tissue, along with massage and passive stretches, for the relief of pain and tension. Treatment decreases swelling and stiffness and increases range of motion. Exercises may be assigned.

BODY-MIND MEDICINE

1. **Art therapy:** Use of basic art materials to discover how to restore, maintain or improve physical and mental health. Through observation and analysis, the art therapist is able to formulate treatment plans specific to the individual.
2. **Color therapy:** The use of electronic instrumentation and color receptivity, according to the work of Jacob Lieberman, to integrate the nervous system and body-mind. It increases well-being and can be helpful for many acute and chronic ailments.

COUNSELING/PSYCHOTHERAPY

A broad category of therapies, which treat individuals as a whole. Treatments and sessions are focused on integrated care on all levels, for individuals, families or groups.

1. **Eye movement desensitization and reprocessing (EMDR)**: An accelerated information processing method using alternating stimuli—either eye movements or sounds—to desensitize and reprocess emotional wounds or install a healthier belief system. EMDR is effective with post-traumatic stress syndrome, childhood trauma, depression, addictions, compulsions, unhealthy patterns and future-oriented solutions.
2. **Guided imagery:** This holistic modality assists clients in connecting with their inner knowledge at the thinking, feeling, and sensing levels, promoting their innate healing abilities. Together, guide and client co-create an effective way to work with—pain, symptom, grief, and stress management; conflict resolution; self-empowerment issues; and/or preparing for medical-surgical interventions.
3. **Hypnotherapy:** The use of a state of focused attention, achieved through guided relaxation, to access the unconscious mind. Hypnosis is used for memory recall, medical treatment, and skill enhancement or personal growth.
4. **Interactive imagery:** Fosters active participation, disease prevention and health promotion, returning the focus of wellness to the individual. See also guided imagery.
5. **Meditation:** A method of relaxing and quieting the mind to relieve muscle tension and facilitate inner peace. There are numerous forms

of meditation, taught individually or in group settings, and it is thought that prayer for the self might have an effect similar to meditation. The nonsectarian form of prayer, which is akin to meditation and used for stress reduction, has long been recognized by clinicians to improve one's sense of well-being. Studies by Dr Herbert Benson of Harvard University have shown that inducing a relaxed state of mind is good both for the health and immune system response. Prayer may work partly in this way.

6. **Music therapy:** An expressive art form designed to help the individual move into harmony and balance. Through the use of music, individuals explore emotional, spiritual and behavioral issues. Musical skill is not necessary as the process, rather than technique is emphasized.
7. **Neuro-linguistic programming (NLP):** A systematic approach to changing behavior through changing patterns of thinking.

PSYCHOTHERAPY

1. **Stress management:** Any therapy or educational practice with the objective of decreasing stress and enhancing one's response to the elements of life that cannot be changed. This broad category may include bodywork, energy work, visualization and counseling.
2. **T'ai Chi Ch'uan:** A movement practice and Chinese martial art, which enhances coordination, balance and breathing, and promotes physical, emotional and spiritual well-being. T'ai Chi is taught in classes or as private lessons and requires home practice to be effective.
3. **Yoga therapy:** The use of yoga postures, controlled breathing, relaxation, meditation, and nutrition to release muscular and emotional tension, improve concentration, increase oxygen levels in the blood and assist the body in healing itself.

BIOLOGICALLY BASED THERAPIES

1. **Biofeedback:** A relaxation technique involving careful monitoring of vital functions (such as breathing, heart rate and blood pressure) in order to improve health. By conscious thought, visualization, movement or relaxation, one can learn, which actions result in desirable changes in these vital functions. Biofeedback is used for medical problems related to stress and for conditions such as incontinence, irregular heartbeat and epilepsy.
2. **Herbal therapy:** The use of herbs and their chemical properties to alleviate specific conditions or to support the function of various body systems. Herbal formulas have three basic functions—elimination and detoxification, health management and maintenance, and health building.

3. **Hydrotherapy:** The use of water, ice, steam, and hot and cold temperatures to maintain and restore health. Treatments include full body immersion, steam baths, saunas, and the application of hot and/ or cold compresses.
4. **Nutritional counseling:** A practitioner who uses diet and supplementation therapeutically as the primary or adjunctive treatment for illness, as well as for maintaining good health. Nutritionists employ a variety of approaches including food combining, macrobiotics and orthomolecular theory.

ENERGY MEDICINE

1. **Chi kung healing touch:** A method of health care involving breath and gentle movements, which follows the Chinese five-element theory and works with the meridian system.
2. **Energy work:** A broad category of body work influencing the seven major energy centers (chakras) and the flow of energy around; and through this field. As the body's energy field is balanced and strengthened, healing occurs simultaneously on the physical and non-physical levels.
3. **Healing touch:** An energy-based therapeutic approach to healing. Touch is used to influence the energy system, affecting physical, emotional, mental and spiritual health; and healing. The goal of treatment is to restore harmony and balance, promoting self-healing.
4. **Magnetic therapy:** The use of magnets to generate controlled magnetic fields, which can benefit the functioning of the nervous system, organs and tissues, and stimulates healing.
5. **Prayer:** Prayer is considered by National Center for Complementary and Alternative Medicine (NCCAM) to belong in the category of putative energy fields (also called biofields). Therapies involving putative energy fields are based on the concept that human beings are infused with a subtle form of energy. This vital energy or life force is known under different names in different cultures such as qui in traditional Chinese medicine, the vital energy or life force proposed to regulate a person's spiritual, emotional, mental and physical health; and to be influenced by the opposing forces of yin and yang.
6. **Reiki:** The use of hands and visualization to direct energy to various parts of the body to facilitate healing and relaxation. Reiki can promote mental, emotional, physical, and spiritual balance.
7. **Therapeutic touch:** A technique for balancing energy flow in the body through human energy transfer. Therapeutic touch is based on the principle that in balance there is health and in health there is growth, order and wholeness.
8. **Touch for health:** A science of energy-balancing encompassing aspects of applied kinesiology, acupressure, massage and nutrition to maximize

physical and emotional health. Touch for health emphasizes the uniqueness of the individual and uses measurement of muscle strength as a biofeedback mechanism to determine the unique needs of the individual.

HOLISTIC NURSING PRACTICE

Holistic nursing embraces all nursing practice that has enhancement of healing the whole person from birth to death as its goal. Holistic nursing recognizes that there are two views regarding holism that holism involves identifying the inter-relationships of the bio-psycho-social-spiritual dimensions of the person, recognizing that the whole is greater than the sum of the parts; and that holism involves understanding the individual as a unitary whole in mutual process with the environment. Holistic nursing responds to both views, believing that the goals of nursing can be achieved within either framework.

The holistic nurse is an instrument of healing and a facilitator in the healing process. Holistic nurses honor the individual's subjective experience about health, health beliefs and values. To become therapeutic partners with individuals, families, and communities, holistic nurses draw on nursing knowledge, theories, research, expertise, intuition, and creativity. Holistic nursing practice encourages peer review of professional practice in various clinical settings and integrates knowledge of current professional standards, law, and regulations governing nursing practice.

Practicing holistic nursing requires nurses to integrate self-care, self-responsibility, spirituality, and reflection in their lives. This may lead the nurse to greater awareness of the interconnectedness with self, others, nature, and God/life force/absolute/transcendent. This awareness may further enhance the nurse's understanding of all individuals and their relationships to the human and global community, and permits nurses to use this awareness to facilitate the healing process.

ROLE OF NURSE IN HOLISTIC NURSING

The goal of holistic nursing is to treat and heal the whole person by recognizing the interconnectedness of body, mind, spirit, and environment. Use holistic nursing as a place to discuss ways to incorporate nursing knowledge, theories, complementary/alternative modalities, expertise, and intuition to guide nurses in becoming therapeutic partners with people in their care, treating their physiological, psychological, and spiritual needs.

The practice of holistic nursing requires nurses to integrate self-care, self-responsibility, spirituality, and reflection in their lives. This may lead the nurse to greater awareness of the interconnectedness with self, others, nature, and spirit. This awareness may further enhance the nurses understanding of all individuals and their relationships to the human and global community, and permits nurses to use this awareness to facilitate the healing process.

Also called complementary health nurses, holistic nurses use alternative medicine, sometimes combined with traditional Western medicine, to care for patients. This field of nursing is based on the premise that you cannot treat a patient's physical health without addressing the 'whole' person—including their mental, spiritual and emotional well-being. This approach to nursing is much different than other, more traditional specialties, and an increasingly sought-after, niche field.

CONCLUSION

Holistic nursing is a specialty practice that draws on nursing knowledge, theories, expertise and intuition to guide nurses in becoming therapeutic partners with people in their care. This practice recognizes the totality of the human being—the interconnectedness of body, mind, emotion, spirit, social/cultural, relationship, context, and environment. The holistic nurse is an instrument of healing and a facilitator in the healing process. Holistic nurses honor each individual's subjective experience about health, health beliefs, and values. Holistic nurses may integrate complementary/alternative modalities (CAM) into clinical practice to treat people's physiological, psychological, and spiritual needs. Doing so does not negate the validity of conventional medical therapies, but serves to complement, broaden, and enrich the scope of nursing practice and to help individuals access their greatest healing potential. The practice of holistic nursing requires nurses to integrate self-care, self-responsibility, spirituality, and reflection in their lives. This may lead the nurse to greater awareness of the interconnectedness with self, others, nature, and spirit. This awareness may further enhance the nurses understanding of all individuals and their relationships to the human and global community, and permits nurses to use this awareness to facilitate the healing process.

SECTION VII
Waste Management

GLOSSARY

1. **Authorization:** Means permission granted by the prescribed authority for the generation, collection, reception, storage, transportation, treatment, disposal and/or any other form of handling of biomedical waste in accordance with these rules and any guidelines issued by the Central Government.
2. **Authorized person:** Means an occupier or operator authorized by the prescribed authority to generate, collect, receive, store, transport, treat, dispose and/or handle biomedical waste in accordance with these rules and any guidelines issued by the Central Government.
3. **Biological:** Means any preparation made from organisms or micro-organisms or product of metabolism and biochemical reactions intended for use in the diagnosis, immunization or the treatment of human beings or animals or in research activities pertaining thereto.
4. **Biomedical waste treatment facility:** Means any facility wherein treatment disposal of biomedical waste or processes incidental to such treatment or disposal is carried out.
5. **Biomedical waste:** Means any waste, which is generated during the diagnosis, treatment or immunization of human beings or animals or in research activities pertaining thereto or in the production or testing of biological and including categories mentioned in Schedule I.
6. **Cytotoxic waste:** The term is commonly used to refer to pharmaceuticals used in treating cancer, e.g. antineoplastics or chemotherapy agents.
7. **Decontamination:** This is a process that removes microorganisms from an object, rendering it safe for handling.
8. **Disinfection:** This is a process that kills most microorganisms but rarely kills all spores. The three levels of disinfection are low level; intermediate level and high level. Disinfectants are substances used to disinfect inanimate objects.
9. **Human blood and body fluid waste:** This consists of human fluid blood and blood products, items saturated or dripping with blood, body fluids contaminated with blood, and body fluids removed for diagnosis during surgery, treatment or autopsy. This does not include urine or feces.

10. **Microbiology laboratory waste:** This consists of laboratory cultures, stocks or specimens of microorganisms, live or attenuated vaccines, human or animal cell cultures used in research and laboratory material that has come into contact with any of these.
11. **Occupier:** In relation to any institution generating biomedical waste, which includes a hospital, nursing home, clinic dispensary, veterinary institution, animal house, pathological laboratory, blood bank by whatever name called, means a person who has control over that institution and/or its premises.
12. **Operator of a biomedical waste facility:** Means a person who owns or controls or operates a facility for the collection, reception, storage, transport, treatment, disposal or any other form of handling of biomedical waste.
13. **Sewage system:** A system for the collection, transmission, treatment or disposal of any liquid waste containing animal, vegetable, mineral, human or chemical matter in solution or in suspension (for purposes of this guideline pump-out systems are excluded as a disposal system for liquids containing untreated biomedical wastes).
14. **Waste sharps:** Waste sharps are clinical and laboratory materials consisting of needles, syringes, blades, or laboratory glass capable of causing punctures or cuts.

CHAPTER

31

Biomedical Waste Management

INTRODUCTION

Proper disposal of hospital waste is of paramount importance because of its infectious and hazardous characteristics. Hospital waste is the waste that is generated from use of medical and surgical facilities, during the diagnosis, treatment or immunization of humans, office and kitchen waste. Hospital waste is a potential health hazard to the healthcare workers, public, and flora and fauna of the area. Hospital acquired infection, transfusion transmitted diseases, rising incidence of hepatitis B and HIV, increasing land and water pollution lead to increasing possibility of catching many diseases. Air pollution due to emission of hazardous gases by incinerators such as furan, dioxin, hydrochloric acid, etc. have compelled the authorities to think seriously about hospital waste and the diseases transmitted through improper disposal of hospital waste. This problem has now become a serious threat for the public health and ultimately, the Central Government had to intervene for enforcing proper handling and disposal of hospital waste; and an act was passed in July 1996 and a biomedical waste (handling and management) rule was introduced in 1998. With concerns about transmission of HIV and hepatitis B on the rise, simple infection control measures were introduced that reduce the risk of transmission of blood-borne pathogens through exposure to blood or body fluids among patients and healthcare workers. These are called 'universal precautions' (Table 31.1).

DEFINITION

1. Biomedical waste (BMW) consists of solids, liquids, sharps, and laboratory waste that are potentially infectious or dangerous and are considered biowaste. It must be properly managed to protect the general public, specifically healthcare and sanitation workers, who are regularly exposed to biomedical waste as an occupational hazard. In hospitals, medical waste, otherwise known as clinical waste, normally refers to waste products that cannot be considered general waste, produced from

healthcare premises, such as hospitals, clinics, doctors offices, veterinary hospitals and laboratories.

2. World Health Organization (WHO) states that 85% of hospital wastes are actually non-hazardous, whereas 10% are infectious and 5% are non-infectious, but they are included in hazardous wastes. About 15% to 35% of hospital waste is regulated as infectious waste. This range is dependent on the total amount of waste generated (Glenn and Garwal, 1999).

Table 31.1: Categories of biomedical waste

Option	Treatment and disposal	Waste category
Cat. No. 1	Incineration/deep burial	Human anatomical waste (human tissues, organs, body parts)
Cat. No. 2	Incineration/deep burial	Animal waste animal tissues, organs, body parts carcasses, bleeding parts, fluid, blood and experimental animals used in research, waste generated by veterinary hospitals/colleges, discharge from hospitals, animal houses
Cat. No. 3	Local autoclaving/micro-waving incineration	Microbiology and biotechnology waste (wastes from laboratory cultures, stocks or specimens of micro-organisms live or attenuated vaccines, human and animal cell culture used in research and infectious agents from research and industrial laboratories, wastes from production of biological, toxins, dishes and devices used for transfer of cultures) waste sharps (needles, syringes, scalpels blades, glass, etc. that may cause puncture and cuts.
Cat. No. 4	Disinfections (chemical treatment/autoclaving/micro-waving and multilation shredding)	This includes both used and unused sharps
Cat. No. 5	Incineration/destruction and drugs disposal in secured landfills	Discarded medicines and cytotoxic drugs (wastes comprising of outdated, contaminated and discarded medicines) solid waste (items contaminated with blood and body fluids including cotton, dressing, soided plaster casts, line beddings, other material contaminated with blood)
Cat. No. 6	Incineration, autoclaving/ micro waving	Solid waste (items contaminated with blood and body fluids including cotton, dressings, soiled plaster casts, line beddings, other material contaminated with blood)
Cat. No. 7	Disinfections by chemical treatment autoclaving/micro-waving and multilation shredding	Solid waste (waste generated from disposable items other than the waste sharps such as tubing, catheters, intravenous sets, etc.)
Cat. No. 8	Disinfections by chemical treatment and discharge into drain	Liquid waste (waste generated from laboratory and washing, cleaning, house-keeping and disinfecting activities)
Cat. No. 9	Disposal in municipal landfill	Incineration ash (ash from incineration of any bio-medical waste)
Cat. No. 10	Chemical treatment and discharge into drain for liquid and secured landfill for solids	Chemical waste (chemicals used in production of biological, chemicals, used in disinfection as insecticides, etc.

Source: The Biomedical Waste (Management and Handling) Rules, 1998

BIOMEDICAL WASTE

NEED OF BIOMEDICAL WASTE MANAGEMENT IN HOSPITALS

The reasons due to which there is great need of management of hospitals waste such as:

1. Injuries from sharps leading to infection to all categories of hospital personnel and waste handler.
2. Nosocomial infections in patients from poor infection control practices and poor waste management.
3. Risk of infection outside hospital for waste handlers and scavengers and at time general public living in the vicinity of hospitals.
4. Risk associated with hazardous chemicals, drugs to persons handling wastes at all levels.
5. 'Disposable' being repacked and sold by unscrupulous elements without even being washed.
6. Drugs, which have been disposed off, being repacked and sold off to unsuspecting buyers.
7. Risk of air, water and soil pollution directly due to waste, or due to defective incineration emissions and ash.

UNIVERSAL PRECAUTIONS

1. Barrier protection should be used at all times to prevent skin and mucous membrane contamination with blood, body fluids containing visible blood, or other body fluids (cerebrospinal, synovial, pleural, peritonea, pericardial, and amniotic fluids, semen and vaginal secretions). Barrier protection should be used with all tissues.

   The type of barrier protection used should be appropriate for the type of procedures being performed and the type of exposure anticipates. Examples of barrier protection include disposable laboratory coats, gloves; and eye and face protection.
2. Gloves are to be worn when there is potential for hand or skin contact with blood, other potentially infectious material, or items and surfaces contaminated with these materials.
3. Wear face protection (face shield) during procedures that are likely to generate droplet of blood or body fluid to prevent exposure to mucous membranes of the mouth, nose and eyes.
4. Wear protective body clothing when there is a potential for splashing of blood or body fluids.
5. Never try to pipette by mouth. Use mechanic pipetting devices instead.
6. Wash hands or other skin surface thoroughly and immediately if contaminated with blood, body fluids containing visible blood or other body fluids to which universe precautions apply.

7. Wash hands immediately after gloves are removed.
8. Avoid accidental injuries that can be cause by needles, scalpel blades, laboratory instruments, etc. when performing procedures, cleaning instruments, handling sharp instruments and disposing of used needles, pipettes, etc.
9. Used needles, disposable syringes, scalpel blades, pipettes, and other sharp items are to be placed in puncture resistant containers marked with a biohazard symbol for disposal.

BIOHAZARD SYMBOL

As we know that waste constitutes an important part of the environment to which man is continuously exposed, which includes refuse or solid wastes, excreta or night soil and sullage. The term 'refuse' is applied to all solid waste from human habitations that is not covered by the sewers, i.e. all wastes other than sullage (waste water or slop water and comprises all liquid wastes including industrial waste, but excluding night soil).

CLASSIFICATION OF HOSPITAL WASTE

1. **General waste:** Largely composed of domestic or house hold type waste. It is non-hazardous to human beings, e.g. kitchen waste, packaging material, paper, wrappers, and plastics.
2. **Pathological waste:** Consists of tissue, organ, body part, human fetuses, blood and body fluid. It is hazardous waste.
3. **Infectious waste:** The wastes, which contain pathogens in sufficient concentration or quantity that could cause diseases. It is hazardous, e.g. culture and stocks of infectious agents from laboratories, waste from surgery, waste originating from infectious patients.

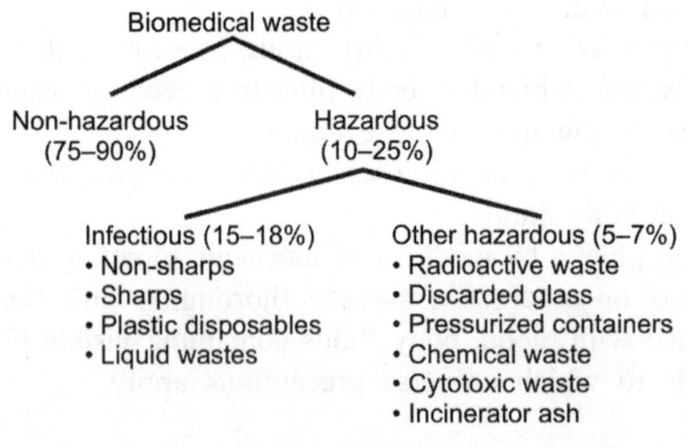

4. **Sharps:** Waste materials, which could cause the person handling it—a cut or puncture of skin, e.g. needles, broken glass, saws, nail, blades, scalpels.
5. **Pharmaceutical waste:** This includes pharmaceutical products, drugs, and chemicals that have been returned from wards, have been spilled, are outdated or contaminated.
6. **Chemical waste:** This comprises discarded solid, liquid and gaseous chemicals, e.g. cleaning, housekeeping, and disinfecting product.
7. **Radioactive waste:** It includes solid, liquid, and gaseous waste that is contaminated with radionucleides generated from in vitro analysis of body tissues and fluid, in vivo body organ imaging; and tumor localization and therapeutic procedures.

APPROACH FOR HOSPITAL WASTE MANAGEMENT

Approach is based on Biomedical Waste (Management and Handling) Rules, 1998 notified under the Environment Protection Act by the Ministry of Environment and Forest (Government of India).

1. **Segregation of waste:** Segregation is the essence of waste management and should be done at the source of generation of biomedical waste e.g. all patient care activity area, diagnostic services areas, operation theaters, labor rooms, treatment rooms, etc. The responsibility of segregation should be with the generator of biomedical waste, i.e. doctors, nurses, technicians, etc. (medical and paramedical personnel). The biomedical waste should be segregated as per categories mentioned in the rules (Table 31.2).

Table 31.2: Type of container and color code for collection of biomedical waste

Category	Waste class	Type of container	Color
1	Human anatomical waste	Chemical waste (solid)	Yellow
2	Animal waste	Chemical waste (solid)	Yellow
3	Microbiology and bio-technology waste	Chemical waste (solid)	Yellow/ Red
4	Waste sharps containers	Puncture proof translucent	Blue/white
5	Discarded medicines and cytotoxic waste	Plastic bags	Black
6	Soiled waste (biomedical waste)	Plastic bags	Yellow
7	Solid (plastic) proof containers	Plastic bag/puncture	Blue/white Translucent
8	Liquid waste		Black
9	Incineration waste	Plastic bag	Black
10	Chemical waste (solid)	Plastic bag	Black

2. **Collection of biomedical waste:** Collection of biomedical waste should be done as per Biomedical waste (Management and Handling) Rules. At ordinary room temperature the collected waste should not be stored for more than 24 hours.
3. **Transportation:** Within hospital, waste routes must be designated to avoid the passage of waste through patient care areas. Separate time should be earmarked for transportation of biomedical waste to reduce chances of it's mixing with general waste. Desiccated wheeled containers, trolleys or carts should be used to transport the waste/plastic bags to the site of storage/treatment.
4. **Treatment of hospital waste:** Treatment of waste is required to:
   a. To disinfect the waste, so that it is no longer the source of infection.
   b. To reduce the volume of the waste.
   c. Make waste unrecognizable for aesthetic reasons.
   d. Make recycled items unusable.

TREATMENT OF INFECTIOUS WASTE MATERIALS

Infectious material is treated by one of the following techniques:
1. **Incineration:** Involves burning of hospital waste like body parts, microbiological waste and soiled dressings at very high temperatures and reducing its volume. However, it generates highly toxic gases like furans and dioxins when plastics are incinerated.
2. **Autoclaving:** This method is used for treating blood and blood products, sharps, body fluids and microbiological waste, but not pathological waste. After treatment with autoclaving, the products are then landfilled.
3. **Treatment with chemicals:** Chemicals treatment using at least 1% hypochlorite solution or any other equivalent chemical reagent. It must be ensured that chemical treatment ensures disinfection.

Table 31.3: Treatment options for infectious waste

Color coding	Type of container	Waste category	Treatment options
Yellow	Plastic bag	Category 1, 2 and 3, 6	Incineration/Deep burial
Red	Disinfected container/Plastic bag	Category 3, 6, 7	Autoclaving/ Microwaving/ Chemical treatment
Blue/White Translucent	Plastic bag/ Puncture proof container	Cateogry 4, 7	Autoclaving/ Microwaving/ Chemical treatment and destruction/ Shredding
Black	Plastic bag	Category 5, 9 and 10 (solid)	Disposal in secured landfill/Biodegradable-vermicomposting/ composting

Note:

1. Waste collection bags for waste types needing incineration shall not be made of chlorinated plastics.
2. Categories 8 and 10 (liquid) do not require containers/bags.
3. Category 8 waste is disinfected by chemical treatment and discharged into drains
4. Category 3 if disinfected locally need not be put in containers/bags.

CONCLUSION

Medical care is vital for our life and health, but the waste generated from medical activities represents a real problem of living nature and human world. Improper management of waste generated in health care facilities causes a direct health impact on the community, the health care workers and on the environment. Everyday, relatively large amount of potentially infectious and hazardous waste are generated in the health care hospitals and facilities around the world. Indiscriminate disposal of BMW or hospital waste and exposure to such waste possess serious threat to environment and to human health that requires specific treatment and management prior to its final disposal. The present review article deals with the basic issues as definition, categories, problems relating to biomedical waste and procedure of handling and disposal method of Biomedical Waste Management. It also intends to create awareness amongst the personnel involved in health care unit.

Note:

1. Waste collection bags for waste types needing incineration shall not be made of chlorinated plastics.
2. Categories 8 and 10 (liquid) do not require containers/bags.
3. Category 8 waste is disinfected with chemical treatment and discharged into drains.
4. Category 3 if disinfected locally need not be put in containers/bags.

CONCLUSION

Medical care is vital for our life and health but the waste generated from medical activities represents a real problem of living nature and human world. Improper management of waste generated in health care facilities causes a direct health impact on the community, the health care workers and on the environment. Everyday, relatively large amount of potentially infectious and hazardous waste are generated in the health care hospitals and facilities around the world. Indiscriminate disposal of BMW or hospital waste and exposure to such waste possess serious threat to environment and to human health that requires specific treatment and management prior to its final disposal. The present review article deals with the basic issues of definition, categories, problems relating to biomedical waste and procedure of handling and disposal method of Biomedical Waste Management. It also intends to create awareness amongst the personnel involved in health care unit.

PREVIOUS YEAR QUESTIONS

I. 2014-APR

LONG ESSAYS

1. a. Define quality assurance.
   b. Explain the role of council and professional bodies in maintaining nursing standards.
2. a. Define nursing process.
   b. Explain the steps of nursing process in detail with suitable examples.

SHORT ESSAYS

3. Tools for evaluation.
4. Factors influencing health and illness.
5. Factors influencing growth and development.
6. Biomedical waste management.

SHORT ANSWERS

7. Types of nursing care plan.
8. Anecdotal record.
9. Primary nursing.
10. Importance of recording.
11. Team nursing.

II. 2013-SEP

LONG ESSAYS

1. Explain the importance of nursing process, discuss in detail the planning phase.
2. Explain the role of theories in nursing practice, discuss the metaparadigm of nursing.

SHORT ESSAYS

3. Progressive patient care.
4. General adaptation syndrome.
5. ICN code of ethics.
6. Problems of adolescent.

SHORT ANSWERS

7. Define nursing.
8. Disposal of sharps.
9. Role of INC

10. Methods of physical assessment.
11. Nursing standards.

III. 2013-MARCH

LONG ESSAYS

1. Explain the extended role of the nurse.
2. Explain the trends influencing nursing practice.

SHORT ESSAYS

3. Concepts of health and illness.
4. Ethical and legal issues in nursing.
5. Developmental stages of an individual.
6. The metaparadigm of nursing.

SHORT ANSWERS

7. Nursing diagnosis.
8. Recording.
9. Nursing audit.
10. Professional bodies.
11. Holistic nursing.

IV. 2012-MARCH

LONG ESSAYS

1. Write in detail regarding the trends and development of nursing in India.
2. Define nursing process, discuss in detail the various steps in nursing process.

SHORT ESSAYS

3. Team nursing.
4. Metapardigm of nursing.
5. Ethical and legal issues in nursing.
6. Expanded role of nurse.

SHORT ANSWERS

7. Cytotoxic drugs.
8. Primary nursing.
9. Development task of old age.
10. Professional conduct for nursing.

V. 2011-AUGUST

LONG ESSAYS

1. Discuss in detail the biomedical waste management.
2. Describe the concept of health and illness.

SHORT ESSAYS

3. Problems solving.
4. Total quality management.
5. Nursing audit.
6. Developmental concept of pre-adolescent.

SHORT ANSWERS

7. Carrier planning.
8. Responsibility of a graduate nurse.
9. Quality assurance.
10. Problems of old age.

VI. 2011-FEB

LONG ESSAYS

1. Discuss in importance of theories in nursing practice, explain in detail Florence Nightingale theory.
2. Discuss the trends influencing nursing practice.

SHORT ESSAYS

3. Problem-oriented nursing.
4. Assessment phase of nursing process.
5. Problems of old age.
6. Total quality management.

SHORT ANSWERS

7. Recordings
8. Nursing care plan.
9. Tools of evaluation.
10. Intensive care unit.
11. Define profession.

VII. 2010-AUG

LONG ESSAYS

1. Define evaluation. Explain the process of evaluation in depth.
2. Explain the needs and problems of old age and role of nurse based on nursing process approach.

SHORT ESSAYS

3. Ethical issues in nursing.
4. Levels of prevention.
5. Describe defence mechanism with suitable examples.
6. Trained nurses association of India.

SHORT ANSWERS

7. Community-oriented nursing.
8. Illness wellness continuum.
9. Define stress and adaptation.
10. Rating scale.
11. Nursing diagnosis.

VIII. 2010-FEB

LONG ESSAYS

1. Explain in detail about professional organizations with suitable diagrams.
2. Define primary health care and explain family-oriented nursing care concept.

SHORT ESSAYS

3. Stress and adaptation.
4. Primary nursing.
5. Principles of growth and development.
6. Formulate philosophy of nursing.

SHORT ANSWERS

7. Functions of professional nurse.
8. Metaparadigm of nursing.
9. Imitative vs guilt
10. Medical diagnosis vs nursing diagnosis.
11. Evaluation.

MULTIPLE CHOICE QUESTIONS

1. A client in the health care arena is a person who:
   A. Is dependent on others
   B. Is guilty of a crime
   C. Seeks specialized care
   D. Needs psychological support

2. Health can be considered as:
   A. Physical health
   B. Mental health
   C. Spiritual
   D. All of the above

3. Health is a state of complete physical, mental, social and spiritual well being not merely the absence of disease given by:
   A. WHO
   B. Pericles
   C. Unicef
   D. HS Hayman

4. PHC, subcentres are responsible for providing which level of health care:
   A. Critical care
   B. Secondary health care
   C. Primary health care
   D. Tertiary health care

5. Nature of illness, characteristics comes under which types of variables:
   A. Internal variables
   B. External variables
   C. Extraneous variables
   D. All of the above

6. Withdrawal, depression, physical changes are characteristics of which stage of illness behavior:
   A. Dependent client care
   B. Assumption of sick role
   C. Symptoms experience
   D. Medical care contact

7. Inflammatory response, phagocytosis are:
   A. First line disease
   B. Second line disease

C. Third line disease
D. Fourth line disease

8. **Any substance when introduced into body is considered as foreign:**
A. Antigen
B. Antibody
C. Complement
D. Supression

9. **The word "Hospital" is derived from:**
A. Latin word hospile
B. French word hospital
C. Both A and B
D. None of the above

10. **Where was the epidemic disease hospital situated?**
A. Chandigarh
B. Delhi
C. Bengaluru
D. Vellore

11. **Illness prevention is expressed in term of:**
A. To maintain present level of health
B. Protecting for actual or potential threats to health
C. Care for sick
D. None of the above

12. **When a mistaken entry is made in charting, the nurse remedies it by:**
A. Striking out the entry, dating it and initialing it
B. Recopying the sheet and destroying the original
C. Using the eraser to remove the entry
D. Painting over the entry with correction fluid

13. **Nurse to the family member it sounds like you are really afraid of what might happen to your husband. This statement reflects:**
A. Empathy
B. Sympathy
C. Trust
D. Respect

14. **The accrediting agency for nursing in India is:**
A. State Nursing Council
B. International Council for Nursing
C. Indian Nursing Council
D. Trained Nurses Association of India

15. Systematic approach to patient care which coordinates medical and nursing intervention is called as:
A. Functional nursing
B. Team nursing
C. Primary nursing
D. Case management

16. The nurse who investigates nursing problems and expands the scope of nursing practice is a:
A. Nurse researcher
B. Nurse educator
C. Nurse practioner
D. Nurse administrator

17. The acts of exchanging thoughts, ideas and sharing of feeling is called as:
A. Relationship
B. Communication
C. Attitude
D. Emotions

18. The type of communication which takes place within a person is called as:
A. Intrapersonal communication
B. Interpersonal communication
C. Public communication
D. Meta communication

19. The communication which takes place between two persons is termed as:
A. Meta communication
B. Interpersonal communication
C. Public communication
D. Intrapersonal communication

20. The element of communication responsible for initiating or motivating the communication process is:
A. Referent
B. Encoder
C. Decoder
D. Receiver

21. The word N in the definition of nurse stands for:
A. Nobility
B. Neatness

C. Both A and B
D. None of the above

22. Nurse should act as:
A. Caregiver
B. Act as an advocate
C. Act as researcher
D. All of the above

23. The word E in the definition of nurse stands for:
A. Efficient
B. Empathetic
C. Economical
D. All of the above

24. The main qualities of a good nurse are:
A. Good listener
B. Good observer
C. Technically competent
D. All of the above

25. Main qualities of a good nurse are except:
A. Obedient
B. Loyal
C. Irrespective
D. Sense of humor

26. Nursing has been defined as:
A. An art
B. A science
C. Both A and B
D. None of the above

27. Members of the health team are except:
A. Physician
B. Nurse
C. Peon
D. Social worker

28. Elements of ICN code of Ethics:
A. Nurses and people
B. Nurses and practice
C. Both A and B
D. None of the above

29. The main categories of values system are:
A. Operative values
B. Terminal values
C. Moral values
D. All of the above

30. 10 months course in Public Health Nursing was started in:
A. 1950
B. 1952
C. 1958
D. 1949

31. The First Registration Act was enacted in Madras Presidency in:
A. 1920
B. 1922
C. 1926
D. 1930

32. Auxiliary nursing services was started in:
A. 1935
B. 1942
C. 1944
D. 1945

33. 1st meeting of INC (Indian Nursing Council) was held in:
A. 1940
B. 1945
C. 1948
D. 1949

34. GNM curriculums were first revised in:
A. 1980
B. 1982
C. 1986
D. 1995

35. The means or ways of conveying the message in communication process is known as:
A. Encoder
B. Decoder
C. Channel
D. Feedback

36. **The personal space or distance for communication at the social zone is:**
    A. 0–18 inches
    B. 18 inches–4 feet
    C. 4–12 feet
    D. Beyond 12 feet

37. **The personal distance between a nurse and client for good interpersonal relationship is:**
    A. 0–18 inches
    B. 18 inches–4 feet
    C. 4–12 feet
    D. Beyond 12 feet

38. **Restating the client's message in the nurse's own words is called:**
    A. Paraphrasing
    B. Clarifying
    C. Focusing
    D. Summarizing

39. **Mechanically repeating the client's words without thinking is called:**
    A. Probing
    B. Parroting
    C. Patronizing
    D. Paraphrasing

40. **A non-therapeutic technique of persistently questioning the client in spite of unwillingness to discuss the issue is:**
    A. Conformation
    B. Probing
    C. Clarifying
    D. Concreteness

41. **A writing method used by the visually impaired is called:**
    A. Sign language
    B. Braille
    C. Jargon
    D. Lonation

42. **Restless leg syndrome, a sleep disorder is medically termed as:**
    A. Cataplexy
    B. Bruxism
    C. Somnambulism
    D. Nocturnal myoclonus

43. The Crimean war took place between:
A. 1854–1856
B. 1550–1850
C. 1618–1648
D. 1800–1825

44. The World Health Day is celebrated every year on:
A. 4th April
B. 5th April
C. 7th April
D. 10th April

45. Emergency admission means admitting the patient for:
A. Treatment
B. Acute conditions
C. Routine examinations
D. None of the above

46. Routine admission means admitting the patients for:
A. Acute conditions
B. Treatment
C. Routine examination
D. All of the above

47. LAMA stands for:
A. Limited access to medical advice
B. Left against medical advice
C. Leave application for medical advice
D. All of the above

48. Admission to the hospital is an:
A. Traumatic experience
B. Excited experience
C. Sad experience
D. None of the above

49. After discharge of the patient:
A. Rooms should be cleaned
B. Windows and doors should be opened
C. Rearrange the room for next use
D. All of the above

50. The dietary department should be informed:
A. After admission
B. After discharge

C. Both A and B
D. None of the above

51. DOR means:
A. Direct order report
B. Direct observation recording
C. Discharge on request
D. All of the above

52. Nurse should identify:
A. Physical needs of patients
B. Social needs of patient
C. Psychological and spiritual needs of patients
D. All of the above

53. Ethical consideration are:
A. Respect
B. Justice
C. Fidelity
D. All of the above

54. Make sure during discharge:
A. Written consent of physician
B. Orally
C. By telephonically
D. None of the above

55. A written law which is formally passed by the government is known as:
A. Act
B. Amendment
C. Legal document
D. Bill

56. A Temporary outline of the act is known as:
A. Agreement
B. Contract
C. Bill
D. Will

57. A false harmful oral report about another person with the intention of hurting his\her reputation is known as:
A. Libel
B. Slander
C. Crime
D. Defendant

58. The person who is accused of his legal rights in a law suite is:
A. Criminal
B. Client
C. Plaintiff
D. Malpractice

59. The party initiating the complaint is called as:
A. Accused
B. Complainment
C. Defendant
D. Criminal

60. Politicians go around influencing the voters. This situation is called as:
A. Tort
B. Lobbying
C. Sue
D. Suit

61. The civil wrong committed against a person or his property to another party is:
A. Battery
B. complaint
C. Tort
D. Accusation

62. The person who gives legal suggestion to an institution is known as:
A. Prosecutor
B. Legal advisor
C. Magistrate
D. Judge

63. Nursing theories are primarily based on:
A. Concepts
B. Philosophy
C. Objectives
D. Process

64. The consensus between two parties to do certain task is known as:
A. Agreement
B. Contract
C. Bill
D. Act

65. Communication is a:
A. One way process
B. Two way process
C. Both A and B
D. None of the above

66. Communication may be:
A. Formal communication
B. Informal communication
C. Both A and B
D. None of the above

67. Based on flow communication is:
A. Downward
B. Upward
C. Horizontal
D. All of the above

68. The elements of communication are:
A. Sender
B. Upward
C. Receiver
D. All of the above

69. Purpose of communication are:
A. To obtain information
B. In influence others
C. To collect assessment data
D. All of the above

70. Non-verbal communication includes all except:
A. Physical appearance
B. body language
C. Vocabulary
D. Gesture

71. Verbal communication includes all except:
A. Vocabulary
B. Eye contact
C. Placing
D. Simple language

72. Communication influenced by these factors:
A. Age
B. Sex

C. Mental state
D. All of the above

73. Barriers of communicate are:
A. Physiological barriers
B. Environmental barrier
C. Psychological and cultural barriers
D. All of the above

74. Physiologic barriers include all except:
A. Difficulty in hearing
B. Difficulty in vision
C. Neurosis
D. Difficulty in expression

75. Psychological barriers include all except:
A. Anxiety
B. Difficulty in expression
C. Neurosis
D. Fear

76. Cultural barriers are:
A. Personality, customs, beliefs, religion
B. Lack of light, extreme light, noise, and congestion
C. Difficulty in hearing, vision, expression
D. Anxiety, fear, ego, stress.

77. Developing helping relationship:
A. Listen actively
B. Be honest
C. Maintain confidentiality
D. All of the above

78. These are the phases of relationship:
A. Pre interaction and introductory phase
B. Working and termination phase
C. Both A and B
D. None of the above

79. Three stages of introductory phases are:
A. Opening relationship
B. Clarifying the problem
C. Structuring and formulating contract
D. All of the above

80. The enema that can be selected for hyperpyrexia and heat stroke:
A. Ice enema (or) cold enema
B. Retention enema
C. Anti-spasmodic enema
D. None of the above

81. The temperature of cold enema is:
A. 80 to 90°F .
B. 27 to 32°C
C. Both A and B
D. 75°F

82. Solutions used for the nutrient enema:
A. Normal saline
B. Peptonized milk 120 mL
C. 2% or 5% dextrose
D. All of the above

83. The therapeutic uses of local hot applications:
A. Promotes suppuration
B. Decreases pain
C. Promotes heating
D. All of the above

84. Therapeutic uses of local cold application:
A. Prevents of gangrene
B. Controls hemorrhage
C. Reduces the body temperature
D. All of the above

85. Medical fomentation/stupes is:
A. Applications of local moist heat
B. Applications of cool on the area
C. Application of the bulb on the area
D. None of the above

86. The amount of drugs administration larger than the maximum dose which will have poisonous effect on the patient:
A. Maximum dose
B. Lethal dose
C. Minimum dose
D. All of the above

87. The drug administration into the spinal cavity is known as:
A. Spinal infusion
B. Intrathecal

C. Intraspinal
D. Both B and C

88. Intraosseous means:
A. Drug administration into bone marrow
B. Injection
C. Dressing
D. None of the above

89. Facies hippocratica is characterized by:
A. Prominent checks and chin
B. Pinched, sharp nose
C. Pale ashy skin, sunker glazed eyes
D. All of the above

90. The stiffening of the body after death is known as:
A. Algormorits
B. Rapid changes
C. Rigor mortis
D. None of the above

91. Autolysis is:
A. A process of hydrolysis of tissues
B. Sterilization
C. Cooling effect
D. None of the above

92. The founder of modern nursing is:
A. Virginia Henderson
B. Mother Therissa
C. Sister Diana
D. Florence Nightingale

93. Florence Nightingale was born in:
A. 1820
B. 1910
C. 1971
D. 1981

94. The following sister was called as lady of lamp:
A. Mother Teresa
B. Sister Nirmala
C. Florence Nightingale
D. None of the above

95. Characteristic of nurse patient relation is except:
A. Empathy
B. Mistrust
C. Mutual respect
D. Genuineness

96. Communication network are:
A. Wheel and chain network
B. Circle and Y network
C. Both A and B
D. None of the above

97. In informal communication:
A. Single strand chain
B. Gossip chain
C. Probability chain
D. All of the above

98. The word nursing comes from the same root word:
A. Nurse
B. Nature
C. Nutritious
D. Nutrition

99. The meaning of etiquette is:
A. Etter
B. Enemy
C. Enginear
D. A code of good manners

100. The use of a spoken (or) written word, which depend on language is called:
A. Communication
B. Community
C. Committee
D. Verbal communication

101. The facial expression, body posture, touch and eye contact is known as:
A. Non-verbal communication
B. Verbal communication
C. Community
D. Committee

102. The nursing ethics was formulated by:
A. INC
B. TNAI

C. ICM
D. ICN

103. The term "Hospes" means:
A. Hope
B. Humming
C. Him
D. Hospital

104. The example of serology laboratory among the following:
A. Hemoglobin
B. Urine routine microscopy
C. Hanging drops
D. VDRL

105. Freedom from infection (or) prevention of contact with micro-organisms is known as:
A. Sepsis
B. Septicemia
C. Anemia
D. Asepsis

106. An agent that will inhibit the growth and development of micro organisms without necessarily killing them:
A. Asepsis
B. Dry-cleaning
C. Antihistamine
D. Antiseptic

107. The cleaning of the articles under the steam under pressure is:
A. Autoclaving
B. Auto cleaning
C. Bleaching
D. Drying

108. The word bacteriostasis is:
A. Bacterial growth is checked without necessarily killing them
B. Kills the virus
C. Kills the bacteria
D. Kills the stasis

109. Bacteriostat is:
A. Improves the bacterial growth
B. Inhibit the bacterial growth
C. Suppresses the virus infection
D. Improves the health

110. Infection transmitted between individuals infected with different pathogenic organism is called as:
A. Infection transmission
B. Infection spreading
C. Infection control
D. Cross infection

111. If a person harbors the pathogenic organisms of a disease in his body without outward signs and symptoms of that disease is called as:
A. Healthy person
B. Sick person
C. Carrier
D. Sender

112. Disinfection meaning:
A. Destroying of all the pathogenic organism
B. Against infection
C. Infection free
D. Infection control

113. The disinfection of the patient's unit with all the articles that is furniture, linen, pillows, utensils, etc. is known as:
A. Sterilization
b. Mobbing
C. Dry wash
D. Terminal disinfection

114. The infection spreads through mouth and nose of one to another person during coughing sneezing (or) speaking:
A. Droplet infection
B. Contagious infection
C. Nasocomial infection
D. None of these

115. The process of disinfection by exposure to the fumes of vaporized germicide:
A. Fumigation
B. Drying
C. Cleaning
D. Sweaping

116. The following is the examples for the portal of entry:
A. Respiratory tract
B. Nails

C. Digestive tract
D. Both A and C

117. The immediate disinfection of all contaminated articles and bodily discharges during the course of disease:
A. Disease
B. Concurrent disinfection
C. Disinfection
D. Comprehensive disinfection

118. After the fumigation of a room with a methylated spirit, can be opened after:
A. 2 hours
B. 24 hours
C. 6 hours
D. 2 days

119. According to Maslow the priority need is:
A. Safely
B. Security
C. Love and belonging
D. Physiological needs (O_2, water, food, elimination, rest sleep)

120. The act (or) faculty of taking notice of something:
A. Observation
B. Knowing
C. Noticing
D. None of the above

121. The art of feeling with the hand is called:
A. Palpation
B. Touch
C. Look
D. None of the above

122. The meaning of inspection is:
A. Observing with eyes and associated with light and seeing
B. Inspiration
C. Both A and B
D. None of the above

123. Among the following, the cardinal signs are:
A. Temperature
B. Look
C. Smell
D. None of the above

124. 1 g of protein gives:
A. 1 g
B. 4 cal of heat
C. 6 cal of heat
D. 4 kilocalories

125. Methods of internal formal communication system:
A. Notice boards
B. Staff meetings
C. Circulars and memons
D. All of the above

126. By which method will nurse assess the quality of the pulse in a patient:
A. Inspection
B. Auscultation
C. Palpation
D. Percussion

127. In percussion, the finger used to strike the body parts is called as:
A. Plexor
B. Pleximeter
C. Tapper
D. Percussor

128. Implementation is a step of nursing process which is:
A. Goal oriented
B. Patient oriented
C. Action oriented
D. Outcome oriented

129. A clinical judgment based on individual's responses to actual or potential problem is known as:
A. Nursing assessment
B. Nursing evaluation
C. Nursing implementation
D. Nursing diagnosis

130. Checking the body temperature in order to evaluate fever is an example of:
A. Subjective data
B. Objective data
C. Demographic data
D. Secondary data

131. The primary biological agents controlling sexual functioning of the females are the following except:
A. Genes
B. Sex organs
C. Menstrual cycle
D. Stature

132. Loss of power of accommodation of the human crystalline lens to a nearby object is called as:
A. Presbyopia
B. Cataract
C. Metropia
D. Glaucoma

133. Name the sense involved in the awareness of the position and movement of body parts:
A. Tactile
B. Gustatory
C. Kinesthetic
D. Stereognosis

134. Inability to understand written or spoken language is called:
A. Complete aphasia
B. Expressive aphasia
C. Receptive aphasia
D. Global aphasia

135. Assessment is:
A. 2nd step of nursing process
B. 1st step of nursing process
C. 3rd step of nursing process
D. 5th step of nursing process

136. Purpose of nursing process is:
A. To protect client from illness
B. To identify the health status of patient
C. Both A and B
D. None of the above

137. Characteristics of nursing process are:
A. Goal oriented
B. Open and flexible
C. Systematic and planned
D. All of the above

138. Assessment phase of nursing process includes:
A. Setting goals
B. Analyzing data
C. Collecting data
D. Synthesizing data

139. Implementation is followed by:
A. Planning
B. Nursing diagnosis
C. Evaluation
D. Nursing assessment

140. Characteristic of nursing process are except:
A. Goal oriented
B. Rigid and non-flexible
C. Problem oriented
D. Dynamic

141. Assessment may be:
A. Initial and focus assessment
B. Emergency and tissue lapsed assessment
C. Both A and B
D. None of the above

142. The main component of assessment are:
A. Collecting data
B. Organizing data
C. Recording data
D. All of the above

143. Secondary sources of data collection are except:
A. Records
B. Patients
C. Reports
D. Family members

144. Observation is the method of:
A. Assessment
B. Planning
C. Evaluation
D. Data collection

145. Methods of data collection are:
A. Interviewing
B. Physical examination

C. Observation
D. All of the above

146. Component of nursing diagnosis is:
A. Problem, etiology, defining characteristics
B. Assessment, diagnose, planning
C. Initial, focused, time-lapse
D. None of the above

147. NANDA stands for:
A. North Australian Nursing Diagnosis Association
B. North African Nursing Diagnosis Association
C. North American Nursing Diagnosis Association
D. All of the above

148. Which of the following taxonomy is used worldwide for stating nursing diagnosis?
A. INC
B. TNAI
C. UNICEF
D. NANDA

149. Hypertension is an example of:
A. Medical diagnosis
B. Nursing diagnosis
C. Actual diagnosis
D. None of the above

150. Actual diagnosis is:
A. Rape trauma syndrome
B. Risk for impaired skin integrity
C. Anxiety related to surgery
D. None of the above

151. During implementation nurse requires:
A. Cognitive skill
B. Ongoing planning
C. Writing skill
D. Cognitive and technical skill

152. Recording is done:
A. After completing of procedure
B. Before completing of procedure
C. Between assessment and implementation
D. Not needed

153. Priorities are set:
A. Nurses condition
B. Hospital condition
C. Client's condition
D. Family condition

154. Activities in evaluation phase are except:
A. Review client goals and outcome criteria
B. Collect data
C. Do not measure goal attainment
D. Revise and modify nursing plan

155. Nursing profession is not 100% profession because it lacks:
A. Autonomy
B. Service
C. Job satisfaction
D. Recognition

156. Hyperesthesia is increased sensitiveness to............... Stimuli:
A. Tactile
B. Visual
C. Gustatory
D. Auditory

157. Mention the medication that can adversely interfere with the effect of anesthesia:
A. Anticoagulant
B. Antipyretics
C. Antidiabetics
D. Anticonvulsant

158. Documents are:
A. Written
B. Verbal
C. Both A and B
D. None of the above

159. Reports may be:
A. Verbal
B. Written
C. Both A and B
D. None of the above

160. Methods of recording are:
A. Narrative charting
B. Source oriented charting

C. Problem oriented charting
D. All of the above

161. Types of reporting are:
A. Change of shift report
B. Transfer report
C. Incident report
D. All of the above

162. Documentation is done:
A. For legal purpose
B. For maintaining consistency in work
C. For minimizing the reputation of block
D. All of the above

163. Anoxia is:
A. Absence of oxygen in tissues
B. Presence of oxygen in tissues
C. Lack of O_2 in tissue
D. None of the above

164. Normal human body temperature is:
A. 98.4°F
B. 100.4°F
C. 95°F
D. 105.4°F

165. Hypoxiemia is:
A. Absence of O_2 in blood
B. Lack of O_2 in tissues
C. Presence of O_2 in blood
D. Lack of O_2 in the blood

166. Tachypnea is respiratory rate:
A. Below 15 per minute
B. Above 20 per minute
C. Above 30 per minute
D. Above 45 per minute

167. Heat is lost by:
A. Conduction
B. Convention
C. Evaporation
D. All of the above

168. Body temperature is regulated by:
A. Kidney
B. Lungs
C. Heart
D. Hypothalamus

169. Normal blood pressure is:
A. 100/70 mm Hg
B. 120/80 mm Hg
C. 180/100 mm Hg
D. 140/90 mm Hg

170. Vital signs include:
A. Temperature
B. Pulse
C. Respiration
D. All of the above

171. Which skill is needed for a nurse for physical examination:
A. Communication skill
B. Objectivity
C. Intact senses
D. All of the above

172. Physical assessment includes:
A. Inspection
B. Objectivity
C. Ausculatation
D. All of the above

173. Abnormal findings during palpation:
A. Bulging
B. Palpation
C. Abnormal sound
D. Both A and B

174. Reflexes are:
A. Primitive
B. Superficial
C. Anterior
D. Both A and B

175. History of present illness includes:
A. Changes in behavior
B. Immunized or not

C. Childhood trauma
D. Any members suffering of disease

176. Characteristics of sound are:
A. Intensity
B. Pitch
C. Duration
D. All of the above

177. Biographic data includes:
A. Age, gender
B. Chief complaints
C. Past history
D. Family history

178. The position used for most of the rectal surgery:
A. Modified Trendelenburg
B. Lateral
C. Lithotomy
D. Trendelenburg

179. Incision and drainage of a wound is an example of:
A. Reconstructive surgery
B. Urgent surgery
C. Required surgery
D. Elective surgery

180. Occurrence of venous stasis in the postoperative period is mainly due to:
A. Surgery
B. Lack of movement of leg
C. Previous history of deep vein thrombosis
D. Antiembolic stocking

181. The instrument used to check the saturation of the oxygen in the body is:
A. Pulse oximeter
B. Spirometer
C. Ventilator
D. Flowmeter

182. The minimum urinary output for an adult with no hour should be:
A. 30 mL/h
B. 70 mL/h

C. 20 mL/h
D. 100 mL/h

183. One of the most important interventions necessary for quick recovery of a surgical client in the postoperative period is:
A. Reducing anxiety
B. Relieving abdominal distention
C. Preventing wound infection
D. Promoting communication

184. The type of anesthesia that cannot be used for anesthetizing the upper part of the body is:
A. General anesthesia
B. Nerve block anesthesia
C. Spinal anesthesia
D. Epidural anesthesia

185. The steps of nursing process was based on:
A. Intellectual model
B. Problem solving process
C. Evaluation process
D. None of the above

186. The hierarchy of human needs was emphasized by:
A. Marlow
B. Erickson
C. Maslow
D. None of the above

187. The terms Athlete's foot is:
A. Irritation characterized by itching, burning skin caused by fungus
B. A sportswoman foot
C. A sportsman foot
D. None of the above

188. The temperature regulating center is:
A. Brain
B. Skin
C. Kidney
D. Hypothalamus

189. The normal range of oral temperature is:
A. 97° to 99.5°F
B. 36° to 37.5°C
C. Both A and B
D. None of the above

190. Rectal temperature is approximately:
A. 1°F higher than oral temperature
B. 1°F lower than oral temperature
C. 2°F higher than oral temperature
D. None of the above

191. Which of the following is called as vital signs?
A. Eye
B. Ear
C. Nose
D. Blood pressure.

192. Aural temperature is:
A. The temperature is measured from the ear
B. Temperature taken from the nose
C. Temperature taken form mouth
D. None of the above

193. All living organisms can be killed by exposure to moist heat at a temperature of:
A. 120°C
B. 121°C for 15 minutes
C. 200°F for 15 minutes
D. Both B and C

194. Raw milk can be disinfected by:
A. Heating milk
B. Cooling milk
C. Pasteurization
D. None of the above

195. Water can be disinfected by:
A. Heating
B. Cooling
C. Bleeching
D. Chlorination

196. Whenever, whatever, whoever the nurse is should maintain:
A. Good body mechanics during the work
B. Good communication shells
C. Both A and B
D. None of the above

197. The common solution that is used in the special mouth care is:
A. Betadine
B. Spirit

C. Dettol
D. Potassium permanganate 1:6000

198. To take the oral temperature the thermometer can kept for:
A. 3 minutes
B. 5 minutes
C. 6 minutes
D. None of the above

199. A cut wound in the continuity of any tissue is called:
A. Wound
B. Infection
C. Inflammation
D. None of the above

200. Phagocytes are known as:
A. White blood cells
B. Red blood cells
C. Nutrition
D. None of the above

201. Which is the pediatrics comfort (or) protective devices among the following?
A. Restraints
B. Repellents
C. Protectors
D. All of the above

202. The specially designed, hazard free rooms used for psychiatric patient:
A. Seclusion (or) quiet rooms
B. Psychiatric cell
C. Rest rooms
D. None of the above

203. The immobility cause the following:
A. Fever
B. Cold
C. Hypostatic pneumonia
D. None of the above

204. The Thomas splint is used in case of:
A. Fractures of shaft of femur
B. Fracture bone

C. Both A and B
D. Skeleton (or) skin traction

205. The splint that is used, in case of fracture of lower leg and the femur just above the:
A. Braun's splint
B. Straight splint
C. Thomas splint
D. All of the above

206. The POP (plaster of paris) bandages are made up of:
A. Crinoline
B. Hydrocarbon
C. Soda bicarb
D. None of the above

207. Plaster of paris consists of:
A. Anhydrous calcium sulphate
B. Carbonic oxide
E. Oxygen
D. None of the above

208. A newly set plaster cast is called as:
A. New cast
B. Green cast
C. Yellow cast
D. None of the above

209. The principle applied in the traction is:
A. Newton's 3rd law of force
B. Johnson's law
C. Newton's 2nd law of force
D. None of the above

210. The example for skin traction:
A. Buck's extension
B. Byant's traction
C. Russel traction
D. All of the above

211. Skeletal traction is:
A. Steinmann pin and Kirschner wire
B. Skeleton
C. Russell traction
D. None of the above

212. After the measurement of oral temperature the thermometer must be cleaned from:
A. Front
B. Front to back
C. From top of stem to bulb of thermometer
D. None of the above

213. Common sites of bed sores are:
A. Sacrum
B. Heels
C. Elbows
D. All of the above

214. These are the steps of back massaging except:
A. Effleurage
B. Kneeding
C. Tapering
D. Tapping

215. Solution used in oral care are except:
A. $KMNO_4$
B. H_2O_2
C. Betadine
D. Lemon juice

216. Strength of $KMNO_4$ for oral care is:
A. 1:5000–1:6000
B. 1:4000–1:2000
C. 1:2000–1:3000
D. 1:5000–1:6000

217. Oral care of unconscious patient is done for:
A. To stinwiate appetite
B. To provide sense of well-being
C. To clean the teeth of food particles, plague
D. All of the above

218. Amputation bed is used for:
A. Fractured patient
B. Operation patient
C. Amputation of part of patient
D. None of the above

219. Mummy restraints are used in:
A. Adolescents
B. Adults

C. Old age patient
D. Small children

220. Elbow and knee restraints are applied to prevent:
A. Abduction
B. Extention
C. Flexon
D. None of the above

221. Chemical agents used for sterilization:
A. Alcohol
B. Savlon
C. Both A and B
D. None of the above

222. Inventory is list of:
A. Books
B. Items
C. Articles
D. Both B and C

223. Gloves are made up of:
A. Rubber
B. Plastic
C. Paper
D. Metal

224. Chemical used to clean the furniture is:
A. Betadine
B. Gluteraldehyde
C. Savlon
D. Both A and B

225. To remove iodine stain from the linen, it should be kept in:
A. Apply spirit
B. Rice water
C. Turpentine alcohol
D. All of the above

226. Following are the restraints:
A. Mummy restraints
B. Elbow restraints
C. Knee restraints
D. All of the above

227. Objective of bed making is:
A. To discomfort the patient
B. To provide comfort to the patients
C. To meet an emergency
D. To gain confidence of the patient

228. Purpose of hand washing:
A. To prevent infection
B. To minimize infection
C. To promote infection
D. Both A and B

229. Common problem of eyes are:
A. Conjunctivitis
B. Cataract
C. Glaucoma
D. All of the above

230. All are the ear problems except:
A. Otitis media
B. Foreign bodies
C. Squint
D. Impact cerument

231. Causes of bed sores are:
A. Friction
B. Moisture
C. Presence of pathogenic organism
D. All of the above

232. The best method used for the sterilization of surgical instrument is:
A. Boiling
B. Hot air
C. Autoclaving
D. Steaming

233. An infection that is not present for a client on admission to a hospital but develops in due course of hospitalization:
A. Nosocomial infection
B. Exogenous infection
C. Endogenous infection
D. Iatrogenic infection

234. The best method to be adopted for preventing the spread of infection in the management of communicable diseases is:
A. Hand washing
B. Immunization
C. Good nutrition
D. Medication

235. When the nurse carries out a surgical dressing for an infected wound. Which method she would adopt?
A. Center to periphery
B. Periphery to center
C. Circular
D. Farther to nearer

236. The effect of any heat application can last for a period of ————minutes.
A. 5–10 minutes
B. 10–20 minutes
C. 15–20 minutes
D. 20–30 minutes

237. The amount of heat loss from the body is directly proportional to:
A. Peripheral artery dilatation
B. Amount of blood that circulates close to the skin
C. Core body temperature
D. The body surface area

238. The type of heat application used for the treatment of decubitus ulcer is:
A. Hot water bag
B. Acquathermia pads
C. Infrared lamp
D. Heat cradles

239. Heat application is a contraindication in all of the following, except:
A. Active bleeding
B. Abdominal distention
C. Localized inflammation
D. Shivering and chills

240. When the temperature raises steeply above the normal, indicates the initial stage of fever?
A. Fastigium
B. Stadium

C. Defervescence
D. Decline

241. Trendelenburg position is used to prevent:
A. Shock
B. Aspiration
C. Dyspnea
D. Backache

242. The volume of air inhaled or exhaled per breath is known as:
A. Residual volume
B. Tidal volume
C. Vital capacity
D. Functional residual volume

243. Immobility may be:
A. Social immobility
B. Intellectual immobility
C. Social immobility
D. All of the above

244. Paralysis includes:
A. Flaccid paralysis
B. Spadic paralysis
C. Quadriplegia
D. All of the above

245. When all four extremities involve. It is:
A. Flaccid paralysis
B. Spadic paralysis
C. Paraplegia
D. Quadriplegia

246. The blood pressure can be measured by:
A. Blood meter
B. Hemometer
C. Sphygmomanometer
D. None of the above

247. The gauge of needle used in intradermal injection:
A. 12G
B. 20 to 26 G and 3/8 of an inch
C. 20 G and 3/8 of an inch
D. None of the above

248. The nurses should remember that the interferon injection could be given as:
A. IV injection
B. Intra-arterial
C. Subcutaneous
D. Z track technique

249. The term gastric lavage means:
A. Aspirating the fluid from stomach
B. Withdrawing of fluid from nose
C. Drawing of blood from blood vessels
D. None of the above

250. While doing the nasogastric tube intubations, if the patient starts chocking the immediate responsibility of nurse is:
A. To secure the tube with tape
B. To aspirate the fluid from stomach
C. Withdraw tube immediately
D. None of the above

251. The position that should be maintained during the nasogastric feeding:
A. High Fowler's position
B. Low Fowler's position
C. Supine position
D. None of the above

252. What type of enema that the nurse can select to clean bowel before going to operation theater:
A. Clearing enema
B. Natural enema
C. Oil enema
D. None of the above

253. The size of nasal catheter used to administer oxygen for women:
A. 10–12°F
B. 10–12°C
C. 10–2°C
D. 12–14°C

254. The drainage system that is used to collect fluid from chest is:
A. Chest fluid
B. Intercostal drainage
C. Intracostal water seal drainage system
D. None of the above

255. When half part of the body paralyzed it is:
A. Paraplegia
B. Flaccid paralysis
C. Opastic paralysis
D. Quadriplegia

256. Lack of coordination includes all except;
A. Ataxia
B. Chorea
C. Waddling gait
D. Dystonia

257. Altered gaits includes all except:
A. Ataxia gait
B. Waddling gait
C. Dystonia
D. Hemiplegic gait

258. Causes of altered mobility are:
A. Trauma
B. Affective disorders
C. Musculoskeletal deficits
D. All of the above

259. Rotation may be:
A. Internal rotation.
B. External rotation
C. Both A and B
D. None of the above

260. Turning the body or body part to face upward is:
A. Inversion
B. Eversion
C. Supination
D. Pronation

261. Turning the feet inward:
A. Inversion
B. Eversion
C. Both A and B
D. None of the above

262. Turning the feet outward is:
A. Eversion
B. Inversion

C. Supination
D. Pronation

263. Fowler's position is given to:
A. To reduce pain
B. To improve circulation
C. To examine rectum and vagina
D. To relieve dyspnea

264. Lithotomy position is given to:
A. To examine gynae patients
B. To relive pain
C. To relieve dyspnea
D. None of the above

265. Sigmoidoscopy is done in:
A. Fowler's position
B. Prone position
C. Knee chest position
D. Lithotomy position

266. Contraindication of hot applications is:
A. Patient with high temperature
B. Patient with malignancies
C. Patient with metabolic disorders
D. All of the above

267. Example of dry heat are except:
A. Heating pad
B. Diathermy
C. Sitz bath
D. Hot water bag

268. Indication of chest drainage is except:
A. Pneumothorax
B. Chest trauma
C. Headache
D. Thoracotomy

269. Indication of giving oxygen inhalation is:
A. To unconscious patient
B. In dyspnea
C. Both A and B
D. None of the above

270. Pulse dosimeters is an:
A. Invasive procedure
B. Non-invasive procedure
C. Both A and B
D. None of the above

271. Suction is a pressure:
A. More than atmospheric
B. Less than atmospheric pressure
C. Equal to atmospheric
D. None of the above

272. Air that develops in the pleural space is referred to as:
A. Pneumothorax
B. Pleural effusion
C. Hemothorax
D. Atelectasis

273. What is the percentage of oxygen reaching the tissue via hemoglobin?
A. 97%
B. 100%
C. 90%
D. 80%

274. Coughing up of blood along with sputum is termed as:
A. Hematemesis
B. Hematuria
C. Hemoptysis
D. Productive coughs

275. The minimum urinary output for an adult within 1 hour should be:
A. 30 mL/h
B. 20 mL/h
C. 70 mL/h
D. 100 mL/h

276. One of the important interventions necessary for quick recovery of a surgical client in the postoperative period is:
A. Reducing anxiety
B. Relieving abdominal distention
C. Preventing wound infection
D. Promoting communication

277. The type of anesthesia that cannot be used for anesthetizing the upper part of the body is:
A. General anesthesia
B. Nerve block anesthesia
C. Spinal anesthesia
D. Epidural block

278. The best method used for the sterilization of surgical instruments is:
A. Boiling
B. Hot air
C. Autoclaving
D. Steaming

279. An infection that is not present for a client on admission to a hospital but develops in due course of hospitalization:
A. Nosocomial infection
B. Exogenous infection
C. Endogenous infection
D. Iatrogenic infection

280. The best method to be adopted for preventing the spread of infection in the management of communicable diseases is:
A. Hand washing
B. Immunization
C. Good nutrition
D. Medications

281. A process by which all forms of microbial life is destroyed using chemicals is:
A. Disinfection
B. Autoclaving
C. Sterilization
D. Cleaning

282. When the nurse carries out a surgical dressing for an infected wound. Which method she would adopt?
A. Center to periphery
B. Periphery to center
C. Circular
D. Farther to nearer

283. Nutrition is:
A. Very important for survival
B. Very important for the growth and development

C. Is primary need of people
D. All of the above

284. Factors affecting nutrition are:
A. Religion
B. Age
C. Lifestyle
D. All of the above

285. Factors affecting nutrition are except:
A. Religion
B. Political system
C. Country
D. Lifestyle

286. Contraindications nasogastric intubation are except:
A. Gastric surgery
B. Fracture jaw
C. Polyps in nose
B. Fracture jaw

287. Indications of nasogastric are:
A. Fracture of jaw
B. Surgery of mouth
C. Both A and B
D. None of the above

288. Methods of nasogastric feeding are:
A. Continuous feeding method
B. Intermittent feeding
C. Bolus feeding method
D. All of the above

289. Complications of catheter insertion are:
A. Arterial puncture
B. Air embolus
C. Pneumothorax
D. All of the above

290. Solutions used for nasogastric irrigation are except:
A. Spirit
B. Plain water
C. Weak solution of sodium bicarbonate
D. Specific antidotes

291. Nutritional assessment includes:
A. Anthropometric measurement
B. Lubrication of joint spaces
C. Both A and B
D. None of the above

292. Functions of the body fluids are:
A. Transportation of nutrients to the cells
B. Lubrication of joint spaces
C. Regulation of body temperature
D. All of the above

293. Total body fluid is:
A. 40% of body weight
B. 60% of body weight
C. 75% of body weight
D. 100% of body weight

294. Cations are except:
A. Sodium (NaCl)
B. Potassium (KCl)
C. Chloride (Cl)
D. Magnesium (Mg_2)

295. Traditionally nursing education adopted the philosophy of:
A. Adults philosophy
B. Modern philosophy
C. Educational philosophy
D. Children philosophy

296. The first BSc nursing was started at:
A. RAK College, Delhi
B. Vivekananda College
C. Lady Reading School, Mumbai
D. MV Shetty Memorial College, Mangalore

297. The boom period in nursing education called:
A. 1893–1913
B. 1820–1840
C. 1190–1200
D. 1900–2000

298. A social anthropologist who encouraged for growth of the nursing education is:
A. Brown
B. Gold mark

C. Charles Dickson
D. Popjan Pal - II

299. Who will be called as father of philosophy of pragmatism?
A. William James
B. Herbert
C. Charles Darwin
D. Mead

300. Needle stick safety and prevention act was passed into law in:
A. November 2000
B. December 1998
C. November 2002
D. April 2010

ANSWERS

1. (A); 2. (D); 3. (A); 4. (C); 5. (A); 6. (B); 7. (B); 8. (A); 9. (C); 10. (C); 11. (B); 12. (A); 13. (B); 14. (C) ; 15. (D); 16. (C); 17. (C); 18. (B); 19. (B); 20. (A); 21. (C); 22. (D); 23. (D); 24. (D); 25. (C); 26. (C); 27. (C); 28. (C); 29. (D); 30. (B); 31. (C); 32. (B); 33. (D); 34. (C); 35. (B); 36. (A); 37. (C); 38. (C); 39. (B); 40. (A); 41. (B); 42. (B); 43. (B); 44. (A); 45. (B); 46. (C); 47. (B); 48. (A); 49. (D); 50. (C); 51. (C); 52. (D); 53. (D); 54. (A); 55. (D); 56. (D); 57. (A); 58. (B); 59. (C); 60. (C); 61. (A); 62. (A); 63. (C); 64. (C); 65. (C); 66. (C); 67. (D); 68. (D); 69. (D); 70. (C); 71. (C); 72. (D); 73. (D); 74. (C); 75. (B); 76. (A); 77. (D); 78. (C); 79. (D); 80. (A); 81. (C); 82. (D); 83. (D); 84. (D); 85. (A); 86. (C); 87. (D); 88. (A); 89. (D); 90. (C); 91. (A); 92. (D); 93. (A); 94. (C); 95. (B); 96. (C); 97. (D); 98. (C); 99. (D); 100. (D); 101. (A); 102. (D); 103. (D); 104. (D); 105. (D); 106. (D); 107. (A); 108. (A); 109. (B); 110. (D); 111. (C); 112. (A); 113. (D); 114. (A); 115. (A); 116. (D); 117. (A); 118. (B); 119. (D); 120. (A); 121. (A); 122. (A); 123. (A); 124. (B); 125. (D); 126. (A); 127. (A); 128. (C); 129. (A); 130. (A); 131. (A); 132. (B); 133. (C); 134. (B); 135. (D); 136. (C); 137. (D); 138. (C); 139. (C); 140. (B); 141. (C); 142. (D); 143. (B); 144. (D); 145. (D); 146. (A); 147. (C); 148. (D); 149. (A); 150. (C); 151. (D); 152. (D); 153. (C); 154. (C); 155. (A); 156. (A); 157. (D); 158. (A); 159. (C); 160. (D); 161. (D); 162. (D); 163. (A); 164. (A); 165. (D); 166. (C); 167. (D); 168. (D); 169. (B); 170. (D); 171. (D); 172. (D); 173. (D); 174. (D); 175. (A); 176. (D); 177. (A); 178. (C); 179. (A); 180. (A); 181. (A); 182. (D); 183. (A); 184. (B); 185. (B); 186. (C); 187. (A); 188. (A); 189. (C); 190. (A); 191. (D); 192. (A); 193. (D); 194. (C); 195. (D); 196. (C) ; 197. (C); 198. (A); 199. (A); 200. (A); 201. (A); 202. (A); 203. (C); 204. (C); 205. (A); 206. (A); 207. (A); 208. (B); 209. (A); 210. (D); 211. (A); 212. (C); 213. (D); 214. (C); 215. (C); 216. (D); 217. (D); 218. (C); 219. (D); 220. (C); 221. (C); 222. (D); 223. (A); 224. (D); 225. (B); 226. (D); 227. (B); 228. (D); 229. (D); 230. (C); 231. (D); 232. (D); 233. (A); 234. (A); 235. (C); 236. (C); 237. (A); 238. (A); 239. (D); 240. (D); 241. (C); 242. (A); 243. (D); 244. (D); 245. (D); 246. (C); 247. (B); 248. (D); 249. (A); 250. (C); 251. (A); 252. (A); 253. (A); 254. (C); 255. (A); 256. (C); 257. (C); 258. (D); 259. (C); 260. (C); 261. (C); 262. (A); 263. (D); 264. (A); 265. (C); 266. (D); 267. (C); 268. (C); 269. (C); 270. (B); 271. (B); 272. (C); 273. (A); 274. (B); 275. (A); 276. (C); 277. (C); 278. (C); 279. (A); 280. (A); 281. (A); 282. (B); 283. (D); 284. (D); 285. (C); 286. (B); 287. (C); 288. (D); 289. (D); 290. (A); 291. (C); 292. (D); 293. (B); 294. (C); 295. (D); 296. (A); 297. (A); 298. (A); 299. (A); 300. (A);

INDEX

Page numbers followed by *f* refer to figure and *t* refer to table.

C

N

O

P

T

U

V

W

Y

Z